Language Learning in Children Who Are Deaf and Hard of Hearing

Multiple Pathways

Susan R. Easterbrooks

Georgia State University

Sharon Baker

University of Tulsa

Allyn and Bacon

Boston ● *London* ● *Toronto* ● *Sydney* ● *Tokyo* ● *Singapore*

To my mother, Norma Plimpton Easterbrooks, who instilled in me a love of writing, and to my husband, Dewey Troutman, and my son William, for their encouragement, support, and patience.—SRE

To my son, Keith Baker, who encouraged me to learn ASL and be part of the Deaf-world, where I have made lifelong friendships, and to my sister, Bonnie White, for her encouragement and support of everything I attempt to do.—SB

Executive Editor and Publisher:
  Stephen D. Dragin
Editorial Assistant: Barbara Strickland
Marketing Manager: Kathleen Morgan
Editorial–Production Administrator:
  Michael Granger
Editorial–Production Service:
  Modern Graphics, Inc.

Composition and Prepress Buyer:
  Linda Cox
Manufacturing Buyer: Chris Marson
Cover Administrator: Kristina Mose-Libon
Electronic Composition: Modern Graphics, Inc.

Copyright © 2002 by Allyn & Bacon
A Pearson Education Company
75 Arlington Street, Suite 300
Boston, MA 02116

Internet: www.ablongman.com

Between the time website information is gathered and then published, it is not unusual for some sites to have closed. Also, the transcription of URLs can result in unintended typographical errors. The publisher would appreciate notification where these occur so that they may be corrected in subsequent editions.

Library of Congress Cataloging-in-Publication Data

Easterbrooks, Susan R.
  Language learning in children who are deaf and hard of hearing : multiple pathways/
Susan R. Easterbrooks, Sharon Baker.
    p. cm.
  Includes bibliographical references and index.
  ISBN 0-205-33100-9 (alk. paper)
    1. Deaf children—Education. 2. Deaf children—Language. 3. Deaf children—Means of communication. 4. Hearing impaired children—Education. I. Baker, Sharon II. Title
HV2430 .E27 2001
371.91′2—dc21   2001031804

Printed in the United States of America

10 9 8 7 6 5 4 3 2 1   06 05 04 03 02 01

Contents

Introduction

It has been said that language is the palette from which people color their lives and culture. Language provides the venue for social movement. According to Falk (1994), "to be human is to be capable of reason, to exercise free will, to have the ability to solve mathematical problems, to possess a visual system that perceives depth, color, and movement in particular ways, but above all, to be human is to have language" (p. 49). Language is central to everything we do. It is the means through which human beings communicate with each other, and it is the bond that links people together.

Yet, in many ways the field of deaf education has denied children who are deaf and hard of hearing from realizing their potential in developing fully functioning language systems. Lack of language has serious repercussions on the development of literacy and on achieving the competencies that enable one to live and work in adult society. Perhaps deaf and hard of hearing students have not fully reached their potential because of the long history of factionalism in philosophies and methods that no other field of education, special or otherwise, can rival. For example, if you put five deaf educators in a room, you will get six opinions on how to teach children who are deaf and hard of hearing. This is the nature of deaf education and, unfortunately, disagreements on ideology have resulted in a lack of uniform efforts toward improving instruction. Controversy can be traced back to the beginning of deaf education in the 1700s with the debates over the best communication approach.

Professionals seem to disagree more than they agree; however, most agree that there is no best method of teaching *all* deaf and hard of hearing children. Hearing losses vary significantly from child to child. In addition, children who are deaf and hard of hearing vary in the way they mediate and encode language. They vary, too, in the way they approach learning. They live in different places, and residency patterns often determine what kind and how often educational services are provided to families. Families also vary in the language choices they make for their children, so to approach deaf education with a one-size-fits-all approach is ineffectual.

In this book we have attempted to take a different approach to language learning than have other texts. We acknowledge that deaf and hard of hearing children represent a heterogeneous population and, therefore, we have created a textbook that will help prepare future teachers to work with this diverse population. We believe that deaf and hard of hearing children learn through multiple pathways. For some the primary language pathway will be auditory as they learn a spoken language (e.g., English or Spanish) by using assistive technology, cochlear implants, or hearing aids. For some students with limited residual hearing the primary language pathway will be the visual pathway. The language map for these children will be American Sign Language with English presented through visual, text-based approaches. And some children will use both a primary pathway and a secondary pathway as they strive to learn language. These children will require management of their auditory potential and visual enhancements to complete what was missed through audition (e.g., Cued Speech or English-based signs).

Current placement procedures into special education programs require teams to look at several aspects of the law, as we will discuss in Chapter 1. Sadly, they rarely consider the primary learning pathway when deciding on the most appropriate educational program for a child. Most often students are enrolled in the program and must adapt their learning to fit the program's philosophy rather than the program adapting to their individual needs. We have presented information in this textbook that, we hope, will change this practice. Future teachers of children who are deaf and hard of hearing need to develop a wide range of expertise in order to meet the diverse needs of the classroom and, therefore, meet each child's individual language needs. We begin with an introduction to deaf education and a discussion of events that bring us to today's practices. In Chapter 2, we discuss what we know about language acquisition in children who are deaf and hard of hearing as well as family and social issues that impact learning. Chapter 3 introduces our philosophy, the Multiple Pathways Approach to language instruction. We see this as a departure from traditional, singular approaches. Chapter 4 presents information pertaining to the issues of assessing the language learning of students who are deaf or hard of hearing. Chapter 5 orients the reader to the theories of pragmatic language development and ways in which language instruction should be situated within authentic contexts. Chapter 6 follows, with information on conversations and questions and how these are interrelated in the language-learning process. And last, Chapter 7 presents the components of English and American Sign Language.

A Discussion of Terminology

In the early writings of the history of deaf education, little distinction was made between deaf and hard of hearing students. Early writings often used "deaf-mute" to describe someone with a hearing loss who couldn't speak. During the 1970s and 1980s, "hearing-impaired" was widely used as an inclusive term for everyone with hearing loss regardless of the severity of the loss or the mode of communication used. It wasn't until the late 1980s that the term "deaf and hard of hearing" became widely accepted as an alternative to "hearing-impaired."

There was growing sentiment at that time that deaf people were not impaired and that being deaf was a difference instead of a pathology. The term "deaf and hard of hearing," while making a distinction that two separate groups of people coexist, is used inclusively in this book to refer to a group of people with hearing losses. Today many Deaf people consider themselves as belonging to a unique cultural group and use a capitalized *D* to indicate group membership. A lowercase *d* is used to indicate physical status of hearing. Where discussion is specific to Deaf culture, the physically deaf, or hard of hearing persons, we identify those groups separately. Otherwise we use the term "deaf and hard of hearing" to refer to the entire group of individuals with hearing losses. In addition, we alternate use of gender pronouns to avoid cumbersome writing.

We have many people to thank for their assistance in the preparation of this book. First and foremost we would like to thank each other for providing consistent effort and mutual support (sometimes with a carrot, sometimes with a stick). Next we would like to thank Cheryl Easterbrooks who graciously spent hours and hours of time reading the book from the perspective of a newcomer to the field. Her comments and suggestions were most helpful in keeping us as reader-friendly as possible. Special thanks go to Keith and Rachel Baker, the second author's son and his wife, who are both teachers at the Texas School for the Deaf, for their input regarding content. Many individuals read parts of chapters or full chapters and gave valuable guidance. Our thanks to Evelyn Dodd (Gallaudet University Ph.D. candidate), Elaine Thagard (Cobb Co. Ga. Hearing Impairments Specialist), Jack Foreman (University of Tulsa), Amy Lederberg and Maureen Smith (Georgia State University), Alan Marvelli (Smith College), Steve Nover (New Mexico School for the Deaf) for reviewing sections pertaining to the Star Schools' Research Project, and to Ruth Strozdas (Oklahoma State University-Oklahoma City), Larry Hawkins (University of Science and Arts of Oklahoma), and the Fall, 2000, Georgia State University graduate class in language learning in children who are deaf and hard of hearing. In addition, Ann Powers (Southwest Missouri State University), David Mercaldo (Idaho State University), and Barbara Strassman (College of New Jersey) gave professional reviews of the final draft. Their valuable time and suggestions provided needed perspective as we refined the book. Our thanks to Gail Lopes for her assistance with the indexing. We also wish to express our gratitude to our editor, Steve Dragin, to Barbara Strickland, his assistant, and to all the other staff at Allyn & Bacon who worked to turn our thoughts into a final product. Finally, to all the deaf and hard of hearing children who have been our friends and students, for they were in our thoughts as we wrote this book. It is all about them.

An Introduction to the Language Instruction of Children Who Are Deaf and Hard of Hearing

What to Expect in This Chapter

In this chapter you will read about people and events in history that have influenced present-day practices of teaching language to children who are deaf and hard of hearing. You will see that many of the concerns of yesteryear confront us still today.

What does the historical record reveal about language acquisition, language learning, and language performance of children who are deaf and hard of hearing? That is the major question posed in this chapter. History reveals that we have made numerous attempts to find *the* one right way to teach all children who are deaf and hard of hearing. You will read in this chapter about certain individuals, methods, and techniques that were highly successful. However, at closer look you will see that while all of these attempts were successful with some children, they were never successful with all children. We know from data over the past half-century or more that there is no single way that is effective with all children who are deaf and hard of hearing. Still, we hold to the notion that there must be one way even though student outcomes prove otherwise. As you read through all that we have done in the name of teaching children to communicate, keep in mind that we must choose from *all* that works in order to meet the needs of *all* children.

Since the inception of deaf education, teaching language to children who are deaf and hard of hearing has been the central focus and primary goal of educational programs. Although there has been a great deal of effort to teach language, the results have been less than acceptable. The literature indicates that there have been low achievement levels and small yearly gains despite twelve to fifteen years of schooling (Paul & Jackson, 1993). Students who are deaf typically gain about one-third of a grade-equivalent in reading comprehension each year (Wolk & Allen, 1984) making it very difficult for them to read typical textbooks. Moores (2000) reported that the overall achievement of the average 17- to 18-year-old student is six to seven years lower than that of his hearing peers. Further, only 10% of students with hearing losses are reading at a 7.5 grade level or better. These numbers have not changed significantly in decades. Despite normal cognitive potential, many children who are deaf and hard of hearing have low academic achievement. According to Moores (2000), we simply have not yet figured out how to teach them effectively. Not only do students have problems with reading, but they also have difficulty with written language (Schirmer, 2000). Without the ability to write, adults with hearing losses may have difficulty in the work environment. Even though the adult might have the ability to communicate face-to-face using some form of signs or spoken communication, writing requires the individual be able to use the English language. Historically, we have emphasized the teaching of rules and drills for mastery of English (McAnally, Rose, & Quigley, 1994), but many now believe that these approaches are not successful in teaching functional communication (Schirmer, 2000).

If deaf educators of the past have placed so much emphasis on language instruction and development, why have deaf children's literacy rates remained low in comparison to the general population? Why have their literacy rates remained low despite changes in philosophies and methodologies and the implementation of early intervention programs and mainstreaming? The answers are not simple and involve many interrelated factors. In addition, what works for one child might not work for other children with similar hearing losses and educational and family environments.

Language Issues within the Context of History

The documentation of the history of deaf people, their contributions to society, and the history of their education are fairly recent events when compared to other historical records. Although early writings have existed for centuries that record historical accounts of deaf people and the education of deaf students, it is only recently that these writings appear in text for contemporary readers. Many scholars point to the absence of the role of Deaf individuals in Deaf history proposing that their lack of acknowledgment and involvement has resulted in marginalization, oppression, and powerlessness (e.g., Lane, 1994; Lane, Hoffmeister, & Bahan, 1996; Plann, 1993; Truffaut, 1993; Wilcox, 1989). However, the past two decades of research, documentation, and publication have provided greater knowledge into Deaf people's lives, the contributions they made, and the systems that educated them.

It is not possible to present the entire history of Deaf education within this section; therefore, we will spotlight individuals, methods, and techniques that made substantial contributions in the area of communication development, tracing events that shaped the history of language instruction. You will find that most of the discussion will be about communication: the way in which language is transmitted.

The Early Records

Throughout the years philosophers have pondered the meaning of intelligence and how intelligence is demonstrated. Aristotle left a profound thumbprint on the lives of deaf people as he believed that innate knowledge could be expressed only through speech (Daniels, 1997). For Aristotle, intelligence was speech. A person without speech could not learn or think so was seen as incapable of reason (Daniels, 1997). The consequences of Aristotle's writings were dire: deaf people who were unable to speak or write were considered less than citizens and were left uneducated and illiterate. Today this ability is often used to measure a deaf person's intelligence (Plann, 1993) by those who lack an understanding of language development and the multiple pathways through which language is developed and expressed.

The Beginnings of Deaf Education

The earliest pioneers in deaf education sought to unlock deaf students' minds. Their primary goal was to make deaf children literate, providing an opportunity for religious salvation (Moores, 2000). According to Daniels (1997), the early pioneers, for religious reasons, worked to improve the ability of deaf people to communicate with each other and with their God. Many of the early teachers generously shared their methods, while others were more secretive, hoping to gain fame and perhaps a competitive hold on the business of teaching deaf children.

Throughout the centuries, the early methods have been borrowed, altered, fine-tuned and replicated. Even today, some of the methods the early pioneers used re-emerge under the guise of a new name or title (Hennon & Ishiel, 2000) but vary little from their original use. Therefore, it is important to know the methods of teaching language that have been used in the past because issues with which the early pioneers were most concerned continue to challenge and perplex the field today.

Tracing the Path of Language Instruction
Using Sign Language

The first school for the deaf began in the mountains of north central Spain in a Benedictine monastery, the San Salvadora de Oña. The Benedictines established schools within their monasteries for religious teachings and established a school for the deaf dedicated to communicating the gift of language (Daniels, 1997). A Benedictine monk, Pedro Ponce de León (1510–1584), is noted in history as being the first teacher of the deaf. During his time, the average man believed that deaf persons were inherently uneducable and that they could not be taught to speak; therefore, when Ponce de León professed to be able to teach speech to deaf students, he was revered and considered quite innovative (Plann, 1993). Among Ponce de León's students were the Valesco brothers, Francisco and Pedro, sons of a wealthy landowner who wanted his offspring educated so that they could receive their inheritance (Moores, 2000). Many of his contemporaries wrote about Ponce de León's methods. He started with the language the children brought with them, then introduced fingerspelling, writing and speech, the ultimate goal being speech (Daniels, 1997; Kisor, 1990). Ponce de León viewed signs as the quickest way to learn language and comprehension.

It would have been natural for him to use signs with his students because the Benedictine monks themselves had used a system of signs for hundreds of years. The monks lived and worked in silence—they communicated by the use of discreet signs. Consequently, a language evolved (Presneau, 1993). Ponce de León knew, from his experiences at the monastery, that language and thought could be communicated silently using signs. The school for the deaf within the monastery of San Salvador de Oña provided an environment where communication flowed freely among all and where learning received a great deal of attention and focus. Plann (1993) theorized that some of Pedro Ponce de León's students had a well-developed signed language because many were from families with histories of hereditary deafness. It is likely that the signs of these children and those of the Benedictine monks together became the manual signs used in instruction.

Thirty-six years after the death of Ponce de León, Juan Pablo Bonet (1579–1633) published the first book of a procedure for teaching deaf students entitled, *Simplification of the Letters of the Alphabet and Method of Teaching Deaf-Mutes to Speak* (Daniels, 1997; Lane, 1989). Some theorists today believe that the manuscript is the work of Pedro Ponce de León, plagiarized by Bonet (Van Cleve, 1987). Regardless of the origins, the publication had a significant impact on the education of deaf students. It was translated into numerous languages and distributed throughout Europe, and teachers of deaf students in other countries adopted Bonet's methods. Hodgson (1953) quotes Bonet as saying:

> A deaf reader literally receives the names of the letters through the eyes in the same way that hearing people secure the declaration of the sound of the letters. In essence, writing is the sound of speech. Mental development is language, nothing less, nothing more. The first duty of a teacher was to secure a student's mental development by any means possible. Sign and gestures were used as long as they were necessary and effective. Speech could not keep pace with the need for lan-

guage, and there was no wish to retard the mental development of a deaf child by slowing down to the pace of speech acquisition. (p. 94–95)

The Spanish contributed significantly to the early education of deaf students. Perhaps their most important contribution is the one-handed fingerspelling alphabet used in Spain in the sixteenth century by deaf students and their teachers. Most early educators, regardless of the communication approach, incorporated this fingerspelling alphabet into their instruction. Although there have been some modifications, the alphabet is essentially the same that is used in the United States and many other countries today.

Although the Spanish were the first to educate deaf students, the most well known teacher of deaf students is the Abbé Charles Michel de l'Epée (1712–1789), a French priest who also sought to save the souls of his students through religious teachings just as his predecessors had done. His interest in teaching deaf students began when he first encountered two deaf sisters while visiting the poor quarters of Paris. De l'Epée, believing the two girls would live and die in ignorance of their religion if he did not attempt some means of instructing them, told the mother to send the girls daily to his home.

Little was known in France during the 1700s about teaching deaf students, but by chance de l'Epée obtained a copy of Bonet's book and it had a tremendous influence on de l'Epée's teaching. The Abbé de l'Epée focused most of his work on language and the mental portion of learning; however, he did not ignore speech as evidenced by his detailed account of methods to teach speech (Marvelli, 1973).

Abbé de l'Epée believed that "it was the want of language, not the want of hearing that affected the apparent intelligence of a deaf person" (Watson, 1809, cited in Daniels, 1997, p. 32). However, most of de l'Epée's students came to the school with an existing sign language (i.e., French Sign Language). He built upon that language by introducing French grammar and adding invented signs based on Latin etymology. He called this approach *methodical signs*. The Abbé de l'Epée's approach to language instruction began by using the fingerspelling alphabet to teach the French letters. Next the students learned to write and label simple nouns and verbs. After the student had an adequate base of sentence parts, methodical signs were taught so that simple sentences could be written. As the students progressed, language instruction involved drills in translating methodical signs into written sentences.

De l'Epée shared his method freely with others. Schools continued to use the methodical sign system invented by de l'Epée for the next fifty years before they eventually abandoned it.

The successor to Abbé de l'Epée was the Abbé Roch-Ambroise Sicard (1742–1822). He accepted the directorship of de l'Epée's school in 1790 and brought his gifted deaf student, Jean Massieu, with him to become head assistant teacher. Massieu was the first deaf person to hold a teaching position at the school. When they arrived in Paris they found conditions destitute, so the

Abbé Sicard immediately went to work to obtain funding that had been promised to de l'Epée earlier. He was successful and that fall the school moved from de l'Epée's home to a new location on the rue Saint-Jacques. In 1815 the Abbé Sicard presented a series of public exhibitions in London and took several students including Massieu and Laurent Clerc with him to demonstrate their skills.

Shortly after the Abbé Sicard dedicated his new school in Paris, Thomas Braidwood (1715–1806) began teaching deaf students in Great Britain. Braidwood's first deaf student, Charles Shirreff, had lost his hearing at the age of three. Under Braidwood's instruction, Shirreff learned to speak, read, and write, and soon Braidwood's success spread throughout Great Britain. Braidwood based his instructional method on the earlier works of William Holder, John Wallis, and Henry Baker, the first professional teachers of deaf students in England (Marvelli, 1973). Both Wallis and Baker emphasized articulation and the use of speech but little is known of their methods because they guarded their work very carefully (Marvelli, 1973). Braidwood's request for public funds to start a school in Edinburgh was turned down, so his family opened a private school with their own funds (Marvelli, 1973). To ensure the stability of his school and to provide a legacy for his family, he hired only relatives to manage his growing business. Those family members were required to take an oath of secrecy, swearing not to reveal the methods to outsiders (Lysons, 1987). Eventually the Braidwoods would establish three schools for the deaf in Great Britain. John Braidwood, grandson of Thomas Braidwood, assumed the directorship of the school in Edinburgh in 1812, but soon after departed to America to establish the fourth school.

In the United States, the young clergyman Thomas Hopkins Gallaudet (1787–1851) became intrigued with the education of deaf children after meeting a young girl, Alice Cogswell, at a neighbor's home in Connecticut. At that time no schools for deaf students existed in the United States. Instead of sending his young daughter to school in Europe, Mr. Cogswell worked with others to start a school in New England. He hoped to duplicate the British model of instruction (Mattingly, 1987) for news of the British model's success had spread to America. They sent Gallaudet to Europe to seek out the most advanced methods for teaching deaf students, and in 1815 he arrived in London. He visited the Braidwood School, which at that time was the most prestigious in Great Britain (Moores, 2000). His visit was met with hesitation by those in charge. First, there was the oath of secrecy (Daniels, 1997). Second, John Braidwood had intentions of establishing the first oral school in America (Marvelli, 1973; Moores, 2000). But Braidwood was an alcoholic and had fled to America after falling into debt while running the Edinburgh school (Marvelli, 1973). Still, his family had hopes that he would be successful at starting a new school in a new place. When Gallaudet made a request to learn the Braidwood method, the family resisted—Gallaudet might become a competitor (Marvelli, 1973). Eventually the Braidwood family realized that although John had good intentions, the school would not come to fruition. Most of John Braidwood's teaching would be on a farm in Fairfax County, Virginia, which, interestingly, has one of the largest public school programs for deaf and hard of hearing students in the United States today.

Gallaudet received permission to learn the Braidwood method at last. However, the Braidwoods insisted on a five-year apprenticeship (Mattingly, 1987). Gallaudet would be required to serve as an assistant and devote several years to learning the techniques, years that he did not have, especially because there were deaf children awaiting his tutelage back home in America. By chance, Gallaudet learned of the public exhibitions that Abbé Sicard had arranged in London. After attending one of the sessions, Sicard invited Gallaudet to serve under his instruction at the school in Paris—there, Gallaudet could learn the methods of Abbé de l'Epée in a few short months. This offer was much more to Gallaudet's liking and was within his available time frame. While at the session he also met a young deaf man, Laurent Clerc, who eventually agreed to return with him to the United States to establish the first school for the deaf in Hartford, Connecticut in 1817 (Lane, 1989). With Gallaudet as principal and Clerc as head teacher, the school flourished using the French method of teaching: methodical signs and the Theory of Ciphers, a structured language approach. The French method looked on the development of articulation as secondary to language. It was not until 1845 that speech and lipreading on an individualized basis were included in the curriculum at the school in Hartford (Fernandes, 1980).

Thomas Hopkins Gallaudet is often given credit for formalizing the instructional plan for deaf education that unfolded during the next decades following the establishment of the American School. However, according to Mattingly (1987) Gallaudet resigned from the American School in 1830 once it was established and went on to other interests. With his departure, the future of deaf education was left up to Laurent Clerc and succeeding generations of reformers such as Isaac Peet, and Edward Miner Gallaudet, the son of Thomas Hopkins Gallaudet.

Tracing the Path of Oral Language Instruction

While many of the early teachers of deaf and hard of hearing students used some form of signs and fingerspelling, the main goal for most was spoken language. Even before de l'Epée, the Oral Method (with minimal use of signs or fingerspelling) began emerging in Europe. Several early pioneers formulated the theories upon which later teachers would base their work.

One early pioneer of oral instruction, George Dalgarno (1628–1687) published *The Deaf and Dumb Man's Tutor* in 1680. This small text had a great influence on others in the field. Dalgarno was a Scot and a teacher in a private grammar school for hearing children in Oxford. He was intrigued with language and the process of language acquisition. Dalgarno believed that the eye could compensate for the lack of hearing if diligence were followed with consistent, persistent, and repetitive exposure to meaningful English (Scouten,

1984). Dalgarno's method used writing and fingerspelling; however, he did not use the Spanish fingerspelling form. Instead he used one he created whereby the twenty-six letters were identified tactilely at points on the open palm. Other than this form of fingerspelling, no other signing was used.

Many early oralists based their approaches on the work of Johann Amman (1669–1724), a Swiss physician, who likened the human body to a machine. Amman hypothesized that if deaf and hard of hearing students could make sounds, they could be taught to speak (Presneau, 1993). Amman's methods for teaching speech and language focused primarily on the mechanics of articulation by teaching elements of speech first, next blending the elements into syllables, forming spoken words, then moving to the written word. Because he was a pioneer in the oral method, Amman is known as the Father of Pure Oralism. Amman may have been the first person to view deafness publicly from a medical perspective rather than as a God-given trait.

Jacob Rodriguez Pereire (1715–1790) was also a noted oral instructor. Pereire was born in Portugal but moved to France in 1733 when he was eighteen. Pereire had a deaf sister and a deaf wife, both of whom inspired Pereire to devote his life to teaching deaf students to speak (Lane, 1976). According to Séguin (Lane, 1989) who wrote a book on Periere's life, Pereire managed to instill in the deaf student a natural voice with correct pronunciation. Because of his talents in teaching deaf students to speak he is referred to as *The Greatest Teacher of Them All* (McAnally, Rose, & Quigley, 1994). In 1753 Pereire opened a private school in Paris with approximately twelve students who came to him from all over Europe. To establish initial communication Pereira used pantomime and the Spanish fingerspelling alphabet. He also invented his own syllable signs. Later language instruction followed a natural approach. From these early beginnings, others came to use the Oral Method.

During the 1750s a young teacher in Germany, Samuel Heinicke (1729–1790), employed the techniques of Amman in order to teach a deaf student to speak. Like de l'Epée he believed that education should be available to all children (Marvelli, 1973). He believed that language was possible only through speech and, therefore, he adamantly believed that deaf students should be taught to speak. Heinicke expanded the method developed by Amman in several ways and formulated his own method regarding language development. According to Scouten (1984) Heinicke believed that deaf students could easily learn language through signs and pictures, but this language would be temporary. He also objected to the introduction of language through the use of print. He believed that learning language through writing was arduous, requiring constant drill and repetition. Consequently, for Heinicke, speech was the only avenue through which lasting language development could occur. Heinicke's method progressed through a sequence of educational events: word study, syllable study, and finally individual sounds and letters (Marvelli, 1973). He also substituted the sense of taste and used various flavors to facilitate students' mastery of vowels during speech drills. Heinicke's method of instructing deaf students became widespread throughout Europe, and today Germany has retained its strong oral emphasis when educating deaf students.

During the later part of the eighteenth century and continuing throughout the nineteenth century, the German oral method of instruction gained support throughout Europe and eventually had a great influence on the education of deaf students in the United States. Approximately fifty years after the American School was established in West Hartford, Connecticut, Bernhard Engelsmann immigrated to the United States with the hopes of establishing a school for the deaf in New York City. Engelsmann had been trained in the pure oral approach at the Vienna Hebrew School for Deaf Children (Mattingly, 1987; Scouten, 1984). It wasn't long before he opened a new school and began teaching students following the German oral method. Today this school is known as the Lexington School for the Deaf.

Within a few months following the opening of the school, a second oral school opened its doors in Massachusetts. In 1867 the Clarke School for the Deaf was established in Northampton, and Harriet Rogers, a well-known and successful teacher, became its first principal (Moores, 2000). The Clarke School for the Deaf holds prominence among oral institutions in the United States. Many early instructional methods and materials developed at the school are still in use today such as the Northampton Symbol System developed by Alice Worcester and Caroline Yale.

Alexander Graham Bell (1847–1922) was perhaps the most influential person to promote the oral method of instruction in the United States. Although he is widely known as the inventor of the telephone, in the field of deaf education he is known as a teacher of speech to deaf students and promoter of the oral method of language instruction. Bell's prestige as an inventor did much to further the rapid acceptance of the Oral Method (Mattingly, 1987). He grew up in Scotland and immigrated to North America in 1871. As a young child he was curious and intrigued by inventions. Because of his mother's postlingual deafness, Bell developed a keen interest in inventions that would help her situation. Thus, some believe he invented the telephone while attempting to invent a hearing device for his mother. In 1871 Bell taught Visible Speech—a method of teaching speech developed by his father—at the Boston Day School for the Deaf and later demonstrated this technique at other schools. Bell based a great deal of his teaching techniques on those of the early pioneer, Dalgarno. He described his teaching methods in the *American Annals of the Deaf* in 1883 after receiving much acclaim for the achievement of his student, George Sanders who, even though prelingually deaf, had an excellent command of the English language. Bell wrote that he divided his method into two areas: articulation and mental development, working on each simultaneously. To develop articulation, Bell first drilled his student in elementary sounds and exercises, then proceeded to words and sentences (although it is noted that he changed his process later in his teaching career). He used the visible speech symbols, displayed on a glove in order to teach tactilely, leaving the student to observe the face of the speaker.

For mental development he believed, as did Dalgarno, that a deaf person should be taught to read and write the same way that all children are taught to speak and understand their mother tongue. Bell believed that everyone should talk to the deaf child just as we do a hearing one, with the exception that the words be addressed to his eye instead of his ear.

The history of Oralism is not complete without recognizing the impact of listening technology (e.g., personal aids, FM systems, cochlear implants, etc.). Life prior to the twentieth century was very different from life today—there were few technological advances, and antibiotics were yet to be discovered. Imagine that you are a parent living in those times and you discover that your child has a hearing loss. Back then your choices were to send your child to a school that was weeks away by buckboard or to keep him at home where his future would be limited. Now imagine that some new, strange, unbelievable device comes along which hints at the possibility of a normal life for your child. Would you not do everything in your power to bring this opportunity to your child? The hearing aid was such a device.

Oral schools began to open in the United States in the 1860s. With a couple of decades of experience with a hearing aid behind them and new inventions such as that of the telephone in 1876, we can understand how the early oralists in America and around the world would be excited. Technology was now available. The increased use of hearing aids in the 1860s and 1870s, and the efforts to ban sign language from schools in 1880, was no coincidence. Oralism emerged as the most prominent educational philosophy used in the instruction of students with hearing loss in the late 1800s and dominated the field until the 1970s. Several factors probably contributed to the dominance of the oralist tradition, including improvements in hearing aid technology, the development of the scientific field of audiology, and the innovative work of individuals such as Groht (1958) and van Uden (1970). [For a comprehensive overview of assistive technology and amplification, see Compton (1998). For an overview of cochlear implant technology, see Beiter and Brimacombe (1998).]

The Path of Contention between Oralism and Manualism

The path of contention between the two philosophies goes deep and has existed since the 1700s when it was brought to the forefront by Heinicke and de l'Epée who were on opposite ends of the oral–manual spectrum. Although the controversy regarding the best communication method to teach language to deaf students probably began much earlier, the disagreements between these two prominent figures escalated the controversy.

In 1783, de l'Epée asked for an impartial tribunal to review the two opposing philosophies and to determine which was superior. The Academy of Zurich was asked to make that determination, and it voted for de l'Epée's approach (Scouten, 1984); however, Marvelli (1973) provides further clarification on the results of the inquiry. "Based on the evidence presented, the judgement was made that neither method was natural, but the manual method was considered better. This decision resulted, in part, from the Abbé de l'Epée's willingness to fully describe his method, while Heinicke was reluctant to share specific information about his method with the judges" (p. 33).

A century later in the United States, Alexander Graham Bell and Edward Miner Gallaudet, the son of Thomas Gallaudet and the founder of Gallaudet University, feuded over the two philosophies. Bell published papers that passionately criticized the manualist system of education of the deaf. He stated that the effect of the system was to isolate deaf people from society and increase the number of marriages among deaf people, which could possibly contribute to a deaf race, something to which Bell was vehemently opposed. In fact he was so opposed to deaf/deaf marriages that he advocated a law forbidding the marriage of congenitally deaf persons (Moores, 2000). To improve the educational system in the United States, Bell (1884) included three recommendations in his papers: eliminate educational segregation in institutions, eliminate the use of sign language, and eliminate deaf teachers who comprised one-third of the teaching force at that time.

Although the backgrounds of Gallaudet and Bell were similar, both having deaf mothers, on the surface they appeared as diametrically opposed as de l'Epée and Heinicke. However, while neither de l'Epée nor Heinicke would compromise his beliefs, Gallaudet began to explore the middle ground between the approaches. Eventually he agreed that the Oral Method might be useful for some students (Mattingly, 1987). The approach Gallaudet conceptualized used American Sign Language (ASL) as the language of instruction, emphasized English through writing and reading, and provided speech lessons to those who could benefit. He called his approach the Combined Method. To some, his addition of speech lessons to the curriculum made him appear more a proponent of the oral method than an advocate for the combined approach. In 1886 he convened a Conference of the Principals of Schools for the Deaf for the purpose of discussing communication methodologies and clarifying the concept of adding articulation and lipreading as a supplement to the present curriculum. He persuaded those in attendance to adopt a resolution calling for all schools for the deaf to embrace the combined approach, thus moving toward the center of the communication debate.

Because of his belief in using all methods, some consider Edward Miner Gallaudet as the first to propose the concept of Total Communication. He wrote for many years about the need for a balanced approach in the use of speech and signs, but his advocacy for a combined system was to stall at the International Congress on Education of the Deaf held in Milan, Italy, in 1888. At the conference, a ban of the use of signs in programs for deaf students was put to a vote (Lane, 1989). So, while in the United States Gallaudet had advocated the inclusion of speech and lipreading into programs that had been historically manual, at the conference in Milan he was put in a position to defend the use of signs. Unfortunately for the field of deaf education, and despite efforts to blend communication techniques in various combinations, this legacy of controversy continues today.

Tracing the Path of the Intuitive Approach to Teaching Language

Early language instruction of deaf and hard of hearing students was quite analytical, using drill and practice to cement concepts into memory. Regardless of whether the students were following a purely oral method or using methodical signs (i.e., those with word order following the sequence of that country's spoken language), memorization was an important part of the instructional technique. Ambroise-Roch Bebian (1789–1839) provided an alternative to these instructional techniques while at the National Institute for the Deaf in Paris. He produced two books: (1) a curriculum guide that provided step-by-step procedures and a sequence for teaching the French language through natural signs; and (2) a book that provided an explanation of the natural signs, which he described through a written system. For example he included characters for handshapes, movements, position, and facial expression. He called his system *mimography* (Scouten, 1984). This was perhaps the first attempt to explain a visual language linguistically.

According to Clerc (Lane, 1989) Bebian was one of the few hearing people ever to become fluent in natural signs. Bebian based his curriculum on the use of natural signs using an approach that he referred to as the Intuitive Method. This method used the printed word to move students from their natural language to written French. Instead of teaching language through drill as de l'Epée and Sicard had done, he taught students to use intuition (e.g., to draw logical conclusions about communication) (Scouten, 1984). He used visual representations such as drawings, illustrations, and pictures to establish a concept for which the teacher would provide the appropriate written and fingerspelled word. After a lesson had been presented, Bebian used a process referred to as Exercises in Assimilation, a series of exercises to reinforce the language principle. Bebian's instructional methodology brought to the field a new approach that was much more natural than the analytical approaches his predecessors used. Some of his ideas could be compared to ASL/ESL techniques used today; however, in the 1800s they were not widely accepted. Bebian eventually left the Paris school to open his own school.

The Swinging Pendulum

In the mid 1800s, the once-prominent school in Paris began to decline. Eventually the school abandoned the use of methodical signs and further restricted the use of natural signs. Other schools throughout Europe followed suit. Schools in the United States that had begun using methodical signs eventually discarded them as well and by 1830 natural signs (ASL) had replaced methodical signs as the language of instruction. The pendulum was to swing again, and by the late 1800s Oralism became the predominant method used in schools.

Language Issues within the Context of Instruction

Instructional practices vary depending on the pathway by which teachers present information. They also vary from a natural orientation to a structured orientation. This next section presents these contexts for language instruction.

Auditory and Visual Approaches Used in Recent Times

Schools in the United States used the Oral Method extensively for nearly a century. Beginning in the 1950s, schools began to experiment with new approaches to language instruction. The Rochester Method, which used fingerspelling to supplement the oral approach, was used in some schools (Scouten, 1984). Another approach that provides a supplement to the Oral Method was Cued Speech, conceptualized by Cornett in the 1960s. "The purpose of this system is to overcome the limitations of pure oral/aural methods without deviating from or compromising any of the objectives that are inherent in the oral philosophy (Scheetz, 2001, p. 129). Cued Speech uses handshapes near the mouth in conjunction with speech; they are neither signs nor the fingerspelling alphabet and cannot be read alone (Heward, 1996). The cues clarify sounds of a spoken language that may be indistinguishable when speechreading. The approach has been successful for students who learn to encode language phonetically through the auditory pathway. Most likely those students for whom Cued Speech provides benefit have usable residual hearing, use hearing aids and other listening technology to take advantage of their residual hearing, and are able to speechread most of what is spoken. Cued Speech is used to ensure that the language code is complete.

In the 1970s, English-based sign systems such as Seeing Essential English (SEE I) (Anthony, 1971) and Signing Exact English (SEE II) (Gustason, Pfetzing, & Zawolkow, 1980) came into prominence. These systems borrowed signs from ASL and attempted to put them in English grammatical order in much the same way as Abbé de l'Epée created methodical signs by putting natural French signs into French word order. Developers of English-based signs created systems by inventing signs, initializing existing signs, and inventing prefixes, suffixes, etc., so that the signs were more representative of English. Some developers avoided the use of fingerspelling because they believed it was too difficult for young children to understand and use (Fischer, 1998).

The 1970s also brought about widespread use of Total Communication, a philosophy focusing on the needs of the individual child. Roy Holcomb first defined Total Communication in 1967 (Evans, 1982; Garretson, 1976). He proposed that it consist of auditory training, speech, speechreading, fingerspelling, and the language of signs (ASL) (Nover & Andrews, 1998). Holcomb felt that Oralism was restrictive and many students failed to develop language under this approach. Many deaf leaders in the field, school administrators, and parents embraced the new philosophy, and new teaching methods began to emerge as the philosophy became integrated into educational practice. It was easy for hearing educators to embrace Total Communication because they could continue using most of their educational practices, only adding signs to their existing instructional repertoire. For this to work, though, they needed a signing system that matched spoken language.

As Total Communication gained in acceptance, the use of oral approaches declined. The new philosophy brought hopes of achieving greater levels of literacy in students who are deaf or hard of hearing. Many university deaf education programs also added sign language to their instructional content although most retained a strong speech-focused curriculum. Total Communication became the most widely used method of instructing deaf and hard of hearing students throughout the United States (Hoffmeister, 1990; Moores, 2000; Nover, 1995; Reagan, 1995; Stewart, 1992). By the late 1970s approximately 65% of all classrooms used Total Communication (Jordan, Gustason, & Rosen, 1976; Jordan, Gustason, & Rosen, 1979). These percentages remained constant until the 1990s (Moores, 2000) when the reporting terminology changed in order to obtain a more functional description. Currently schools indicate that 51% use speech and sign, 42% use oral/aural only, and 5% use sign only.

While Total Communication brought hope to parents, it failed to produce desired outcomes for many students. The underlying assumption of Total Communication was that if children were exposed to English visually in the form of signs, they would learn English naturally in the same way that hearing children do. However, many children with hearing losses never achieved this goal. Perhaps it was not the philosophy of Total Communication itself that failed, but the way it was put into classroom practice. Most teachers at the time had been trained in oral methods and many had never taken a sign language course; therefore, they were most often learning signs on-the-job. In addition, most programs equated Total Communication with speaking and signing simultaneously or *sim com*. According to Johnson, Liddell, and Erting (1989), there are inherent problems in depicting English, an auditory language, through signs. They found that most of the signs used by teachers did not match their spoken output. English is an auditory, sequential language while ASL is a visual, spatial language, so blending the two languages into a clear language code is challenging. Those students who have usable residual hearing or have postlingual losses may benefit from English-based signs because they are able to fill in information gaps through their residual hearing and speechreading skills. However, English-based signs provide an incomplete language code for profoundly deaf children who rely solely on vision to access information.

Total Communication did not increase literacy levels as the founders had hoped. Deaf and hard of hearing students who were educated in the 1970s and 1980s did not read or write English significantly better than students who had been educated orally. "Disappointing results from these approaches may stem from the fact that none represents a complete language system in itself to the deaf child (Strong, 1995, p. 119).

The *Bilingual-Bicultural* philosophy began to appear in the 1980s due to dissatisfaction with the outcomes of deaf education. The philosophy developed from a growing body of research in child language development, cognitive science, and sign language linguistics. These studies reported that deaf children who had deaf parents and were exposed to ASL were superior to deaf children of hearing parents in academic achievement, literacy, English usage, and social-emotional development (Meadow, 1967; Stuckless & Birch, 1966; Vernon & Koh, 1970). The Bilingual-Bicultural philosophy is founded on the premise that deaf children learn more efficiently through their unimpaired visual channel than through their impaired auditory pathways. The most efficient visual language for deaf students is ASL. Through learning ASL, the brain develops the plasticity and connections upon which a second language (English) is learned. English is taught through print in written form. According to Finnegan (1992), bilingualism involves the ability to function linguistically in two different language communities. It doesn't, however, imply equal skill and proficiency in both languages. Bilingual-Bicultural methods use ASL as the first language of a deaf child and English as a second language, understanding that because of the shared language, a culture of Deaf people coexists with the majority culture. There is growing acceptance and recognition of this approach in the education of deaf children both in residential and local schools.

The Bilingual-Bicultural philosophy requires different communication and instructional approaches, practices, and techniques than have been used in the past; therefore, transitioning from Total Communication approaches to Bilingual-Bicultural approaches is much more challenging. One of the greatest challenges is the retraining of current teachers who must often break out of old ways of thinking, remove old prejudices, and learn new ways of teaching language. For example, teachers who were trained in oral methods and English-based signs must become fluent in ASL and learn visual strategies for teaching language. (See Nover & Andrews, 1998; 1999 for more information on the Bilingual-Bicultural philosophy).

Auditory Verbal Therapy has been showing promising results. This therapy is a form of aural rehabilitation similar to the Acoupedics approach promoted by Pollack in the 1970s. According to Pollack (1964) a child who is taught to speechread or sign will rely on the visual channel and may not develop his listening potential. Deaf students educated in this method are dissuaded from using their vision in order to develop their listening to the greatest extent possible. While many of the teaching strategies used in Auditory Verbal programs are similar to those used in the 1970s, advances in technology, specifically cochlear implants, have made this approach appropriate for many children. Auditory Verbal therapists provide a habilitative environment for children with implants, focusing on the development of the child's auditory skills and oral language development. The difference between Auditory Verbal techniques and a traditional oral program is that the latter permits the use of vision to supplement audition and occurs in the classroom while the former restricts input to the auditory channel during one-to-one therapy. For example, a student in a traditional oral program may use visual strategies such as speechreading or Cued Speech to supplement residual hearing. Teachers of deaf students utilizing the Auditory Verbal method require specialized training in the development of auditory skills but are not required to be proficient in a signed language because no manual communication is used.

The Auditory Verbal method of instruction is growing in momentum for several reasons. The most important reason is advances in the technology used in cochlear implants. As the technology becomes more sophisticated, success rates are increasing. In addition, children who are candidates for cochlear implants are being identified earlier due to increased efforts in infant hearing screening by hospitals. The earlier children are implanted, the more successful the results (Connor, Hieber, Arts, & Zowlan, 2000). As success rates are increasing, the procedure is becoming more common, physicians are recommending it more often, and insurance companies are approving the procedure, thus making this option more readily available to families.

Structured, Natural, and Combined Approaches

Language instruction for children who are deaf or hard of hearing had a different meaning in the past than it does today. Before, language instruction most often meant teaching English grammar using visual tools to show English structure. Several approaches, often building on one another, were developed and used with students with a variety of outcomes. Often there were disagreements among educators regarding the extent to which structured approaches should be used; however, most early teachers agreed that in order for children who are deaf or hard of hearing to develop competence in written English a structured approach was necessary. Some educators taught language through drill and memorization using structured approaches as the central part of their language instruction. Some used structured approaches to reinforce language patterns presented through language experience activities. For example, Fitzgerald emphasized the need to develop language through classroom experiences while using the Fitzgerald Key as a tool for constructing and reinforcing written language. The Fitzgerald Key (Table 1.1) is the most commonly mentioned example of a structured approach. Others used structured language programs for older students to help them refine written language production. Structured approaches have been used in a variety of ways and combined with natural approaches in varying degrees depending on the school's language curriculum. We

TABLE 1.1 *The Fitzgerald Key*

Model	Who:		What:	Whom:		For…:	How far:	
						With…:	How often:	
	Whose:			Whose:	Where:			When:
						How:	How long:	
	What:	=	Whom:	What:		Why:	How much:	
Example	William plays				outside	with the puppy		after school.
	Mom	gives	him cookies		under the tree	for a snack		sometimes.

have included approaches typically referred to as combined approaches because they evolved from other structured approaches. Table 1.2 reveals that as structured approaches matured, the rigidity with which teachers used them diminished and developers integrated more natural elements into their systems and practices.

During the 1950s natural approaches emerged as an alternative to the rigid structured approaches that often used memorization and drill. Advocates of natural approaches to teaching language believed that structured approaches were overused and devoid of meaning. They believed that language should be taught through incidental occurrences especially to young children. Although often associated with the oral philosophy, natural approaches model early language interactions between a parent and child and are widely used today regardless of communication methodology.

As we progressed in our understanding of how students learn to communicate, many other programs developed that were a hybrid of structural and natural approaches. These are referred to as *combined approaches* and are commonly used across the nation. These are included in Tables 1.2 and 1.3 as they are outgrowths of the other approaches. For example, Anderson, Boren, Kilgore, Howard, and Krohn (1980, 1999) refined the language structures to be taught into ten basic sentence patterns and published a series of workbooks called the *Apple Tree*, which is an acronym for "A Patterned Approach for Linguistic Expansion Through Reinforced Experiences and Evaluations." In addition to ever-changing combinations of structured and natural approaches, many different instructional materials were developed and published for use in teaching language (Table 1.4). For example, McCarr (1980) developed *Lessons in Syntax*, and Gallaudet University Outreach (1985) developed a *Structured Tasks in English Practice* series. These tended to be in the form of workbooks that were primarily useful as tools for reinforcement.

One departure from the typical approaches used in language instruction was *A Process Approach to Developing Language with Hearing Impaired Children* by Reed and Bugen (1986). This program stressed the importance of understand-

TABLE 1.2 *The Evolution of Structured Approaches to Language Instruction and Associated Combined Approaches*

Individual	Year	Approach	Conceptual Foundation
Abbé Sicard, used by Clerc and Gallaudet	1800s	Theory of Ciphers—Coding system of columns and numbers to form language patterns.	Students could learn to construct sentences by means of a grammatical system.
Peet	1844	Peet's Language System—System that used color codes to represent the structure of English sentences.	Believed ideas should precede words. Lessons presented in small, sequential steps. Concepts presented one at a time.
Jacobs	1858	Primary Lessons—Highly structured and systematic plan for language instruction illustrations. Lessons were presented in small, graduated steps.	Language instruction should begin early proceeding from the alphabet to writing.
Teachers at the American School for the Deaf	mid 1800s	The Hartford System—Based on the Theory of Ciphers, a set of diagrams or line drawings to represent grammatical relationships and syntactic rules of English.	A visual system of English is necessary to provide students with a foundation in language.
Storrs	1880	The Storrs System refined and adapted the Hartford System to become a more scientific method where students memorized 300 conversational patterns. Forty-seven box-like figures were used to help children fill in the grammatical formula.	Deaf children unable to learn complexities of grammar through the natural method could memorize formulas of grammar to serve their daily communication needs.
Wing	1883	The Wing Symbols—Symbols were placed over words when analyzing the grammar of English sentences.	Prior to this method students memorize grammatical structures. Designed to help students develop a sense of grammar.

Barry	1893	Barry Five Slates—A five-slate system built on the Theory of Ciphers that used five columns each representing the subject, verb, direct object, preposition, and object of the preposition. A sixth slate was used to expand sentences.	Visual patterns of grammar used to assist deaf children in developing sight rules of language just as hearing children rely on auditory rules of language.
Fitzgerald	1926	Straight Language System or the Fitzgerald Key—An elaboration of the Barry Five Slates, the system used five columns each labeled with words and symbols to indicate grammatical structures and functions. A popular system used by most schools from 1926–1970s.	Deaf students can not be taught English as one would a foreigner. Gave students a tool to learn syntactic relationships and rules of English when constructing written language. Although "Key" was highly structured, Fitzgerald suggested natural, experience-based situations.
Pugh	1955	Steps in Language Development for the Deaf—Built on the Fitzgerald Key, designed for younger children than Fitzgerald had targeted, the curriculum presented a sequence for presenting language structures and concept development.	Prior to this program, little was known about the sequence of language development. This curriculum emphasized language form and correct word order.
D'Arc and Buckler, St. Joseph's School for the Deaf	1958, 1968	The Patterned Approach to Connected Language—Built on the Fitzgerald Key. e.g., Verb + What Verb + Where Verb + Adjective Verb + Whom	Built on the work of Groht, the model blended natural and structured approaches and used command forms, requests, and questions with basic and expanded patterns within natural settings and functional situations.
Streng	1972	Streng's Applied Linguistics—Based on Chomsky's transformational-generative grammar, is a structured approach to teaching language in a natural manner.	Students need a more directed approach. Should not be taught the rules, but teachers should provide situations in which they discover rules inductively.

(continued)

19

TABLE 1.2 *Continued*

Individual	*Year*	*Approach*	*Conceptual Foundation*
Anderson, Boren, Kilgore, Howard, & Krohn	1980, 1999	A Patterned Program for Linguistic Expansion Through Reinforced Experiences and Evaluations (Apple Tree), a commercial curriculum that focuses on the development of ten basic sentence patterns after a basic vocabulary has been established. e.g., N1 + V N1 + V + Adjective N1 + V + N3 + N2	Through a sequential, spiraling system of instruction that includes presentation of concepts in natural settings, instruction in various sentence patterns, manipulation of word cards that form sentence patterns, and completion of workbooks, students achieve competency in the use of specific language patterns outlined in the program
Reed & Bugen	1986	The Process Approach to Developing Language with Hearing-Impaired Children—A systematic program of language instruction designed to assist older students in developing the sense of language through pragmatics and semantics while practicing target language structures. e.g., Since_____, the_____.	Language learning in the classroom is based on student/teacher interactions. Teachers facilitate language acquisition through shared experiences, stimulation, and discussion. Language instruction is a process teachers follow when planning and presenting language lessons.

Sources: Anderson, Boren, Kilgore, Howard, & Krohn, 1980, 1999; McAnally, Rose, & Quigley, 1994; Moores, 2000; Streng, 1972; Reed & Bugen, 1986.

TABLE 1.3 *The Evolution of Natural Approaches to Language Instruction and Associated Combined Approaches*

Individual	Year	Name of Approach	Conceptual Basis
Hill	mid 1800s	Mother's Approach	Experience before expression.
Greenberger (Green)	1880	Mother's Method—Built on the concepts presented by Hill, instruction centered around learning language through daily activities in the context of the situation and needs of the children.	Found memorization of rules meaningless. Encouraged development of language through experiences based on need for expression rather than through imposition of expression externally.
Groht	1958	The "new" Mother's Method or the Natural Approach to Teaching Language—Based on the work of Greenberger and Hill, used a natural approach through real experiences. Artificial exercises and drill absent of personal meaning were avoided.	Language evolves and develops through natural interactions and occurrences for real purposes in the environment rather than as a subject to be mastered. Deaf children need to be exposed to language through communication in natural settings.
van Uden	1970	The Maternal Reflexive Method—Continued the work of Groht by expanding the natural approach to include naturally structured conversations emphasizing receptive language. Conversations were recorded in writing.	Language develops through natural communicative interactions. Contrived experiences and language patterns are not successful in teaching language.
Moog, The Central Institute for the Deaf	1971	CID Language Program—A natural approach that teaches language in the sequence in which hearing children acquire language.	Children with hearing losses are innately capable of learning language and should proceed through the natural stages of development.

(continued)

TABLE 1.3 *Continued*

Individual	Year	Name of Approach	Conceptual Basis
Blackwell, Engen, Fischgrund, & Zarcadoolas, The Rhode Island School for the Deaf	1978	The Rhode Island Curriculum—Based on the theories of Chomsky and Piaget, a grammatically structured method of teaching language within a natural framework. Presented at four levels: exposure, recognition, comprehension, and production. Complexities build on basic sentence patterns.	Deaf children have the innate ability to acquire language through conversation, interactions, modeling, and imitation. Stresses the use of content from the humanities (social studies and literacy) as information to be communicated.
Schleper	1980–present	Whole Language or Literacy Based Approach—Emphasizes language development through integration of all aspects of language instruction (spoken and signed communication, writing, reading). Emphasis is on communicative competence and learning English through text in a print-rich environment.	Language is acquired within authentic contexts in a natural way. Language is presented as a "whole" not broken down into isolated parts. The emphasis of the whole language approach is on literacy and students learn English through writing and reading about their experiences or topics that intrigue them.

Source: Groht, 1958; McAnally, Rose, & Quigley, 1994; Moores, 2000; van Uden, 1970.

TABLE 1.4 *Remedial Language Programs*

Individual	Year	Approach	Conceptual Basis
Costello and Watson Gallaudet University	1975	Structured Tasks in English Practice—A syntactic structures series of workbooks that provide practice in language structures.	A remedial program for students in secondary and post-secondary programs.
Kretschmer and Kretschmer	1978	One of the first models to stress the three-dimensional nature of communication including cognitive, linguistic, and pragmatic aspects of English language usage. Specifically designed for children who have an established English language base, the program assesses children's spontaneous use of language (signed, spoken, written) in a variety of natural settings and conditions.	Language instruction should focus on the interrelationships among the various aspects of language including structural organization and pragmatic intent. Planning for language intervention requires several decision-making steps included in the program.
Quigley and Power	1979	Test of Syntactic Abilities Syntax Program—A set of supplemental programmed exercises used to reinforce the language experiences and instruction in the classroom. Materials provided drill and practice in several linguistic structures.	Developed as remedial materials for students ten years and older who were having trouble with English language structures.
McCarr	1980	Lessons in Syntax—Consists of workbooks and uses a programmed linear approach to learning syntax through drills and practice.	A remedial program for students at the intermediate through post-secondary levels to help students develop English syntax.

(continued)

TABLE 1.4 *Continued*

Individual	Year	Approach	Conceptual Basis
Phelps-Terasaki & Phelps-Gunn	1988, 2000	Teaching Competence in Written Language—Based on the Fitzgerald Key, a program to teach written expression that uses a visual cue system to generate sentences, elaborate and expand sentences, and organize paragraphs.	Students with learning disabilities and language disorders have special problems with written language and need a structured writing process in order to acquire this skill.
Fokes	1982	Fokes Sentence Builder System—Built on the Barry Five Slates system, uses five grammatical categories. A colored box containing pictures represents each category. Children arrange the pictures to form sentences.	Provided a structured program for language-disordered children.
Peter	1984	Learning Sentence Patterns with Jack and Julie	A remedial program for elementary students that used illustrations to bridge to written English.

Source: Fokes, 1982; McAnally, Rose, & Quigley, 1994; Moores, 2000; Paul & Quigley, 1994; Phelps-Terasaki & Phelps-Gunn, 1988, 2000.

ing the semantic and pragmatic sense of why we use a particular language structure in the real world before we actually use the structure. Most approaches used today stress the importance of pragmatics and semantics as the basis for language acquisition. Whether or not we follow old approaches or new approaches, we can no longer view the language acquisition process as a simple mastery of a set of rules. As teachers you need to know these rules yourself so that you can arrange real-life experiences that bring these skills to life, but mastery of a set of grammatical structures can only make sense if we place them within the context of meaningful experiences and practical purposes. This book stresses the importance of situating language instruction in the real world.

Language Issues within the Context of Technology

While professionals in the education of children who are deaf and hard of hearing often disagree about instructional approaches, most agree on the potential of technology in increasing literacy in students who are deaf or hard of hearing. Already there have been tremendous advances in technologies that have created opportunities for such students to access information (e.g., closed captioning and the Internet). Classrooms have more computers and educational software and teachers are integrating technology into their instruction to a greater extent. According to Johnson and Dilka (1999) teachers are reporting that students are more interested in reading when technology is incorporated into the lesson. Technology often presents information through graphic images and text, and students become more motivated when learning to read via highly visual means. The challenge for schools and teachers is to keep up with fast-changing technologies, equipment, and skills. Hirsch (1987) stated that "advancing technology, with its constant need for fast and complex communications, has made literacy ever more essential to commerce and domestic life" (p. 3). Thus, we have a double-edged sword. The technology that may make it easier for students to learn to read will also demand that these students have better reading skills.

In addition to technology that enhances the development of literacy and communication, advances in medical technologies are occurring at a rapid pace. In 1993 the National Institutes of Health (NIH) along with other agencies and organizations held a consensus development conference on early identification of hearing loss. At that time only eleven hospitals reportedly screened infant hearing. By the time this book was being written, thirty-two states had passed some kind of legislation mandating universal newborn hearing screening. Identifying infants with hearing losses during the first few weeks of life allows medical interventions and specialized services to begin earlier and, therefore, increases the likelihood that infants and families will receive benefit. Two sources of information on the statistics regarding states' responses to universal newborn hearing screening are the websites of the National Center for Hearing Assessment and Management at Utah State University (http://www.infanthearing.org) and the Developmental Disabilities website section of the Centers for Disease Control in Atlanta (http://www.cdc.gov).

In addition to universal infant hearing screenings, advances in the technology used for cochlear implants is making the surgery an option for many families. For some children the implant has been successful (e.g., those children who are traditionally advantaged). For other children, especially those who were older when implanted or those who were unable to attend the extensive post-surgery therapy sessions, implants have not provided benefit and in some cases have actually contributed to language delays. There are still unanswered questions regarding who these are most likely to benefit (Easterbrooks & Mordica, 2000). Nevertheless, new technologies are appearing rapidly that will make hearing loss a non-issue for many children. For example, voice recognition technology may make it possible for one to speak to a deaf individual who can then read what the speaker has said on a computer screen.

All of this is very exciting and the possibilities are endless, but they are not here yet for all children. We face a similar problem of equal access to technology and services today as the poorer deaf children of Spain faced in past centuries. Not all children have equal access to technology, not all children have great enough hearing losses to be candidates for cochlear implants, and not all children have a sufficient foundation in literacy skills to access the text-rich Internet. As with all aspects in this field, technology may not be the magic pill.

Language Issues within the Context of Culture

Current research into language acquisition places language development squarely within pragmatic or social contexts. It is within the culture of the family that children learn to communicate. Devoid of this cultural milieu, communication cannot develop normally. In nearly all descriptions of transmission of culture and the acquisition of language, it is assumed that children have access to adult language models. Children who have families who provide a comprehensible language and who are active in their language development have access to this cultural cradle whether they use a spoken or signed language. Children whose parents are not active in their language acquisition develop language mechanically devoid of cultural connections, purpose, and meaning. Culture is a critical aspect of language acquisition for it is the context for communication. To understand language one must understand culture.

Culture has been defined as "a set of learned behaviors of a group of people who have their own language, values, and rules for behavior and traditions" (Padden & Humphries, 1988, p. 4). Culture defines the way of life of a social group, thus culture is a human-made environment—dynamic, complex, and ever changing (Banks, 1994). The most distinguishing feature of Deaf culture and that which separates it from other disability groups is the aspect of a shared language. The shared language of Deaf people in North America is American Sign Language. ASL accommodates language acquisition by the eye and is highly valued among Deaf people for it is this unique visual language that affords them complete communication access and allows them to form a social identity. Older Deaf people often sign CHERISH to describe their feelings about ASL, perhaps because it is their true or natural language. Neissar (1983) wrote that Deaf people have a deep biological bias for the language of signs and that speech is never natural and never automatic for them.

Most likely, though, ASL is cherished because of what comes with the language: communication, social relations, and group identity. Although in the past ASL was believed to have negative effects on English language acquisition (Scouten, 1984), efforts to eliminate ASL have been fruitless. ASL is a resilient language; it has survived even the most ardent attempts to prohibit its use. Even when banished from educational programs in the late 1800s, Deaf people continued to use ASL in social clubs, in residential school dormitories, and in the privacy of their homes. Equally as resilient, for they are inextricably linked, is the culture of Deaf people. That "[Deaf culture] has endured, despite indirect and tenuous lines of transmission and despite generations of changing social conditions, attests to the tenacity of the basic human needs for language and symbol" (Padden & Humphries, p. 121). "Much of the impetus for changes in how society in general views deaf individuals has come from the work of linguists" (Akamatsu, 1998, p. 28) whose research validated ASL as a formal language based on linguistic principles. After the formalization of ASL, the concept of Deaf culture came to the fore, however, it was over two decades before the positive aspects of Deaf culture were mentioned to educators. In 1988, the Commission on Education of the Deaf (COED) recognized that deaf and hard of hearing students have cultural needs.

> Culture is knowledge that gives individuals a shared understanding of what are accepted behaviors and values. It enables the world to become expected and anticipated; individuals can gauge their place in it. Differing cultural standards, when not recognized, can interfere with the learning process in the classroom in a major way. (p. 23)

Even though the COED identified positive benefits of Deaf cultural affiliation, understanding this concept is extremely challenging for hearing parents. Deaf culture is foreign to them. In addition, cultural affiliation necessitates learning a signed language and tragically, most hearing parents never achieve the level of skill necessary to hold a sustained conversation with Deaf adults (Marshark, 1997). Perhaps parents feel trepidation towards Deaf culture due to the way it is presented (or omitted) early on. Further research in this area is necessary in order understand hearing parents' views and to develop strategies when working with families of young deaf and hard of hearing children.

Not only are there cultural issues among the families of deaf and hard of hearing children, there are also cultural issues due to the great diversity of the United States. The United States is comprised of people from many culturally and linguistically diverse groups and Deaf people reflect this great diversity. The term *cultural pluralism* is used when the cultural differences that make up a society are mutually respected and the differences are encouraged by all the members of the larger society. According to Janzen (1994) the goal of cultural pluralism is to keep ethnic groups intact so that their ways of knowing and acting will be respected and continued. Assimilation, on the other hand, accepts the importance of understanding multiple beliefs, but has as its primary goal the amalgamation of all groups into the American mainstream (p. 9). Embracing the theories that relate to positive aspects of cultural pluralism is a recent phenomenon. Prior to research studies that revealed the positive aspects of cultural pluralism on students' outcomes, the cultural assimilation view (i.e., melting pot theory) was commonly held. With this view students were expected to assimilate into the majority culture leaving behind their heritage, traditions, and native language. School placement decisions for many Deaf and hard of hearing students have been made in an effort at amalgamation or inclusion into hearing society.

Deaf and hard of hearing children from culturally and linguistically diverse backgrounds represent an additional dimension of the Deaf experience (Christensen, 1993). As the number of language categories represented in the United States increases (the U.S. Census in 1990 identified 380 language categories), we can expect the diversity and complexity of each child's experiences to increase. Some Deaf and hard of hearing children have dual group membership (i.e., hearing family, Deaf community). These children often operate in a bicultural environment. Students who are Deaf and hard of hearing representing diverse groups (e.g., African American, Latino, Native American, and Asian/Pacific Islander) operate from a trilingual/tricultural perspective, often compounding their role confusion and identity crises (Cohen, 1993). In order to understand these children, one must consider the home language and culture, the school language and culture, and the visual language and culture of the Deaf community (Christensen, 1993).

Language Issues within the Context of the Law

Children who are deaf and hard of hearing live in most communities throughout the United States. They attend schools that, unless they are private and receive no public support, must follow laws, mandates, rules, and regulations, most of which address the broader category of disabilities in general. As goes regular and special education, so goes deaf education. In some cases these laws have allowed us to make many gains on behalf of children with hearing losses.

In others, it has caused setbacks. This next section looks at the impact of legal issues on communication development in deaf students.

Prior to the 1970s parents of children with hearing losses had two options: keep their children at home or send them to a special school for deaf students. Each choice had repercussions on the family. In some instances families with deaf children relocated to be near a school for the deaf so that their children could live at home. In other instances, deaf children either remained in the home or attended public schools with support that varied from little to none.

During the seventies and eighties, federal laws changed the education of people with disabilities including deaf children. The Rehabilitation Act of 1973, Section 504, prohibited discrimination based on handicapping condition. It requires provision of auxiliary aids (e.g., interpreters for deaf students). The law worked almost identically to the Civil Rights Act of 1964, which prohibited discrimination based on race, color, or national origin. In 1975 Public Law 94-142, the Education for All Handicapped Children Act (EHA), required local school systems to provide a free, appropriate, public education (FAPE) to all children and to write Individualized Education Plans (IEPs). In 1986 PL 99-457 extended that law down to the early childhood years, requiring schools to write Individualized Family Service Plans (IFSPs) on preschoolers. Congress reauthorized the EHA in 1990 and retitled it the Individuals with Disabilities Education Act (IDEA). IDEA was reauthorized again in 1997, and the amendments included specific provisions for students with hearing losses.

When the first regulations were disseminated in 1977, the local public schools geared up for a mass integration of children with disabilities and began implementation of the legal requirements of the law. Children who were deaf and hard of hearing were now being mainstreamed into the public schools, some with more success than others. At issue was access to communication. Many deaf and hard of hearing children were eventually mainstreamed into classes where they did little more than occupy seats. Even though schools were meeting the requirement of PL 94-142 by providing classrooms for deaf and hard of hearing students, most programs, especially in rural areas, were lacking. There just was not an adequate supply of highly skilled specialists to work with the children in mainstreamed settings. In addition, the issue of Least Restrictive Environment (LRE) was very controversial. According to the law, LRE means that, to the maximum extent *appropriate*, students with disabilities are educated with their non-disabled peers. Separate classes, special schooling, or other removal of students from the regular class environment occurs only when the nature or severity of the disability is such that education in regular classes with the use of supplementary aids and services cannot be achieved satisfactorily. In the more narrow interpretation, LRE means attending the same neighborhood school a student would attend if not disabled. Unfortunately, many individuals assume that this means that the regular classroom is more appropriate. In fact, it is for some, but for a large majority of students with hearing losses, especially those who are deaf, the regular education environment can be very restrictive.

The issue of placement, or where deaf children should attend school, is very controversial. As we begin this century, most children who are deaf or hard of hearing are being educated in their neighborhood schools. This differs greatly from two decades ago when the percentage of children attending special schools for the deaf was greater than the number attending public school programs (Marshark, 1997). This reversal in enrollment trends is directly attributable to federal and state statutes that support children's education in their neighborhood schools. Providing deaf and hard of hearing students with appropriate services is indeed complex because of the great variance from child to child, and public schools often have difficulty understanding the unique needs of deaf children (Bowe, 1988; Easterbrooks, 1999; Siegel, 2000).

An example of this occurred in 1982. The case involved a deaf student's right to have an interpreter at the neighborhood school she attended. The U.S. Supreme Court ruled that the school district was not required to provide an interpreter because the student was receiving educational benefits (i.e., making satisfactory progress) without one. With this decision school districts throughout the country began quoting the Rowley Decision to override Section 504 of the Rehabilitation Act of 1973 and to justify denying educational interpreter services for deaf students who were mainstreamed. This was an unfortunate misapplication of the ruling. At issue was the definition of the law's use of the word *appropriate*. In this case the courts decided that the student's program was appropriate because she was making satisfactory progress. With the passage of the Americans with Disabilities Act of 1990 and reauthorization of IDEA in 1997, the responsibility of schools to provide interpreters was reaffirmed, and today, schools that fail to provide equal access leave themselves open to legal action.

During the 1990s some families whose children had profound disabilities lobbied for the rights of their children to be included physically in the regular education classrooms for socialization purposes, even if they could not compete academically. Known as *full inclusion*, this philosophy appealed to most individuals because they felt it was ethical for students with disabilities to be educated in the same school they would attend if not disabled. However, full inclusion did not appeal to all parents of children with hearing loss as it limited choices (Hawkins, 1993; Hawkins & Harvey, 1995; Hawkins, Harvey, & Cohen, 1994). Some deaf and hard of hearing children were able to attend their neighborhood schools with limited support. Some needed to be in self-contained classrooms with deaf education specialists. Others needed to attend special schools in order to have direct communication access with everyone and to have the opportunity to learn in these highly specialized environments. Yet, the volume of all the united representatives of other disability groups eclipsed the voices of parents of deaf and hard of hearing children. At the center of the debate was the LRE. When placing children into educational programs, IEP teams typically gave placement preference to the neighborhood schools because they were viewed as the least restrictive placement and many came to view special school placement as a last resort rather than an opportunity for full communication. For deaf and hard of hearing students this often meant that the students' needs for communication access were overlooked. The irony of this is that inclusion in schools with non-disabled peers often ended up being exclusion for many deaf students because of the lack of a shared communication system. It took the efforts of Robert Davila, deaf himself, to clarify this issue. From 1989 to 1992 Davila held the position of Assistant Secretary for Special Education and Rehabilitation Services in the United States Department of Education. During his term he was able to provide guidance on the issue of the education of deaf students. The report, *Deaf Students Education Services Policy Guidance*, published in the Federal Register (1992), provided clarification on the issue of educating deaf and hard of hearing students and their unique educational needs, which, in many ways, cannot be compared to those of other children with disabilities. Since the publication of this policy guidance greater choices in school placement are available to parents of deaf and hard of hearing students. During the 1990s several charter schools for deaf and hard of hearing students, using a bilingual-bicultural philosophy, were established in metropolitan areas (e.g., The Metro Deaf School, St. Paul; The Denver Magnet Deaf School; The Laurent Clerc School, Tucson; The Jean Massieu Academy, Dallas; The Jean Massieu School, Salt Lake City; and the J. Schuyler Long Academy of the Deaf, Oklahoma City).

When the IDEA was reauthorized by Congress in 1997 provisions were included specifically for deaf and hard of hearing students. Perhaps the most important addition is the reference to deaf students' needs for direct communication with others. In other words, instead of always going through an interpreter or being required to write in order to communicate, the children should have direct access to individuals with whom they have a shared communication system. Today, schools must identify on the IEP how they address this issue.

Summary

In this chapter we have attempted to spotlight people and events that have influenced language development of deaf and hard of hearing students. The early records indicated that four countries were influential during the early endeavors to teach deaf and hard of hearing students: Spain, France, Great Britain, and Germany. We know more about the French method of instruction because its teachers shared their methods freely with others and maintained written documentation of their activities. However, we continue to learn more about other countries as historians and researchers uncover new information and documents that describe early efforts. The early pioneers were indeed dedicated to the betterment of deaf and hard of hearing students and most dedicated their entire lives to this effort. They have provided a foundation upon which we continue to build today. Early pioneers found themselves often in conflict with one another over which communication method was the most efficacious when instructing deaf and hard of hearing students. This question is still debated today.

Comparing communication methodologies and approaches to language instruction that have been used historically to those currently used, it is apparent that many have been recycled. For example, communication methods that were used in the eighteenth century were used again in the twentieth century. Our challenge is to continually improve what we do, whether the work is based on existing theories or new ones, and to remain cognizant of the past so that we do not make changes merely for the sake of change. Historical trends also reveal that early educators of the deaf developed methods and techniques for teaching grammar and written language. Many of these techniques were based on the earlier work of others, often revealing a systematic effort at improving language instruction. However, as we look at student outcomes it is apparent that while structured, natural, and combined approaches worked for some, they did not work for all.

During the past decade, researchers have proposed new theories and new approaches to teaching language that are based on theories of first and second language acquisition and new technologies (Nover & Andrews, 1998). In addition, the fields of neuroscience and ASL linguistics are contributing to what we know about language learning. Other innovative techniques, treatments, technologies, and advances are occurring in many fields. These will continue to have an impact on the field of deaf education. However, what is considered "cutting edge" today will be obsolete tomorrow, and teachers will need to rise to the challenge of continually updating their base of knowledge and skills.

Questions for Critical Thinking

1. Why do cycles occur? Why do we seem to keep recycling old approaches?

2. How are the main approaches described similar and how are they different?

3. Why have educational outcomes for students who are deaf and hard of hearing remained substandard?

4. What is wrong with the "one size fits all" approach to teaching language to deaf and hard of hearing students?

5. Why do individuals have such difficulty embracing new techniques and approaches?

2

Language Acquisition in Children Who Are Deaf and Hard of Hearing

What to Expect in This Chapter

In this chapter you will read about language acquisition in hearing students and in students who are deaf and hard of hearing. You will learn about the challenges that face students who are deaf and hard of hearing and their parents as they learn to communicate.

Most children are born with an innate ability and desire to learn to communicate. Usually this learning occurs within the nurturing environment of the home. Normal language development follows a predetermined sequence that is similar across most cultures. Depending on geographical, cultural, and familial circumstances, a hearing child will become a native speaker of at least one language through the natural supports that facilitate language growth intuitively, not by direct instruction. The language development of deaf or hard of hearing children also follows a predetermined sequence; however, delays in development occur that may range from mild to severe. These delays are a direct result either of their inability to process auditory input or a lack of sufficient exposure to visually encoded language (Spencer & Meadow-Orlans, 1996). Delays in hard of hearing children result from their inability to comprehend a complete message through audition. As a consequence, the most debilitating aspect of deafness is not the hearing loss, but the lack of language that results from insufficient visual or auditory input.

How do deaf and hard of hearing children for whom auditory input is distorted or absent learn a language? Is there is a biological basis for language? In the past researchers posited that deaf children were concrete thinkers who lacked the ability to think abstractly. This is a limited view and is incongruent with what we know currently. Language development in children who are deaf and hard of hearing is complex and multifaceted. To best explain the process of language acquisition in deaf and hard of hearing children, you need to understand how typical language develops and the social context within which children learn to communicate. This chapter presents various aspects of language development and how they relate to language learning in children who are deaf and hard of hearing. We present current research on language development in children who are deaf and hard of hearing and explore the critical issues that confront our field today.

The Nature of Language

Language is a very complex field of study, therefore we begin this chapter with the universal aspects of language. Although in the past there was a belief that speech was language, we now know that speech is simply a tool or a mode of transmission and is distinct from the cognitive system that underlies language. According to Meier, "Human linguistic competence is in some sense deeper than the mode of expression" (1991, p. 6). Language, therefore, goes deeper than any communication mode. Meier further stated, "We are biologically equipped to use language, we are not biologically limited to speech" (p. 6). While language can be represented by speech, there are other modes by which language can be conveyed. Language can be conveyed through signs, which use a visual-gestural mode to convey linguistic information. Both modes, auditory and visual, are reasonable vehicles by which people share complex ideas through-the-air. Language resides in the brain and mind of the communicator, and as you will discover, the brain shows no preference for one pathway over the other when processing language input. If language is more than the mode of transmission, then what else is language? Certain universals have been identified that all languages have in common.

Language Has Form

In 1965, Chomsky stated that "Language is a system of rules that in some explicit and well defined way assigns structural descriptions to sentences" (p. 8). Chomsky's work ushered in a new wave of theories and concepts pertaining to speech, language, and communication. Bloom and Lahey added to the definition of language and stated that language is the "code whereby ideas about the world are represented through a conventional system of arbitrary signals for communication" (1978, p. 4).

Language Involves Representation

Language is the means by which we share our thoughts and ideas with others. According to theories that have held over time (Bruner, 1990; Bruner, Goodnow, & Austin, 1956; Muma, 1998), language involves representation. The objects and experiences of the world are too numerous for the brain to process; therefore, we put information into meaningful chunks or categories. The categories we create are deeply steeped in cultural context. In order to share mental categories with another person, we must represent them in some manner. We do this in several ways. The easiest, least arbitrary way to represent ideas is through *enactive representation* whereby we enact or re-enact an object or event. A child with no language might growl like a dog, make a biting gesture, then point to teeth marks on his leg to represent the idea that something within the category of animal bit his leg. The second level of representation is *iconic representation* whereby we use visual organization to present a concept or category. A stop sign is an icon that represents the action of stopping. An outline of a person is an iconic representation of that person. In other words, the linguistic form is an icon or picture of some aspect of an entity or activity (Valli & Lucas, 1995). The third level of representation is arbitrary *symbolic representation*. Languages include symbols that users manipulate to produce meaning in a systematic, rule-governed way. English has a written equivalent; however, ASL does not have a written symbolic system.

Piaget (1970) discussed the nature of language stating that children between the ages of one-and-a-half and eight go through a period when sensory-motor intelligence is internalized at the level of representation. He explained that representation takes many different forms. Spoken language is not the exclusive means of representation, in fact, spoken language is only one aspect of symbolic functioning that includes gestures, either idiosyncratic or, as in the case of signed languages, systematic. Symbolic functioning also includes deferred imitation (i.e., imitation that occurs when the model is no longer present). It includes drawing, painting, modeling, and mental imagery. In these cases there is a signifier, which represents that which is signified. All of these ways that language can be represented are used by children in their passage from intelligence that is acted out to intelligence that is thought. Language is but one aspect of symbolic functioning; however, in most cases it is the most important of all.

Battison (1992) provided an example of the systematic properties of ASL. He proposed that ASL sign formations were based on two conditions: a symmetry condition and a dominance condition. The symmetry condition states that in a two-handed sign, if both hands move, then they will have the same handshape and type of movement. The dominance condition states that in a two-handed sign, if each hand has a different handshape, then only the active hand can move. In English, symbols are used to represent sounds and combinations of sounds that form words. Words form phrases, sentences, etc. In other words, it is productive. Language shows the relationship among symbols through a grammatical system. English prepositions are used to show the relationship between other words (e.g., The sandwich is on the table). In ASL the relationship is shown by using classifier predicates (Valli & Lucas, 1995).

Languages Are Arbitrary

The words or signs that make up a language are mostly arbitrary: There is little logical or natural relationship between the sounds of the word or the handshapes of the sign and the object or action represented. In spoken languages there are onomatopoeic words such as "moo" representing the sounds of a cow; however, most spoken words have no such relationship. The same is true for American Sign Language. Research into the structure of ASL reveals that it is mostly arbitrary (Jannedy et al., 1994), although there are a number of signs that are iconic (i.e., visually onomatopoeic). Linguists have identified three levels of iconicity for signs. Transparent signs have the greatest degree of iconicity and are easily understood by a naïve observer. Translucent signs are less iconic, but retain some recognizable relationship to the referent. And opaque signs have no recognizable relationship to their referent (Jannedy et al., 1994). Children learning ASL often do not perceive the iconic elements of the sign. In fact, they perceive it as a fully arbitrary language (Meier, 1991). Further, an adult signer may not perceive the iconic origin during normal conversation, just as a hearing person does not perceive word etymology during spoken conversation.

Languages Are Shared

Members of a community share the same communication system. For example, ASL is a language that is shared by the Deaf community and although there are regional variations (Valli & Lucas, 1995), users of ASL have a common communication base through which they share ideas and thoughts. ASL, however, is not a universal language—an Esperanto—as some believe. Communities around the world have their own signed languages, which, most often, are very different from ASL.

The Elements of Language: Form, Content, and Use

Bloom and Lahey (1978) created a model that is used widely in education and psychology to describe the components of language. They divided language into three areas: form, content, and use. Form is the surface structure (i.e., phonology, morphology, and syntax). Content is what we know about the world and how we describe it (i.e., semantics). Use refers to the way language functions as a social mediator (i.e., pragmatics). Valli and Lucas (1995) provided a linguistic analysis of ASL, which we will compare to spoken English in the following discussion. They used capital letters to *gloss* or represent the English equivalent of a sign. We use glossing throughout this book.

Phonology. Phonology in spoken languages is the study of the linguistic rules governing a language's sound system and how particular sounds form an integrated system for encoding information. Phonemes are the smallest elements of speech and include vowels and consonants. Phonologic rules reveal how sounds are sequenced and combined. (For a well-developed discussion of speech refer to the works of Calvert and Silverman, 1980; Easterbrooks, 1986; Ling, 1976; Subtelny, 1980.) Linguists who study signed languages use the term phonology to refer to the smallest contrastive units of language and the study of how signs are structured and organized; however, because ASL is a multidimensional language, it has phonologic features that do not occur in spoken languages. ASL signs have five basic parts: handshape, movement, location, orientation, and nonmanual markers (Valli & Lucas, 1995). Phonology in ASL also includes the study of hold segments and movement segments. "A hold segment has handshape, location, and movement segments, and likewise, a movement segment has handshape, location, orientation, and nonmanual features" (Valli & Lucas, 1995, p. 50). Phonologic holds and movement segments, when studied in isolation, have no meaning.

Morphology. Morphology is the study of how the basic units of meaning (morphemes) are combined to form meaningful units. Morphemes are the smallest *meaningful* units of a word or a sign and dictate how we structure what we say or sign. Spoken English as well as ASL are comprised of two types of morphemes, free and bound. A free morpheme is essentially any independent unit (*cat* is an example of an English free morpheme and CAT is an example of an ASL free morpheme). Bound morphemes are dependent and must be attached to a root in order to impart any meaning (e.g., the English plural "s" as in *cats* has no meaning when presented in isolation. In ASL, the 3-handshape in THREE-MONTHS is a bound morpheme) (Valli & Lucas, 1995).

By studying morphology we see how words and signs are produced, how compounds are formed, how new words are created, and how language changes over time. Morphology is related to syntax in that a morpheme may change the grammar of a word or the acceptable placements of that word within a sentence (e.g., in English "quick + ly" changes the adjective to an adverb). Morphology is related to semantics in that the entire meaning of a sentence can be changed by one morpheme (e.g., English verb tense). In English "sweet + ness" is made of seven phonemes and two morphemes that form the lexical item, "sweetness."

The English morphological system is particularly difficult for many deaf or hard of hearing children to master. Hard of hearing students may minimize the morphological aspects of language during speech (e.g., *runnin'* instead of *running*). Even though hearing children learn the morphological aspects of English through simple exposure, the signed grammatical morphemes added to

English-based sign systems were not acquired by deaf and hard of hearing children in the same way (Schick & Moeller, 1992). This may occur because signed English morphemes are not used with enough consistency. However, "research has shown that when deaf children are given such a slow system in lieu of a natural language, they quickly pare off many of the artificial structures of the code and create their own grammatical system (Jannedy et al., 1994, p. 403). It appears that a great deal of English morphemes such as "ed" and "ing," while simple to construct in a spoken language, are awkward in a visual mode. Deaf and hard of hearing children learning English as a second language must learn the morphological aspects of English as well as those of ASL, which are represented differently than spoken or signed English (e.g., pluralization represented by sign reduplication).

Syntax.   Syntax is the system of rules and categories that allows words/signs to form sentences. It forms the grammar of a language and includes phrase structure rules, transformational rules, and morphological rules (Muma, 1978). Syntax refers to the structure of sentences, the word or sign order, and the changes that take place in that word/sign order. It is the glue that holds a sentence together. The syntactical systems of ASL and English differ significantly because they are two very separate and distinct languages. Deaf and hard of hearing children who learn a native language on schedule (whether ASL, English, or another spoken or signed language) typically acquire syntax automatically. However, the majority of deaf and hard of hearing students do not have this opportunity and face a lifelong struggle to master grammar.

Semantics.   The purpose behind language is to communicate a meaningful message. Part of linguistic competence involves one's ability to determine the meaning of sentences. Semantics is the study of meaning and how words and sentences are related to situations they describe or to real or imaginary objects to which they refer. Semantics deals with the denotative (e.g., *fishy* = a little fish) and connotative (e.g., *fishy* = strange) meanings of words. The study of semantics in ASL is the same as the study of semantics in any spoken language. It begins with the study of meaning at the basic lexical (i.e., word) level and proceeds to more complex structures.

Pragmatics.   Language is not only represented by isolated structures but also by rules that guide exchanges between people. *Pragmatics* is the study of how we use language to communicate, express our intentions, and get things accomplished in the world (Gleason, 1993; Owens, 1996). Pragmatics can be defined as the set of sociolinguistic rules that are situational and that one knows and uses in determining who says what to whom (Muma, 1978). Pragmatic issues are those which surround the appropriateness of communication. Language occupies a central role in social learning and in determining appropriate and inappropriate ways of acting and interacting. Pragmatics is culturally based. Ways of communicating vary depending upon what is culturally accepted and appropriate in certain situations. For example, Native American children often have very little eye contact with elders or non-family members. In their culture, this is perceived to be a sign of respect. However, for many children who are deaf or hard of hearing, vision is critical to learning, so to be Native American and deaf presents conflicts that involve pragmatic issues (Baker, 1996).

Theories of Language Development

Many investigators have defined language over the years, and as our knowledge base has increased, so have our perspectives on language. Every new theory has spurred the development of new interventions. Today we understand that language is very complex, involving multiple systems and multiple processes. We also know that good intervention takes into consideration the best from each theory and weaves this into an integrated approach. Our job as teachers is to take the best from each theory and to use this in our interactions with children who are learning language. This book assumes that the reader has a basic familiarity with linguistic theory. Rather than providing a review, we summarize the operational principles you should keep in mind when developing language programs and activities.

Principles of Language Instruction

1. Multiple Influences Principle. Physiological, psychosocial, intellectual, motivational, and environmental circumstances influence language. We must take into consideration the deaf or hard of hearing child's degree of hearing loss, age, emotional development, ability, attending and organizational capabilities, home situation, hearing status of parents, and peer relationships when determining an approach to language development.
2. Meaning and Ideational Principle. Language is the symbolic way in which we represent, express, and share what we mean with other people. There are any number of ways that we can represent meaning and ideas (e.g., vocalizations, icons, signed language). The way we represent ideas must never become more important than the actual ideas themselves.
3. Categorization Principle. Language allows us to categorize the objects, events, experiences, feelings, and thoughts which occur daily so that we may express what we mean, store it, or share it. We cannot possibly remember every little fact, bit of information, color, hue, nuance, or variation on a theme, so we think in terms of categories of experiences. Words do not refer directly to objects or events in the world but rather to our categories or cognitive organizations of the world. We must help deaf

and hard of hearing children see the way the world is organized so that the system they use to represent the world, whether auditory, visual, or tactile, facilitates their interactions with others.

4. Relationships Principle. In the real world meaning occurs from relationships, and interactions occur among objects, events, experiences, or categories. In general, a particular word is meaningless unless it relates to something else. We express ideas and relationships through language and the various structures within it. However, before we teach a student a grammatical structure, we must first demonstrate how the words are related in the real world.

5. Systematic Rules Principle. Language is comprised of a system of rules that specify how we understand and produce utterances. These rules or codes exist in the areas of phonology, morphology, syntax, semantics, and pragmatics. They are found both in English and ASL. They are too numerous to teach one at a time, so the better you as a teacher understand what these rules are, the better able you will be to integrate these into ongoing instruction to maximize your teaching time.

6. Socialization Principle. Language is both dependent upon and reflective of socially and culturally prescribed experiences. Effective users of language understand the subtleties and nuances of social interaction (e.g., body language, clique slang, intonational innuendoes). The major reason we communicate is to meet our needs within the context of other human beings. We want something, so we communicate. In order to meet our needs, we have to have someone to communicate *with*. Language does not develop in a vacuum. This means that conversation should play a major role in our involvement with students who are deaf and hard of hearing.

7. Integration Principle. Language requires smooth integration of principles 1–6. Highly sophisticated coordination of all the systems and principles must occur rapidly and smoothly in order for the magic of language to happen. If any of these principles is not adhered to, disruptions in communication may occur. That anyone learns to communicate is truly remarkable when we consider the degree of complexity involved. That students who are deaf and hard of hearing learn to communicate given the challenges they face should remind us of the indomitable nature of the human spirit.

Stages of Language Development

Normal language develops through several stages or phases that are not completely discrete but flow one into the other. We will discuss normal development and then discuss language acquisition of children who are deaf or hard of hearing.

Prelinguistic Stage in Infants Who Are Deaf or Hard of Hearing

Infants who are deaf or hard of hearing respond to their environment in much the same way hearing infants do (Table 2.1). They eat, sleep, and cry when they are hungry or uncomfortable. The difference between the two infants, though, is in how each responds to environmental stimuli. Infants with hearing loss do not usually respond to loud noise unless it is accompanied by vibration. In addition to vibration, they are sensitive to other environmental stimuli such as lights, shadows, and smells. Hearing infants are also aware of these stimuli, but they rely more on their auditory sense to understand the world around them. As the infants mature, there is little difference in the way each responds. Both will reach early developmental milestones at approximately the same time; however, the infant with a hearing loss often misses a critical precursor to language development: sharing linguistic input with caregivers.

New research on brain development has identified optimal windows during which the brain is open to learning different skills (Huttenlocher & Dabholkar, 1997). During the prelinguistic stage of development some parts of the brain, including the visual cortex, are wired rapidly. Others such as the auditory cortex explode with new connections after birth and maintain this activity until age twelve. Most synaptic connections are formed randomly, becoming stable only after they have been activated by sensory input (touch, sight, hearing, smell, or taste). Connections that are used repeatedly during a child's early years become the foundation for the brain's organization. Synapses that are not activated by sensory input are eventually discarded and do not become incorporated into neural networks. Consequently, the world in which a child is born greatly influences how the brain forms and functions—that is, environment is central in shaping the brain.

During the baby's first year, sensory input shapes the brain's organization and the baby becomes sensitive to the idiosyncrasies of her particular language (Hendricks, 1998). Hearing infants are particularly sensitive to sounds of a language in the first few months of life and by eighteen months they can detect sentences with grammatical inconsistencies (Jusczyk, 1997). Infants with hearing losses are sensitive to visual input and touch. All infants, however, participate in early visual interactions with caregivers.

Beyond these basic visual interactions, infants with hearing losses need to have early visual experiences that form the basis of later language acquisition (Table 2.2). However, most are at risk during early brain development because they lack access to sensory input that creates the connections upon which language is formed.

Communication through the Sense of Touch. Studies of tactile contact with infants have presented interesting information regarding the role of touch in

TABLE 2.1 *The Typical Sequence of Language Development in Hearing Children*

Stage of Development	Age	Receptive	Expressive
Early prelinguistic	0–6 months	Infants turn toward the speaker, attend closely to sounds of an unfamiliar voice, and respond to comforting vocal tones. Infants in this stage are highly sensitive to touch.	Infants will share sounds with their parents (coos and reflexive babbling of vowel-like sounds in various combinations). Infants use different sounds or cries to communicate contentment or discomfort.
Later prelinguistic	6–12 months	Listens when spoken to and turns and looks when name is called. Recognizes names of familiar people and objects (*daddy, keys, eyes, kitty*). Begins to respond to requests and questions. Discovers the fun of games, finger plays, and nursery rhymes.	Babbling becomes more complex and includes more consonants and long and short vowels. Babbling approximates words (*mama, dada*) and are reinforced by caregivers. Infants use sounds (other than crying) to get and hold your attention. Later in this stage children begin to produce strings of utterances that vary in stress and intonational patterns of adult speech. Known as jargon—children appear to be talking, but will say few distinguishable words.
Single sign/word	12–18 months	Understands and responds to basic communication.	First words appear that are often in the form of reduplication of consonant–vowel combinations—*mama, daddy, bye-bye.* Jargon continues as children practice the intonational patterns of adult language.
Early word combinations	18–24 months	Points to pictures in books or body parts when named. Can follow simple commands and understand simple questions. Likes to listen to simple	Child is developing vocabulary at a rapid pace and will combine two words into simple sentences and questions (e.g., *daddy work; more juice*). Begins

		stories and nursery rhymes and enjoys singing songs.	to use one-word attributes (*dirty*). Two-word utterances form the beginning of syntax and semantics.
Multiword combinations	24–36 months	Children understand complex sentences. They can understand commands that require two acts and understand contrastive meanings of words such as *hot/cold*. Fast-mapping occurs as the brain reorganizes language operations to the left hemisphere.	Vocabulary is exploding. Children learn 2–4 new words each day. Sentences include combinations of multiple words that are mostly incoherent, but that caregivers understand. Uses attributes to describe nouns such as *big dog*. Jargon disappears. Pragmatically children establish topic–comment relations resulting in rigid adherence to subject–verb–object word order.
Expanded grammar	3–4 years	Understands complex language forms including the syntactic rules necessary to use "wh" questions.	Sentences and questions are becoming longer and more complex. Ninety percent of sentences are grammatically correct. Semantic development includes talking about experiences that happened away from home or that will happen in the future.
Adult-like language development	5 years	Has mastered a complex syntactic system to go along with an extensive vocabulary. Enjoys stories and can answer questions about them.	Can construct long and detailed sentences. Tells long and involved stories using adult-like grammar. May tell fantastic, tall stories and engage strangers in conversation.

Source: Bever, 1961; Brownlee, 1998; Dale, 1972; Hendricks, 1998; McAnally, Rose, & Quigley, 1994; McNeill, 1970; Menyuk, 1971; Tranthan & Pedersen, 1976.

TABLE 2.2 *Early Visual Interactions*

Deictic gazing	Child "points with his eyes."
Mutual gaze	Visually signals increased attention
Joint reference	The parent and child share a common focus on one entity.
Facial expressions	Communicate affective dimensions of language; facial expressions of deaf mothers typically do not include the morphological features of ASL until their infants reach two years of age.
Gestures and signs	Promote early language experiences and communicate an intent

Sources: Bateson, 1979; Collins, 1977; Owens, 1996; Reilly & Bellugi, 1996.

communication. Field (1990) found that infants are extremely responsive to touch as a vehicle for communication. Koester, Brooks, and Traci (2000) stated that "touch plays an important role in the development of interactive dialogues between caregiver and child" (p. 128). Koester et al. (2000) provided information regarding ways parents touch their babies and used these elements to construct a coding system for research on deaf mothers of deaf children.

- Duration—the longer the duration the more time the body has to perceive and process the sensory stimulation.
- Threshold level—the body is more sensitive to touch in different areas of the body.
- Regionalization—stimulating more regions (i.e., parts of the body) causes the infant to have different perceptions.
- Intensity—the degree of intensity (e.g., playful, comforting, arousing, soothing) influences the child's interpretation of the experience.

Koester et al. (2000) found that both deaf and hearing mothers tended to use touch as a natural part of intuitive parenting. This system is mutually regulated by the infant and the parent with the parent providing appropriate visual and vocal strategies to elicit and maintain the infant's attention and engage in shared interactions (Koestner, Papoušek, & Smith-Gray, 2000). Both mothers used tactile strategies to elicit and maintain their child's visual attention in order to communicate with them. Even though there were apparently no differences in the quantity of tactile stimulation, there were differences in the quality of interactions. Formation differences became apparent when comparing the child and mother's hearing status (i.e., matched dyads and mismatched dyads). For example, there were differences in intensity, type, and location of touch. Deaf mothers used greater intensity of touch than hearing mothers. Both mothers used short duration initially and increased their use of moderate duration as the infant's age increased. However, when comparing the extent of longer duration, only the deaf mothers increased their use of tactile contact with older children.

Overall, hearing mothers tend to incorporate more vocalization (i.e., vocal games, nursery rhymes, etc.) while simultaneously moving the infants' body parts (e.g., cycling legs, clapping hands). Deaf mothers use touch to elicit visual attention, to alert the infant that a signed communication is forthcoming, to assist the child in emotional regulation, or to continue communicating when eye contact has been broken. To do this they often use the "tap/sign" strategy (a brief tapping on the infant's body, usually the legs or arms) to alert the infant to watch for a sign. Deaf mothers also employ other tactile strategies when communicating with their child. For example, the mother may reach out and sign on the body of the child (e.g., touching the child when signing YOU and HUNGRY).

Nonverbal maternal behavior incorporating touch may be important for the development of an infant's expressive communication. Koester, Papoušek, and Papoušek (1989) found in a study of the maternal interactions with hearing three-month-old infants that the tempo of playful tactile stimulation accompanied by maternal vocalizations was 2.64 bps, a similar rate of infant cononical babbling that appears later. This indicates that nonverbal maternal behaviors may influence infants' expressive communication capacities.

Motherese. When hearing adults communicate with hearing infants they alter their speech patterns in order to maintain the child's attention. This form of modified speech is referred to as *motherese*. Cross-linguistic studies conducted in several languages have found that motherese may have universal linguistic and prosodic features. Erting, Prezioso, and O'Grady-Hynes (1994) studied motherese used by deaf mothers for whom ASL was their first language to identify attributes of motherese in ASL. They found that deaf mothers placed the signs closer to the infant, oriented the palm so that the full hand was visible to the infant, maintained full-face visibility, directed eye gaze to the infant, and lengthened signs by repeating the same movement. The conclusion of the study was that parents use special articulatory features when communicating with infants, including parents who use a signed language for communication.

Motherese is characterized by modifications such as simplified language structure, more repetitions, and clearer articulation. It also contains prosodic features, including higher pitch, longer duration of speech sounds, slower rate, and longer pauses (Ratner & Pye, 1984). Masataka (2000) compared motherese of deaf mothers and hearing mothers in Japan and found that the motherese of Japanese deaf mothers was analogous to spoken motherese. She found that sign motherese was parallel to speech motherese in varying prosodic patterns indicating that the "specifically patterned linguistic input that is expressed by motherese might enhance the infants' acquisition of the basic forms of the languages equally in the signed or spoken modalities" (p. 5). Because motherese occurs equally in the manual and vocal modes, at least in regard to prosodic elements, then does motherese in a signed language enhance a deaf child's acquisition of the basic units of language? Hearing babies have been known to show preferences for exaggerated prosodic features as young as two days of age (Cooper & Aslin, 1990), thus babies can begin learning about their native language from a very young age. Masataka found that hearing infants were attracted to signed motherese. Therefore, it appears that infants are predisposed to attend to motherese whether it is spoken or signed.

Babbling. It is well accepted that during the first year of life, hearing or auditory perception has a tremendous influence on speech production. Table 2.3 provides a comparison of deaf and hearing infants based on the stages of vocal development during the first few months of life.

As the infants mature, there is little difference in the way each responds to its physical environment. Both will reach early developmental milestones at approximately the same time. The hearing child for whom the auditory feedback is fully functioning will eventually babble and practice all the sounds of the spoken language of the home. Later they will form words due to reinforcement and prompting from caregivers. The deaf child's babbling, even though it begins in much the same way it does in hearing children, will soon diminish because verbal feedback from caregivers is not comprehensible. Clement and Koopmans-van Beinum (1996) found that deaf infants showed a dramatic decrease in babbling during the later stage. In fact, marginal babbling disappears quickly because of lack of auditory feedback. Another phenomenon that occurs at the onset of marginal babbling is rhythmic manual activity. Ejiri (1998) found that

TABLE 2.3 *Stages of Vocal Development*

Stage	*Age*	*Comparison of Deaf Infants with Hearing Infants*
Phonation	0–1 months	No significant differences between the infants
GOO	2–3 months	No significant differences between the infants
Expansion Marginal babbling	4–6 months	At approximately 6 months of age both infants produce vocalizations characterized by rhythmic vocal play, some with familiar sounds (e.g., *mama*, *dadda*). Both infants' vocalizations have slow, but well-formed consonant and vowel production.
Canonical babbling	6–7 months	Hearing infants begin producing rapid consonant–vowel productions; however, the deaf infant's babbling decreases dramatically.

Source: Oller, 1978.

75 percent of marginal babbling was accompanied by rhythmic manual activity in hearing babies, but as the hearing infant proceeds to canonical babbling, the rhythmic manual activity decreases dramatically. Ejiri further found that deaf infants' marginal babbling frequently co-occurs with rhythmic manual activity. Caregivers who reinforce rhythmic manual activity in the same way that babbling is reinforced in hearing babies may facilitate early sign acquisition in their children.

Of significant interest to researchers has been the question of whether deaf children of deaf adults babble in sign language. Petitto & Marentette (1991) analyzed manual babbling in deaf and hearing children and concluded that deaf children produced many more "manual babbles" than hearing children. Marschark (1997) referred to this as manual babbling or *mabbling*. He stated that manual babbling consists of simple production or repetitions of the basic components of a sign, such as isolated handshapes or movements. One example provided by Marschark was the hand movements for the sign MILK, made by opening and closing the hand into a fist. Deaf parents respond to these mabbling attempts in the same way as hearing parents respond to babbling, thus reinforcing the production. Mabbling changes into meaningful signed communication in the same way as babbling changes into spoken words and communication. A distinction needs to be made between gestures and mabbling. Gestures are used to communicate an intent while mabbling does not. Infants practice mabbling and babbling components of a language, and when reinforced, these components eventually interconnect to form a whole word or sign.

While gestures are not considered mabbling or babbling, gestures play a role in early communication and are an important part of early communication. Hearing children use gestures to accompany words and phrases and assist in clarifying communication. Deaf children use gestures also, especially during early stages of language development before a formal language is acquired. Sometimes the gestures that deaf and hard of hearing children use form a homesign or idiosyncratic communication system through which they communicate with others on a limited basis. Researchers agree that gestures are an important part of emergent language and may actually facilitate language development. Schirmer (2000) presented five aspects of symbolic gesture development in children.

- Both infants who are hearing and infants who are deaf use symbolic gestures to communicate.
- Symbolic gestures appear approximately at the same time as spoken words in hearing children.
- Symbolic gestures seem to be used for requesting before they are used for labeling.
- Gestures and words are both used first in routinized activities.
- Gestural communication is an important stage in the acquisition of language. (p. 7)

Single-Word/Single-Sign Stage

Hearing children say their first word at around twelve months of age (Gesell, 1940; Menyuk, 1971). McNeill (1970) referred to this as the holophrastic stage. In children's first year they have heard all the sounds in their environment. Caregivers, siblings, and extended family members have participated in vocal play and encouraged them to speak. As with hearing children, deaf children with signing parents reach the one-sign stage at about twelve months, although there have been reports of children signing much earlier (Spencer & Lederberg, 1997). Newport and Meier (1985) found that at twelve months of age, deaf children produce isolated signs drawn from the vocabulary of the adult language. Children in the single-word stage add new categories almost daily to their semantic repertoire. An important characteristic of words at this stage is that they must be able to assist the child in causing change (Nelson, 1973). Words such as *tree* or *chair* are not very common in early vocabularies because a child's use of the words is not likely to bring about much change. However, words like *milk*, *blanket*, and *car*, are more likely to cause others to perform some kind of action.

Spencer (1993) conducted research on deaf and hearing infants between twelve and eighteen months of age. Her findings revealed that deaf and hearing infants who had access to linguistic information communicated in similar ways. She concluded that both deaf and hearing infants in the early stages of prelinguistic development seem to be developing two important language developmental prerequisites: (1) intentional communication and (2) referential and symbolic gesture.

The Pointing Gesture.   The pointing gesture has been found to fill an important role in children's transition from single-word to multiword utterances. According to Spencer and Lederberg (1997) the first pointing gesture is redundant (e.g., point to and say/sign *dog*). Children are merely naming the object to which they are pointing. The second pointing gesture that emerges is the nonredundant gesture and it appears immediately before multiword productions, signaling a readiness for expression of relations between symbolic actions (e.g., point to a frog and sign/say *jump*). Hearing children and deaf children have been found to develop the pointing gestures (redundant and nonredundant at approximately the same age (Spencer & Lederberg, 1997). Newport and Meier (1985) indicated that deaf children acquiring ASL from their deaf parents begin to combine single signs with pointing to clarify meaning.

Fingerspelling.   Deaf parents with deaf children use fingerspelling as a natural part of communicating with their children. Studies of young deaf children indicate that they are able to recognize fingerspelled words without knowing the printed letters (Kelly, 1995). Fingerspelling is a critical component of language development in children who are deaf or hard of hearing, and although adults learning fingerspelling often have difficulty producing and reading finger-spelling, children acquire the skill quite readily. According to Padden and Ramsey (2000) skill in fingerspelling interacts with reading achievement.

Development of Vocabulary.   By eighteen months children will have approximately fifty words in their vocabulary. After eighteen months of age, vocabulary growth is rapid. Even though some deaf children of hearing parents acquire first words at the same rate as hearing children, they typically fall progressively behind their peers in vocabulary growth (Spencer & Lederberg, 1997).

Lederberg, Prezbindowski, and Spencer (2000) provided a unique look into deaf and hard of hearing children's development of vocabulary, based on the research of novel mapping strategies (Merriman, Marazita, & Jarvis, 1995). While the child developing his first word attaches labels to objects he and a caregiver are looking at together, the older child (two-and-a-half to four years of age) attaches new words to unfamiliar objects. That is, if there is something in his environment that is novel and the adult uses a word that is novel, the child will associate that word with the novel object (e.g., a wrench versus a shoe or spoon). The child is able to do this even without explicit clues. Further, the child will apply the new word to other examples of the category (i.e., other wrenches) without explicit feedback from the caregiver (Golinkoff, Hirsh-Pasck, Bailey, & Wenger, 1992).

In Lederberg, Prezbindowski, and Spencer's (2000) study, nonce signs (i.e., nonsensical invented signs that follow phonological rules but have no legitimate referent) were presented to deaf and hard of hearing children attending a special school for the deaf. They examined novel mapping and rapid word-learning strategies (where the researcher made the nonce sign/referent connection explicit) of nineteen subjects between the ages of three years two months and six years ten months. Lederberg et al. refer to the two categories of novel mapping and word-learning strategies as *fast mapping*. They found that twelve of the nineteen children (called *novel mappers*) used a novel word-learning strategy to learn the label for a novel object. Sixteen of the nineteen children were successful in learning new words during the rapid word-learning task. The researchers postulated that "there appears to be three levels of word learning abilities: *novel mappers, rapid word learners,* and *slow word learners*" (Lederberg et al., 2000, p. 23).

Next the researchers grouped novel mappers and novel nonmappers for the purpose of further study and found that the novel mappers had larger vocabularies than the novel nonmappers. Additionally, they followed the subjects over time and found that all subjects proceeded through the same sequence of stages and that the slow learners' vocabularies remained smaller than the other subjects' vocabularies. The researchers concluded "the atypicality of these children's language learning environment did not prevent them from developing the strategy" (p. 27) of novel word mapping.

Early Word Combinations

After the child has developed a basic vocabulary, he begins putting these into simple word combinations. By two years of age, most hearing children use two-word utterances frequently in their speech (Wells, 1985). These combinations are referred to as semantic-syntactic pairs because they focus on meaning yet contain our first glimpse at word order. At this stage, it is often hard for the parents or caregiver to figure out meaning unless the context is clear. Children will also use stress to help clarify meaning. For example, *my shoe* might stress the possession aspect of the comment whereas *my shoe* might stress the object aspect. By eighteen months many deaf children of deaf parents have begun to put two signs together. Early sign combinations often occur without the morphological inflections of ASL, much as the hearing child leaves off English morphology (Spencer & Lederberg, 1997). Deaf children of hearing parents proceed along the same path of language acquisition, but most often they are severely delayed.

Snyder and Yoshinaga-Itano (1998) studied specific play behaviors and the development of communication in children with hearing losses. They found that the development of certain play behaviors correlated highly with children's understanding of simple phrases. The two behaviors that correlated most highly were *symbolic substitution play* and *sequenced symbolic play*. Symbolic substitution involves using one object to represent another. For example, the child might use a block as if it were a toy car. Sequence symbolic play involves engaging in two actions related in time such as taking a diaper off of a baby doll then putting a new one back on. Play allows children to explore their environment, to see how objects interact, then to represent both objects and actions. Representational play in space is a necessary precursor to the use of language as a means to represent experiences.

Multiword Combinations

Uninflected verbs (verbs with no tense markers) are a notable characteristic of the early word combinations state. When hearing children begin to combine words, they leave off all the structures of the auxiliary system of the verb. The auxiliary system is comprised of morphological elements, which determine tense, noun-verb agreement, and other modifications of the verb. They also leave off the determiner system (e.g., *a* and *the*). The child, therefore, will say, "Baby fall down" or "Puppy chase car."

In hearing children the auxiliary system develops during the period from eighteen months to three years, along with the negation system, the determiner system, and the question system. During both early combinations and multi-word combinations, the child overgeneralizes the use of structures he has just learned (Owens, 1996). For example, although the child begins to use specific irregular verbs at a very young age, he often overgeneralizes the use of the regular marker, "-ed," as in *runned* for *ran, bringed* for *brought*, and *hided* for *hid*, and will even add an "-ed" to some irregular forms producing *satted* for *sat* or *sawed* for *saw*. Children will overgeneralize plural forms as in *foots, mouses*, or *mans*, comparatives and superlatives, as in *biggerest*, and other morphological components.

Wilbur (2000) stated that "what differentiates deaf children's use of overgeneralization from hearing children's is its long-term persistence and its extension to larger syntactic domains" (p. 84). While hearing children overgeneralize words for which there are exceptions, deaf students overgeneralize due to several factors. The first is limited input. Deaf and hard of hearing children often have limited experience with English syntax rules and they often learn the rules incorrectly. The second factor is that structures are taught in isolation, which does not provide students with sufficient experience with the structure to learn all the different ways it can be used. Teaching structures in isolation, as some structured approaches recommend, often creates an instructional situation that becomes more rigid and syntax-based rather than retaining its focus on pragmatic intent. The third factor provided by Wilbur is that only certain structures are taught. For example, a teacher may select certain structures to teach, omitting others in hopes that they will be taught in subsequent years. Without a sequential curriculum and ways of monitoring students' acquisition of structures, some may not be taught to students thus creating a skill deficit. Unfortunately, certain aspects of English grammar remain a mystery to deaf and hard of hearing young adults, many of whom never develop proficiency (Moeller, Osberger, & Eccarius, 1986).

"Hearing children learning spoken English and deaf children learning ASL exhibit similar development of syntax: The signed utterances of deaf children are much like hearing children's spoken utterances. Thus modality of language has little impact on structure of the earliest word or sign combinations, even though the structure of signed languages and spoken English are different in later stages" (Spencer & Lederberg, 1997, p. 223). Deaf children of hearing parents who are exhibiting difficulties with multiword acquisition most likely have deficiencies due to an incomplete language model. They most likely will experience slow growth of syntactic abilities. Spencer and Lederberg (1997) stated that by school age, "as a group deaf children with hearing parents display significant language deficits, having limited vocabularies as well as difficulties with English syntactic structures" (p. 204).

Early Semantic Development in Children Who Are Deaf or Hard of Hearing.
Yoshinaga-Itano, Snyder, and Day (1998) and Snyder and Yoshinaga-Itano (1998) studied early language development in children with hearing losses. They found a high degree of relationship between symbolic play (as previously discussed) and language development. Not only did the symbolic play skills of their subjects correlate highly with early word combinations, but they also correlated highly with the number of words understood and produced. When a

child plays, he sees comparisons of similar objects, preparing him to understand descriptive vocabulary. When a child plays, he places one object in relation to another, preparing him to understand the meaning of basic prepositions. Play allows the child to develop the ability to represent objects, actions, their descriptions and their relationships as a precursor to representing these through language.

Early Pragmatic Development in Children Who Are Deaf or Hard of Hearing. Research into pragmatic development of hearing children has revealed that children begin acquiring these skills in early childhood and reach conversational maturity at approximately eight to ten years of age. From a review of existing literature, the authors provided a schedule of development based on hearing children's sequence of acquisition (Table 2.4).

In order to determine conversational aspects of pragmatic skill development in deaf students, Jeanes, Nienhuys, and Rickards (2000) studied students from eight to seventeen years of age. The students were deaf and either used oral communication or English-based signs. Their results were compared to hearing students in the same age group.

The ability to request clarification is a fundamental skill in effective face-to-face interaction. These researchers found that oral deaf students made requests for clarification more often than did hearing students or deaf students who sign. They concluded that these students recognized communication breakdowns and sought to repair them more often than the others; however, the oral deaf students may have used this strategy to gain additional information because their ability to receive clear communication was less precise. They also investigated the ability to make specific requests for clarification during com-

TABLE 2.4   *Sequence of Acquisition of Pragmatic Skills in Children*

Age	Pragmatic Skill
In early infancy	Infants exhibit early emerging skills essential for smooth conversation (e.g., turn taking).
By age two	Children respond to natural requests.
By age three	Children respond to clarification.
By age four, five	Children improve and revise their original message in response to listener feedback.
By age five	Children begin to appraise the quality of speakers' messages.
By age seven	Children show early skills at disambiguating messages.
By age eleven	Children make specific and nonspecific requests for clarification.

munication and found that hearing students made far more specific requests than did deaf students as a group, with the signing students making the fewest. When required to respond to a specific request for clarification, all three groups responded appropriately and at the same rate.

In order for communication to have positive outcomes speakers must provide appropriate responses that keep communication going. Confirmatory responses are often used to provide feedback to the other communicators thus serving to keep the conversation flowing. Oral deaf students used this skill; however, the signing students were less likely to do so. They, instead, most often simply repeated their original communication. Perhaps they do this because they perceive the communication breakdown as resulting from failure to understand their signing rather than a misunderstanding of the message.

The overall findings of this research revealed that both oral and signing deaf students were more immature in their communicative interactions than were hearing students. Deaf students "showed evidence of immaturity in their skills in maintaining smooth face-to-face conversational interaction" (p. 245). They have "difficulty in using appropriate, productive pragmatic behaviors when requesting clarification, when responding to requests for clarification, and at times of communication breakdown" (p. 246). The reasons for this lack of pragmatic development are multifaceted; however, most likely pragmatic deficits are a direct result of delayed language because most students with hearing losses have less opportunity to communicate with fluent communication partners. As the researchers noted, deaf students' pragmatic development may be correlated to their stages of language development in general. In order to facilitate pragmatic development in deaf students they need to experience meaningful face-to-face interactions with fluent communicators early because it is through natural conversation that pragmatic skills develop.

Adult-Like Language Skills

Along with the development of semantic categories, the verb system, the auxiliary system, determiner, negation, and the question system, hearing children begin to use basic phrase structures. The hearing child is able to use noun phrases (e.g., *the big dog, my mommy's car*), verb phrases (e.g., *was running, slipped and slid*), adverbial phrases (e.g., *in the car, with a clean fork*), and the adjectival system (e.g., *big and strong, clean and pretty*). Language systems develop in an ebb and flow, with some systems leaping past others, then others catching up. The syntactic, semantic, and pragmatic systems are closely interwoven (Shirai & Andersen, 1995). The child puts sentences together into basic sentence patterns and continually combines these in new and novel ways, adding more and more phrases until full sentences abound. The hearing child developing on schedule uses all the forms and structures mentioned by the age of five (Menyuk, 1969). Thus, it requires only a few years from the time the hearing child is uttering single-word sentences until he uses complex systems that approximate adult form. These complexities include advanced nuances of the verb system, complements, relative clauses, subordination, and a host of other skills.

The child may be able to put words together into sentences, but it takes many more years before he will comprehend all the semantic variations, innuendoes, and complexities that comprise adult language. The semantic system that develops from this point on includes not only word meaning but sentence and discourse meaning as well. Language users deal with a whole host of abstract language issues including literal and figurative meanings of words, phrases, sentences, and discourse.

Language and Literacy.   The most important change that occurs at the stage of adult competence is that we begin to read and write the language that we know. Deaf and hard of hearing children who did not receive early access to a complete language exhibit the deficit that began in infancy. By the time the child is eight years of age the deficit is so severe that generally a crisis occurs. Third grade is a pivotal point when many language-dependent skills come together on the road to literacy. By third grade a foundation in reading, writing, and mathematics creates opportunities for later learning. Standardized testing usually begins at the end of third grade, and these scores often reveal a deaf or hard of hearing child functioning well below hearing peers (Moores, 2000). Some have reported that standardized tests are biased against children from diverse linguistic backgrounds, and while this is undisputedly true, most deaf and hard of hearing children's backgrounds could be described more as linguistically impoverished than linguistically diverse. Linguistic diversity implies a functional native language other than the language of the standardized test (e.g., Spanish as the native language; English as the test language). Deaf and hard of hearing students often do not have native language competency; therefore, this argument is questionable. Without a well-formed language base, literacy development is compromised.

Deaf and hard of hearing students face tremendous challenges when learning to read and write English. While some may believe that ASL impedes reading development, others disagree (Wilbur, 2000), pointing out that any effort that helps students develop a solid language base, whether signed or spoken, is likely to improve the ability to read. Tur-Kaspa and Dromi (1998) reported that students with hearing losses tended to produce simple complement structures in spoken language whereas students with normal hearing tended to use more relative clauses. "Dative, question, negation, conjoined, and elliptical clauses appeared significantly more in the spoken language; subject verb object (SVO), coordinated, and uncodable clauses, on the other hand, appeared significantly more in the written language samples" (p. 192). Further, "about 15 percent of the spoken clauses and about 10 percent of the written clauses of the students with hearing loss included either subject omission or main verb omission" (p. 194). In general, the English language skills of students with hearing losses remain a large contributing factor to the difficulties they experience in reading and writing.

The Critical Period for First Language Acquisition

One of the most important hypotheses about language acquisition is the critical-period hypothesis. According to Lenneberg (1967), the critical period of language development is the period from around two years of age to thirteen or the onset of puberty. After the onset of puberty it is extremely difficult to acquire fluency in a first language. For deaf and hard of hearing children the critical-period theory has serious implications and could possibly explain why language development for most deaf children, specifically those with hearing parents, is a slow and arduous process (McAnally, Rose, & Quigley, 1994).

Through the years researchers have tested Lenneberg's hypothesis by looking at rare instances of delayed exposure to a first language. The first well-known case, Victor, the Wild Boy of Aveyron, was described by Lane (1976). Victor was abandoned as a young child in 1800 and taken to the National Institute for the Deaf in Paris. Jean-Marc Itard attempted to teach him to speak, but Victor could not exceed the use of simple words and sentences. More recently, researchers studied Genie, a young girl who had been isolated by an abusive father until the age of thirteen (Curtiss, 1977). Genie eventually learned a great deal of English vocabulary and produced simple sentences, but she failed to acquire the more intricate complexities of the English language. Delayed exposure to a first language is common among deaf and hard of hearing children with hearing parents, although severe cases of isolation and deprivation are rare. Many communicate with their families in a homesign system (Stokoe, 1995) that provides a form of communication, albeit a primitive one. Studies of severe isolation, however, provide our best glimpse into the nature of deprivation and how it impacts language acquisition in deaf and hard of hearing students.

Grimshaw, Adelstein, Bryden, and MacKinnon (1998) discovered two case studies of deaf children who were linguistically isolated until after the critical period of language acquisition. One case involved a fifteen-year-old male instructed orally and another involved a sixteen-year-old female instructed in ASL. Both had acquired a homesign system prior to formal instruction. After four years of therapy the student taught orally had integrated speech with his homesign system; however, his language remained severely delayed with deficits comparable to Genie's. The student learning ASL readily acquired the basic structures of the language in a short period of time, but she had difficulties with syntactic features.

These cases indicate that first-language acquisition in puberty does not progress as rapidly as first-language acquisition in the younger years.

Lenneberg (1967) attributed this to loss of neural plasticity. Newport (1990) indicated that cognitive processes might develop during adolescence that inhibit language development.

Many deaf children with hearing parents receive little exposure to either spoken or signed languages during early childhood (Meier, 1991). Newport and Supalla (1990) studied adult deaf subjects to determine the effects of delayed exposure to a first language on this population. The researchers found that knowledge of basic ASL word order is not dependent upon one's age at initial exposure. However, as the complexity of the language increases, the age at exposure becomes a predictor of success. Apparently deaf children may gain a certain degree of skill with ASL no matter when they begin to learn the language, but to develop native competence in a language they require exposure to that language during the critical period (Meier, 1991).

Research establishes that age of acquisition is one of the best predicators of ASL fluency among the deaf adult population. Other studies (Newport, 1991; Newport & Supalla, 1990) also showed that on average the fluency of deaf adults who learned ASL early (before age six) was indistinguishable from that of native ASL signers (deaf adults who were born to ASL-using deaf parents) on various tests of production and comprehension of ASL grammatical structures. Newport and Supalla's research provides clear direction: If deaf children are to have full mastery and native competence in ASL, exposure must begin as early as possible. If deaf and hard of hearing children of hearing parents are taught ASL in preschool, they would most likely tap the biological potential to reach native-like competence in ASL (Singleton, Supalla, Litchfield, & Schley, 1998).

Further evidence of a critical period for language learning in students who are deaf or hard of hearing has been documented. In 1979 the first schools for the deaf were established in Nicaragua bringing together children from all around the country. Each child brought a unique set of homesigns to the school and as the children interacted, their homesigns blended into a pidgin language. Pidgin languages are simplified languages derived from two or more languages. Sometimes pidgins are referred to as *contact languages* and are used by people in a given geographic area who do not share a common language. The structure of a pidgin language is very simple and its use is limited. Most often pidgin languages die out; however, when a pidgin is used over an extensive period of time and when children learn the language, something happens to the language that is quite remarkable. Usually the complexity of the language increases, syntax develops, and the vocabulary becomes more robust. As the language undergoes this refinement, native speakers (children) acquire it as their first language. In this process the language has evolved from a pidgin to a creole.

The signed language of the young children at the only primary school in Nicaragua was beginning the process of creolization (creolization is the formalization of a pidgin language into a new language with its own grammar). In 1986 Shepard-Kegl, a linguist who studies language and the brain, came to Nicaragua to evaluate the signed language phenomenon. She eventually documented the birth of this modern-day signed language. In the process of documenting the Nicaraguan Sign Language (NSL) she discovered aspects of language acquisition that support the earlier works of Chomsky (1965) relating to the biological basis for language, of Pinker's (1984) language instinct, and of Lenneberg's (1967) theories of the critical period for language acquisition.

Shepard-Kegl found that the adolescents and adults in the vocational school were only able to engage one another in rudimentary conversation in their pidgin language. However, at the primary school a different story was unfolding. The primary-age students came to the school with a homesign system just as diverse as that of the older students, but their communicative interactions were quite different from those of the older students: the children "pulled grammar out of their heads and put it into their signs" (BBC, 1996, p. 3). Their homesign system became a pidgin signed language and then was creolized into a fully grammatical language. The children spontaneously created their own language, consistent from person to person, with a rich grammar and vocabulary. Why did the younger, second generation of students develop a grammar for their language while the older, first generation students did not? The answer may lie in the age at which these students began to learn the new language.

Shepard-Kegl's research suggests the brain is open to a signed language until the age of twelve or thirteen, then the opportunity begins to diminish. The younger children were brought together when their biological instinct for language acquisition was strong. Conversely, the older students were brought together as the door to language instinct was closing. The older students developed a pidgin, but did not develop a grammar. Apparently children are born already programmed to understand the basic notions of subject, verb, object, and the rules of grammar that relate to them; however this ability diminishes with age. In addition to learning language early it appears that the language instinct needs a catalyst: a certain minimum amount of raw material. For the children of Nicaragua, homesigns became the raw material. " 'I'm convinced that language is in the brain, but I'm also convinced that language needs a trigger,' stated Shepard-Kegl. That trigger is communication" (Pelley, 2000, p. 3). "We used to think that if you took a child and you put him into a nurturing environment and they had parents that fed them, interacted with them, and socialized with them that language would come into being because language is some sort of instinct. From observing families where there's a deaf child with hearing parents, I'm convinced that a deaf child left in the home will remain languageless" (p. 15).

What are the implications of Shepard-Kegl's research on deaf children? Her research emphasizes that development of fluency in a first language must occur during the first years of life when children have the innate capacity to develop knowledge of syntax and grammar effortlessly. This innateness diminishes as children get older and children deprived of the opportunity to develop first-language fluency may end up languageless, operating in a primitive form of a pidgin language.

Factors That Contribute to Language Acquisition

Many authors have summarized the literature on the development of language in deaf and hard of hearing children and concluded that language acquisition in deaf or hard of hearing children follows along the path of normal language development, proceeding through the same stages that hearing children go through. However, language acquisition in children with hearing loss is usually delayed and occurs at a much slower rate than in children with normal hearing (McAnally, Rose, & Quigley, 1994; Schirmer, 2000). Several factors lead to this delay, factors that if not changed may cause children with hearing losses never to catch up, remaining impoverished for a lifetime. We discuss these factors next.

Early Exposure to Language

Even before a hearing child is born, the maturing fetus hears the sounds of the fetal environment. After the infant is born, some are soothed by sounds to which they became accustomed in the womb (e.g., a particular piece of music or their mother's voice). Through hearing the child listens to environmental sounds and begins to make sense of the sounds of language. For a child deprived of hearing the situation is quite different. A child with a hearing loss may live in a linguistically rich environment; however, access to language may be severely restricted.

Prior to the 1970s researchers in the field of psychology, linguistics, and communication disorders explored deaf and hard of hearing children's language development because it seemed to provide an intriguing and unique opportunity. The deprived environment, devoid of sound, seemed to provide a unique opportunity to study language acquisition removed from the influence of communication. Early research (Furth, 1969) explored the question: Can deaf children think without language? Researchers studied deaf children with the hopes of discovering more about language learning in general and how the lack of auditory input impacts thought processes.

Many researchers believe that language is an innate human trait. Lenneberg (1967) postulated that humans have a Language Acquisition Device (LAD) that exists internally and orchestrates the burst of language acquisition in childhood. There are certain prerequisites for this to happen. The child must have the capacity to learn and the child must have access to language. A biological predisposition for language is wasted unless a child has access to a comprehensible language system, and for language acquisition to continue on schedule it must be fueled by communication with caregivers. Quite possibly language acquisition occurs on schedule in as few learners as 10%, those being deaf children of deaf parents who provide a rich language environment in which language acquisition occurs naturally and spontaneously. The benefits of early language access are obvious with this population. Similarly, some very young cochlear implant recipients who receive early and consistent auditory input are learning to communicate (Fryauf-Bertschy, Tyler, Kelsay, Gantz, & Woodworth, 1997).

In recent years a great deal of information has been gathered in the field of neuroscience regarding brain development during infancy and beyond. This research is significant to language acquisition in that it provides insight regarding what happens to the brain when language exposure is delayed. Aoki and Seikeuitz (1988) found that the young infant's brain is quite plastic and malleable. As the infant takes in stimuli, language develops because the brain is establishing neural connections and pathways. Neural pathways grow at an explosive rate in children who are able to receive information from their environment. The implications for infants who cannot hear the sounds of their environment are that we must provide sufficient information to build the brain's infrastructure. Such information might be presented auditorally or visually, but the message must be complete.

Mother–Child Interactions

Language development in most cultures begins immediately at birth. Mothers (being the primary caregiver in most cultures) use natural, intuitive parenting that facilitates language acquisition. Several research efforts have compared deaf children with hearing mothers to deaf children with deaf mothers in order to identify those aspects of the mother–child relationship that were beneficial and those aspects that were atypical or detrimental to a deaf child's development (Lederberg, 1993; Meadow-Orlans & Steinberg, 1993; Pressman, Pipp-Siegel, & Yoshinaga-Itano, 1998) (Table 2.5). Assumptions have been made that the deaf child with a hearing mother is at a disadvantage to the other dyads in most areas. Meadow-Orlans (1997) found that the quality of interactions between deaf mothers and deaf infants and between hearing mothers and hearing infants was similar; therefore, it is not the children's deafness that impacts maternal behavior, but rather the mismatch between the mother's and infant's hearing status.

Spencer and Lederberg (1997) summarized the literature on hearing mother's interactions with their deaf babies. They noted that families tend to change communication modes over time, which complicates the ability of researchers to isolate factors that influence language development. Most frequently, families choose an oral approach, and then switch to a signing approach at a later date (Stredler-Brown, 1998). Whether a family chooses to sign or to use an oral approach, speech accounts for the bulk of linguistic input especially during the first three years of an infant's life. The situation in which a hearing mother of a deaf child finds herself is one that is extremely emotionally and linguistically challenging. As she struggles with understanding the meaning of her infant's hearing loss, she is also struggling with learning to communicate in a way that is totally new to her.

TABLE 2.5 *Mothers of Children Who Are Deaf*

Deaf Mothers of Deaf Children	Hearing Mothers of Deaf Children
Respond intuitively to their child's affective needs during early development. They cuddle the baby, use touch to console or comfort the child, and respond to the child's needs.	Respond in the same way as deaf mothers to their child's affective needs during early development. They respond intuitively to their child's needs and support typical growth in many areas of development.
Use strategies to support the learning of a visual language. They will sign near an object with which the child is playing or wave a hand to draw the child's attention towards them.	With little experience in a visual language, hearing mothers use insufficient visual accommodations for language to develop.
Use exaggerated facial expressions when communicating with their baby.	When attempting to sign, use few facial expressions with their baby.
Communication is visual. They use visual motherese to facilitate language growth.	Regardless of the communication approach chosen, hearing mothers use speech predominately to communicate with their infant.
Use modifications to hold and maintain attention span, allowing for greater time to process language input (e.g., they will sit and wait for their infants to look at them before beginning to sign).	Because the infant cannot hear the mother's voice, attention is most often on an object or event instead of what is being communicated.
Modify their signs: use signs that are larger, slower, and have more exaggerated movements. Signs are strong rhythmically with frequent repetitions.	Simplify their speech and use simple patterns of syntax. Use less prosodic and intonational changes to their speech.
Sign in a fluent, rich manner. Communication occurs naturally and results in frequent interactions.	Sign in a stilted, impoverished manner. They often make errors and experience communication breakdowns resulting in fewer interactions.
Communication facilitates language development.	Lack of communication disrupts the child's development.

Sources: Erting, Prezioso, & O'Grady Hynes, 1994; Lederberg & Mobley, 1990; Lederberg & Prezbindowski, 2000; Masataka, 1992; Spencer & Lederberg, 1997.

Hearing mothers of deaf children appear to be uncomfortable and unnatural in their communication interactions. In some instances their natural instincts for communication are so altered that they will even whisper to the child rather than use a natural voice (Spencer & Lederberg, 1997). They are, indeed, at a severe disadvantage when learning to communicate with their baby. Because they do not share the same language, a mismatch occurs that creates an unnatural situation. Hearing mothers tend to be less responsive to their deaf children's visual needs compared to deaf mothers of deaf children. In addition, hearing mothers with deaf children show increased intrusiveness and directiveness, which results in decreased reciprocity (Spencer & Gutfreund, 1990). Fiese (1990) noted that mothers' intrusive attempts to redirect children's play tended to lower instead of raise the child's cognitive level.

Although research has shown that mother's educational level influences outcomes of hearing children, Calderon (2000) found that maternal communication skill proved to be a more significant indicator for language development, early reading skills, and social-emotional development in children who are deaf or hard of hearing than did the mother's educational achievement. She found that even mothers with higher levels of education might struggle with communicating effectively with her child. "Mothers [with deaf or hard of hearing children] who demonstrated better communication skills had children with higher language and reading scores and less behavior problems. . . . (p. 151).

Language Uptake

Goodwyn and Acredolo (1993) found that the quantity of linguistic input directly related to increased early language development in children. In other words, the greater the input the greater language gains children exhibit. To test this hypothesis, Lederberg and Everhart (1998) conducted a study of communication and language development in twenty deaf children. When comparing mother–child interactions, speech remained the dominant method of communication. Even though the majority of the children were enrolled in Total Communication programs and parents had access to sign language classes, the mothers used signs on an extremely limited basis. Hearing mothers of deaf children seem to be able to facilitate nonlinguistic communication; however, the results of this study indicate that they are unable to help their child acquire language beyond this basic level.

In this study the deaf children were language delayed despite the amount of input the mothers presented. Gallaway and Woll (1994) found similar conclusions, that is, the rates of speech of deaf children's mothers compared to hearing children's mothers were approximately the same. Mothers of deaf infants talk to them just as much as a hearing mother talks to a hearing infant. Both sets of mothers used spoken motherese regardless of their children's hearing status. Gallaway and Woll (1994) make a distinction between the amount of language in the environment (input) and the amount of language the deaf child comprehends (uptake). In most deaf children, uptake is extremely limited. Consequently, the amount of input has little to do with the amount of uptake deaf children experience. The study by Lederberg and Everhart (1998) revealed that deaf children of hearing mothers were severely language delayed with some deaf three-year-olds using less language than hearing twenty-two-month olds, and some producing no language at all. In fact, the research revealed that deaf children communicated primarily through nonlinguistic vocalizations with increasing use of gesture.

We have incontrovertible evidence that deaf and hard of hearing children must learn a complete communication system before they start formal schooling (i.e., traditional kindergarten and first grade) or they will struggle to gain communication proficiency. It does not matter to the brain whether it is spoken English developed through technologically enhanced residual hearing or if it is American Sign Language. There is also some evidence that early exposure through visual enhancements such English-based signs or Cued Speech (Luetke-Stahlman, 1988) can result in age-appropriate communication in some children. Others have discussed the incompleteness of English-based signs (Johnson, Liddell, & Erting, 1989). The important point to remember is that comprehension or uptake depends on the availability of a complete language system. If children are receiving incomplete information, they will not develop a complete language system. Even though input may be abundant, uptake is the critical factor in language development. Children with limited uptake will have impoverished language skills. "If no uptake is possible, no formal language will develop" (Spencer & Lederberg, 1997, p. 225). Language acquisition must occur early. If not, during the remainder of the student's school years, the student will find language-learning a challenging task.

Deaf children of hearing parents present the most challenge. Singleton, Supalla, Litchfield, and Schley (1998) concluded that deaf students of hearing parents, when given the opportunity to master ASL before the age of six have systems of grammar similar to those of deaf students whose parents are also deaf. Therefore, it is possible for both groups (i.e., deaf children of hearing parents and deaf children of deaf parents) to learn a first language and enter school with a fully functioning language on which all future learning is based. Wilbur (2000) identified the advantages of having a fully developed first language. First, knowledge of ASL is beneficial because it taps normal capacities at the appropriate stage of development. Second, knowledge of a first language facilitates learning of a second language. Knowledge of a first language serves to reduce the complexity of the second language and, therefore, reduces need to teach particular syntactic structures. Last, a fully developed first language serves as a bridge to literacy in the second language. All of these factors are critical in the development of advanced literacy skills in deaf and hard of hearing students.

The Influence of Bilingualism on Deaf Education

When cultures come into contact, changes to the language of each culture occur. Dialects, pidgins, and creoles may develop. In North America we are experiencing a rapid increase in the diversity of languages among the population. At least ten out of every thirty school-age children are from language minority families (McLaughlin & McLeod, 1996). In some states there are over one hundred different languages used in the homes of American school children. This means that a large portion of the school-age population will be either bilingual or in the process of learning English as a second language. The increase of bilingualism has provided insights into language acquisition processes that have caused the field of deaf education to rethink some of its fundamental premises (Nover & Andrews, 1999). One concept that has vast implications for deaf education lies in the comparison between new language learners and heritage/home language learners. A *heritage language* is that language which the hearing child hears at home (Valdes, 1995). Children newly arrived in North America have varying abilities and proficiencies in their heritage language (National Standards for Foreign Language Education Project, 1996). The same may be said for children who are ASL users; varying abilities and proficiencies in the heritage language exist.

Hearing students with weak knowledge of their heritage language need opportunities to maintain, retrieve, and/or acquire language competencies (National Standards for Foreign Language Education Project, 1996). The same may be said for deaf children whose developing skills in ASL would benefit from programs of maintenance, retrieval, and/or acquisition. The field of bilingual education (e.g., Spanish/English; French/English) has several models from which to choose as well as a body of research that presents data regarding model effectiveness. For example, much as been written about simultaneous acquisition of the heritage language (L1) and the new language (L2) and successive acquisition of L1 and L2 (Grosjean, 1980). Many researchers believe that simultaneous acquisition is more beneficial (Cummins, 1980) as it allow us to avoid several problems. One serious problem is that when instruction is presented in L2, the student may not have the necessary language facility to learn through the medium of that language. While models of bilingualism exist in the education of students who have normal hearing, few exist in deaf education.

In addition to the lack of models of instruction, we do not have a comprehensive K–12 program for the ASL heritage language learner. Presently there are no curriculum guides or textbook series that have been developed for deaf and hard of hearing children to learn ASL as a first or heritage language. Recently, some states have begun to develop curricula to teach ASL to hearing students (e.g., Texas and Georgia). They have developed standards for teaching ASL as a foreign or second language to high school students. Until deaf children have equal access to learning about their language, the potential of ASL to ESL programs may fall short of the mark.

The greatest amount of longitudinal data we presently have comes from Sweden and Denmark. Bilingual programs for deaf and hard of hearing students have been in existence since 1981 when the Swedish Parliament passed a law stating that deaf people need to be bilingual in order to function successfully in families, in school, and in society (Mahshie, 1995). This law required all education of deaf and hard of hearing students in Sweden to be bilingual using Swedish Sign Language (SSL) as the first language and spoken Swedish as a second language. The goals of the program were to achieve grade-level achievement, full participation in society, and fluency in both the language of the majority and the language of the Deaf community and the home (Mahshie, 1995). The first students to receive this bilingual approach are in their late teens or early twenties and the results of their achievement testing provide longitudinal evidence of the positive benefits of bilingual education. "Upon graduation, achievement of the students in the bilingual class in Copenhagen was at or above grade level and all passed their exit exams on time—tests that had previously been considered unattainable for deaf students" (Mahshie, 1995, p. 21). There are obvious differences between the cultures and policies of Sweden and those of the United States. For example, Sweden's population does not reflect the wide diversity that we have in the United States. In addition, they do not adhere to the concept of full inclusion in early education. In Sweden deaf and hard of hearing students attend specialized preschool programs and specialized regional programs for deaf and hard of hearing students long before they enter the regular education classrooms. Students first have the knowledge and, most importantly, the language base to support learning in that environment. "In Sweden today deaf children are exposed to sign language from very early in life. Their hearing parents sign, their preschool teachers, both hearing and deaf, sign. They watch sign language in children's programs on television and later on, when they enter schools for the deaf, they are instructed in sign language. In school sign language is also an independent subject. Sign language is regarded as the mother tongue even if it is a second language for most parents" (Ahlgren, 1994, p. 55).

In the United States the Star Schools Project (Nover & Andrews, 1999) is beginning to provide similar evidence regarding ASL/English bilingualism. The project staff is creating a bilingual model (ASL, ESL) based on extensive research conducted at schools for the deaf.

The bilingual movement has its critics. In support, Andrews (2000) explained that "Many hearing people erroneously believe ASL will interfere with a child's learning of speech or written language. Further, they often think the deaf child will rely too much on signs and refuse to learn English, and that a deaf teacher will negatively affect their children's speech and language development" (p. 56). Actually, the opposite occurs. ASL does not interfere with the acquisition of speech or written language. Instead, it serves as a bridge to learning another. Moreover, deaf teachers have positive instructional results because they are fluent in the language, while often hearing parents and teachers are not. Deaf teachers are a critical component in any bilingual program.

Hard of Hearing Children

Hard of hearing children remain among the least well-served subgroup of this population because they are frequently overlooked and their needs are often misunderstood. Although there are multiple fail-safe mechanisms in place within the system-wide procedures to prevent children from falling through the cracks, if there are such cracks one can expect hard of hearing children to fall through them. Because they hear some things they may not be referred for testing until later. In addition, their amount of hearing may be misjudged. Because of their hearing loss they often misunderstand what is going on around them, and they are often misplaced within the educational system. They may have been retained a grade. The accumulative effect of years of misunderstanding may have resulted in an ability-achievement gap that qualifies them for services in an interrelated classroom with a teacher who has no knowledge of the needs of students with mild hearing losses. They are at risk socially because they miss the nuances of the social substrata of the hallways, the cafeterias, and the basketball courts. They are accused of laziness, not caring, and worse yet, stupidity. Those whose loss is not severe may deny that their hearing loss exists at all, which has implications for socio-emotional development later. The issues and challenges of students with mild and moderate hearing losses are indeed complex and often result in severe implications to many areas of development.

The hard of hearing school-aged population is becoming more heterogeneous. This has a significant impact on how children with hearing losses should be served. Parents, teachers, and administrators often misunderstand students' needs because they do not understand the implications of heterogeneity. Teachers must assist others in developing a broader perspective on the needs of the population.

Summary

In this chapter we have described several factors that influence the language learning of deaf children. Of all of the factors presented, perhaps environment is the most crucial aspect of early language development. It is within the context of the family that language develops naturally even if that language is not the family's heritage language. Learning a first language through the normal process of language acquisition is such a powerful developmental requirement that it influences many areas including cognition, communication, parent–child attachment, socio-emotional health, and the future development of second-language literacy. In order for all these areas to come together a first language must be acquired as early as possible because the window of language-learning opportunity is most responsive in the first few years of life. Of the total population of deaf and hard of hearing children, 10 percent have families who are deaf. For those children, language will develop naturally in the same way that hearing children learn a spoken language. They will mediate language primarily through visual pathways. These deaf children of deaf adults develop first-language competency in American Sign Language and learn English as a second language. The remaining 90 percent of children who are deaf or hard of hearing have hearing parents and, because of many complex factors, the repercussions are severe, most often resulting in delayed acquisition of a first language unless family support and appropriate interventions begin early. When early language acquisition is delayed, language must then be acquired in sterile school settings that were meant instead to provide instruction in reading, writing, math, etc. That force behind all of human development, whatever you believe it to be, never intended us to learn language in school settings. It intended us to learn language and to learn to communicate at our mama and papa's knees.

Questions for Critical Thinking

1. What factors do you believe have the greatest influence on language learning in children who are deaf or hard of hearing?

2. What needs to occur for children who are deaf or hard of hearing to learn language on schedule?

3. How does learning a language visually compare to learning a language auditorily?

4. Describe the accommodations that hearing mothers must learn in order to facilitate language growth in their children who are deaf.

5. Why is teaching language to children who are deaf or hard of hearing such a difficult task?

3

Multiple Pathways to Language Learning

What to Expect in This Chapter

In this chapter you will read about our philosophy of language acquisition in children who are deaf and hard of hearing, which embraces multiple languages and multiple means of acquiring these. The first part of this chapter describes theoretical underpinnings. The second part places this in the context of real children. You will see that teachers need to develop a broad perspective on language acquisition.

This chapter explores the ways in which children who are deaf and hard of hearing understand communication. We begin with a look at various models, or pathways, by which the brain takes in information, uses it, stores it, and allows us to retrieve it. This information is the foundation for understanding the idea of multiple pathways. Next we explain why teachers and parents must embrace the notion of multiple pathways; the population is heterogeneous. So many factors surround a hearing loss that it is better to think of each child as a population of one than to think of deaf and hard of hearing children as one population.

How Children Learn Language

Three theories that hold prominence in the field of language today are the *information/linguistic processing theory* (Owens, 1996; Torgeson, 1996; Borkowski & Burke, 1996), the *neuropsychological theory* (Bachevalier, Malkova, & Beauregard, 1996; Denckla, 1996), and the *cognitive-socialization theory* (Bruner, 1981, 1990; Nelson, 1985, 1996; Muma, 1998). Each theory helps us understand how children who are deaf and hard of hearing think and learn.

Linguistic/Information Processing Theory

The information processing model was proposed by Osgood (1957) to describe how humans receive information, manipulate it in their heads, and express their thoughts to others. The linguistic processing model (Luria, 1966) is based upon Osgood's model. We treat them here as one entity because they are so closely related. The linguistic/information processing model views the human brain as a computer. The computer receives information (called input, intake, or receptive communication) from various sources such as a microphone, scanner, or keyboard (i.e., auditory, visual, or tactile sources) that are external to the system (i.e., the actual computer itself). The information enters a program on the desktop (i.e., working or short-term memory) where we are able to manipulate it in many ways. For example, we can cut and paste our sentences so that *The girl hit the boy* becomes *The boy was hit by the girl.* We can search the system's thesaurus to find just the right word we need, and we can even generate a map to get us from one place to the next. After we have worked with the information getting the message we mean into the form we want, we can save it into long-term memory on the hard-drive. If we want to share this information with someone, we find the appropriate file (search our memory), retrieve the information (open the file), then transmit it via the sound card, words, pictures, or a hard copy (i.e., in some auditory, visual, or tactile manner), variously called expressive communication or output.

Owens (1996) identified the major components of information processing as attention, discrimination, organization, memory, and transfer. Table 3.1 provides definitions of the vocabulary used by information/linguistic processing theorists. Information/linguistic processing proponents focus their attention on input, processing, and output modes (i.e., receptive language, inner language, and expressive language), forms that language takes across these modes (i.e., listening, speaking, reading, writing) and the sensory modes that convey information (i.e., auditory, visual, and tactile stimulation and processing). For example, we might use this theory to explain why a hard of hearing student might need an interpreter. While the student may be able to hear and understand the teacher in a one-to-one situation, that same student may not be able to understand the teacher in a noisy classroom. She might benefit from receiving English through the visual mode (i.e., English-based signs) when in the regular education setting.

Regarding the development of students who are deaf and hard of hearing, the linguistic/information processing theory has been used to describe differences between the major philosophies (Oralism, Total Communication, Bilingualism-Biculturalism) with regard to languages (English and ASL) and modes (auditory and visual). Consequently in the literature we see reference to English in the auditory mode and English in the visual mode. Most psychoeducational testing is based on this philosophy. Most studies of memory processes in students who are deaf and hard of hearing have followed this model as well. For example, Bebko (1998) noted that "memory for spatial or simultaneous information tends to be

TABLE 3.1 *Definitions of Linguistic/Information Processing Concepts*

Concept	Definition
Active processing	New information coming in is actively compared with information existing in the system. Also referred to as Top-Down Processing.
Passive processing	Unfamiliar information enters in bits and pieces until there are enough pieces to make sense. Also referred to as Bottom-Up Processing.
Attention	The process of focusing on and maintaining interaction with information. Involves awareness of a stimulus array (orientation), *selective attention* to the most relevant stimulus, *encoding* of the stimulus so that the system can manipulate it and ultimately store it, *sustained attention* to the stimulus over time, *maintenance* of attention in the face of competing stimuli, and *redirection* of a stimulus when it is no longer meeting a need.
Discrimination	The process of differentiating between or among stimuli based on some dimension or scheme. *Auditory discrimination* involves differentiating between auditory stimuli, *visual discrimination* between visual stimuli, and *haptic/tactile* discrimination between stimuli we feel or touch. We also discriminate stimuli that we perceive with our senses of taste and smell.
Organization	The process by which information that has been discriminated is categorized or chunked in a manner that will both maintain memory space in the system and allow us to represent those categories as concepts.
Memory	The ability to recall information that has been previously learned or experienced. *Working* (short term) memory is that memory process by which we hold information for active attention and processing, either auditorily via a *phonological feedback loop* or visually on a *visuo-spatial sketchpad*. After sufficient *rehearsal* of the stimuli, whereby it is situated within various phonologic (either English phonology or ASL phonology), semantic, syntactic, morphologic, and pragmatic, locations and associations in the brain, *encoding* has taken place, and the information is now in *long-term* memory. There are many types of memory, but *successive* (serial) memory and *simultaneous* (parallel) memory are most often associated with this theory. Successive memory is memory for information in sequences and is often related to auditory information, but not exclusively so. Simultaneous memory is memory for information presented holistically and is often related to visual information, but not exclusively so.
Transfer	The process of *generalizing* new information to novel situations.
Metacognition	The process of using one's awareness of information processing skills to learn new information.

Sources: Baddeley, 1986; Owens, 1996; Torgeson, 1996.

at least equivalent among deaf and hearing samples" at the same time noting that deaf individuals had greater difficulty "with sequential processing, tasks typically handled by hearing individuals with verbal encoding" (p. 4). Lack of sequential processing skills influences the ability to grasp grammatical order as well as those memory tasks that require rehearsal. When language is delayed and sequential processing is limited, activities that assist memory by placing information visually in a spatially oriented array are needed to take up the slack.

Opponents of the information processing model express concern over the pervasive emphasis on modality. They feel that concern with input and output modes is a simplistic view of what happens during the process of communication.

Neuropsychological Theory

The neuropsychological or neurocognitive theory (Shaywitz et al., 1997; Shaywitz & Shaywitz, 1996) places human learning and behavior in the brain and central nervous system. Neurolinguistic theorists seek to identify those locations within the brain that are directly responsible for specific language activities. To understand the literature on neurolinguistics and its implications, you need to know the basic structures of the brain and central nervous system and their hypothesized functions. You will find definitions of basic structures that neurolinguists might discuss in Table 3.2.

The brain has specific locations that are more or less related to various aspects of the language task (Fiez et al., 1996; Habib, Demonet, & Frackowiak, 1996). These areas are widely dispersed among lobes and across hemispheres. For example, language impairments occur in the presence of left hemisphere damage (Corina, 1998) and right hemisphere damage (Rehak et al., 1992).

The neurolinguistic theory sees the human brain and language learning as more like the Internet than like a computer. When logging on to the Internet, you may have several purposes in mind:

1. to find and understand new information (i.e., to comprehend),
2. to locate specific information you have dealt with before (e.g., remember),
3. to use the information in some creative way (i.e., think), and
4. to put it in some form to share with others (e.g., write, speak, or sign).

We encode new concepts and the words that refer to them in many areas of the brain. Some areas of the brain encode grammar, some encode meaning, and some encode pragmatic intent. This sets information up in the brain in a system of interconnected neural networks, much like the network of the Internet. For example, if you were to do a web search for the Council on Education of the Deaf, you might get to the website by any number of means. You might type in the URL and go directly to the site. Or, you might find the site as a link

TABLE 3.2 *Terminology Associated with the Neurolinguistic Theory*

Term	Definition
Arcuate fasciculus	A fibrous bundle of nerves that communicates between the receptive and expressive language centers of the brain.
Broca's area	That part of the left frontal lobe of the brain that coordinates speech output.
Central nervous system (CNS)	That part of the nervous system which is made up of the brain and spinal cord.
Corpus callosum	A large bundle of nerve fibers that run between the left and right hemispheres of the brain, allowing the two sides to communicate with one another.
Cortex	The outermost, gray portions of the brain.
Lobes	Major paired brain masses including the frontal (front), parietal (top), and temporal (side) lobes, and the occipital lobe (back).
Hemispheres	Two sides of the brain, anatomically separated from one another and connected via the corpus callosum.
Heschl's gyrus	Areas of the auditory cortex in each hemisphere that receive incoming auditory information.
Myelination	The process of developing a protective protein and fatty coating around the nerves.
Neurolinguistics	The study of the anatomy, physiology, and chemistry of the brain associated with language development, comprehension, and use.
Peripheral nervous system	Those components of the nervous system that are outside the protective skull and the spinal cord.
Reticular formation	That part of the brain thought to be responsible for sensory integration and inhibition of information. Acts like a dispatcher.
Thalamus	Location higher in the brain stem that relays information to appropriate places in the brain for analysis (relay station).
Wernicke's area	That location in the left temporal lobe of the brain responsible for analyzing incoming information and organizing outgoing information.

Sources: Perkins & Kent, 1987; Owens, 1996.

from another organization such as the American Society for Deaf Children. You might even get to the website by going through three or four different links. The same holds true for information coded in language. If you are watching a popular game show and the contestant is asked, "How many miles is it from Earth to the sun?" your first attempt would be to remember the fact straightforwardly. Lacking an immediate grasp of the information, you might search your memory, hoping that that would jog loose the information. Or perhaps you recently helped your son study for a science test. You think of *son*, which makes you think of *sun*, and you remember that while helping him study for the test you learned that the sun is approximately ninety-three million miles from Earth.

As with the Internet, there are many different pathways for getting to the same piece of information in your brain. This is because information is stored in a number of places in the brain as traces of grammar, as memory of sensory information, or as memory of emotion. This, in fact, leads us to a very important tenet of instruction: The more variety you use to represent information (demonstrate, show, make pictures, discuss, role play, etc.) and the greater experiences a student has with information (i.e., enactive, iconic, and symbolic), the more places in the brain he will store the information. This will allow him to access that information through a variety of mental addresses and links.

The last decade has produced some very exciting research that gives us a glimpse into the way that deaf people's brains function. This research has the potential to change the way we think about language relative to children who are deaf and hard of hearing.

Corina (1998) summarized the works of Hickock, Bellugi, & Klima (1996) and others in two areas:

1. the effects of brain damage on the understanding and use of language by people who sign, and
2. the results of neuroimaging studies.

He found some interesting information. First, no matter whether a person is deaf or has hearing, when there is damage to the left hemisphere of the brain, language functioning is impaired. Second, when there is damage to the right hemisphere, nonlanguage issues such as social use, discourse, and visuo-spatial use (e.g., directionality and facial expression), are impaired in both deaf and hearing individuals. He reported disturbances in phonology, morphology, syntax, and semantics. This occurs in both English and ASL.

Corina (1998) described similarities in the brain responses of hearing and deaf subjects when exposed to open-class (meaningful) words (e.g., nouns, verbs) but differences in brain responses when exposed to closed-class (non-meaningful) words (e.g., *a, the, of*). Meaning-based information results in similar responses between deaf and hearing language users, but non-meaning-based information does not. He felt that the "neural systems that mediate formal languages [are] independent of the modality through which language is acquired" (p. 42). He further stated that "there are strong biological constraints that render these particular brain areas well suited for the processing of linguistic information, independent of the structure or the modality of the language" (p. 45). In addition, he indicated that neural activity in users of spoken English and ASL is more similar than the neural processing of users of signed English and spoken English because users of spoken English and ASL are processing a language, not a visual or auditory pattern. In other words, it does not matter which language you use, English or ASL. The brain seems to code information in similar ways *if* the brain has a complete language, and these ways are more consistent and stable when the information given has meaning. This has important implications for instruction in multipathways classrooms. Language lessons must be meaningful. The old notion that the brain would atrophy if it did not receive auditory stimulation is simply false. To the brain, information is implications. It is only to society that the difference between auditory and visual pathways is relevant.

Cognitive-Socialization Theory

Cognitive-socialization theory holds that communication is a social process (Brown, 1956; Bruner, 1973,1975,1981,1990; Halliday, 1975; Muma, 1998; Nelson, 1974,1981,1985,1996; Piaget, 1964; Vygotsky, 1962) based on the following ideas:

1. certain cognitive structures (e.g., reversibility) must first be in place as a result of maturation, and
2. once in place the child can understand corresponding linguistic structures (e.g., passive voice).

Cognitive-socialization theorists believe that there is a normal, natural rate and sequence to the development of language and that social interaction is the impetus for maturation. Cognitive-socialization theorists believe that the intent of a message forms the basic tool for learning to use and understand language, and that this intent determines the way in which we converse (Muma, 1998). Early theorists focused on *speech act theory*, which contends that our communication intent (what we want the other person to know or do) influences the words we choose, the grammar we choose to tie our words together, and the means by which language is conveyed (speech or signs).

The first component of this theory has to do with the basic thought processes involved in mastering world knowledge. *Categorization* is the tool by which we organize information about the world. The brain cannot possibly respond to every discrete piece of information that it takes in, so it chunks or groups this information into categories, and we respond to members of a category in similar manners. For example if Fluffy the cat scratches six-month-old

Timmy, then the next time he sees a cat he will pull away from it. He does not need to wait for Friskie the cat to scratch him before he pulls away. Timmy responds to the category of *cat*, not to each individual instance. He learns to represent that category via the word *cat*, which he may say or gesture or sign, depending on his own language pathway. Timmy is able to infer the action of one animal to the next. Based on that inference, he can solve problems, such as how not to get scratched again. He develops a *possible world* (Bruner, 1986) that makes sense to him based on his past perceptions (Glasser, 1998), and he responds to information in the future from the perspective of his *situated mind* (Nelson, 1996), a frame of reference that is situated within a set of sociocultural experiences. The way a child carves out the world, labels it, and invests it with social purpose and meaning, and the way the important people in his world do this with him is the fundamental base upon which all the rest of communication lies.

A second component of this theory is that the child applies a code of language implicitly and explicitly. For example, he may say or sign, "Thanks for my present," giving the explicit content, or he may do so in the context of a negative tone of voice or a scowling face, giving the implicit, or implied, meaning. As our brain subconsciously decides on the implicit and explicit messages and how we will say/sign it, it does an amazing thing: it pulls all the pieces together (construction), then plans and executes the speech/sign act. This higher level of functioning is quite complex including the cognitive skills of categorization, representation, planning, constructing, using, and executing.

We used the analogies of the computer and the Internet to describe the previous theories, and we attempt another here. The cognitive-socialization theory is more like a time-traveling machine. We enter the time machine not knowing what we will find and are transported onto a ship of angry pirates about to attack us. "Mommy!" would not be an appropriate explicit term to use if our intent were to dissuade our attackers rather than seek sympathy. "AARRGGHHH!" might be a better choice, letting the attackers know that we are not afraid of them (even if we are). In our attempt to convince them that we are one of them, we would not use vocabulary and grammar such as, "Hey, dudes. This is a righteous ship, and your weapons are awesome!" We would search our memory of swashbuckling movies and try to use words, grammar, and accents that would let them know we are not strangers. Whether our time machine spits us out onto a pirate ship, in front of a firing squad, or in some twenty-fifth-century version of harm's way, we must carefully convey that we mean no harm and hope no harm will come to us.

Muma (1998) wrote that we need to move past the information processing model and into the CCCE model: cognition, codification, communication, and expression. Cognition refers to how the mind works, including its ability to categorize, represent, attend, plan, and execute its tasks. Memory is a key component of cognition. Schachter (1996) detailed several kinds of memory states that have implications for learning. New research on explicit memory, implicit memory, semantic memory, episodic memory, procedural memory, and state-dependent retrieval, among other memory forms, is giving us clearer direction regarding how best to help students learn. Memory is very complex, and there isn't just one way to help children retain information.

Codification refers to the process of turning our intent into a form someone else will recognize. If the brain doesn't care what that code is, then that opens up many pathways to children who are deaf and hard of hearing. That pathway might be auditory, it might be visual, or it might be tactile. Each student's brain is seeking some code, any code, just as long as it receives one, and it must be complete. The choice of which code to support must be made carefully. We suggest you ask the following questions.

1. Do the parents understand, through careful observation, the brain-based pathway most appropriate for their child?
2. What is the likelihood that the child will receive sufficient support for a complete code during the critical period for language learning?
3. Does the child have access to auditory information, either due to an implant, an aid, or because he has a hearing loss that does not exceed the severe range? If not, a visual code is needed.
4. Will the child attend a school or school system consistently over time or move from school to school and teacher to teacher?

Next in the CCCE model is communication. By this Muma meant the pragmatic arena. He built a strong case for the centrality of intent (p. 8) in all communication. By moving away from rote drill and instruction of discrete grammatical structures and lexical items in contrived classroom experiences and toward an examination of vocabulary and grammar as they serve pragmatic intent, educators are more closely approximating how the brain wants to learn communication. Intent is the growing medium, and social interaction is the fertilizer. We agree that pragmatic intent is central to language learning. Pragmatic intent forms the basis for our chapter on theory to practice.

The fourth component of the CCCE model is expression, a component largely overlooked by other models. By expression Muma is referring to affect or emotion. A great deal of pragmatic intent is conveyed in the way we express ourselves. We express affect or emotion through inflection and tone of voice in spoken English and through facial expression and other body indicators in ASL. We know that the right hemisphere of the brain is engaged in both hearing and deaf individuals when facial expression is used for affective purposes (Corina, 1998). We use affect both to express emotional content of communication and to capture the listener/watcher's attention. Bloom, Beckwith, Capatides, and Hafitz (1988) felt that language is acquired to express the contents of states of mind and to interpret the states of mind of others. States of mind include, for example, sadness, euphoria, fear, and agitation, and each state is expressed via the affective components of communication. These are often far more powerful than words. Have you ever been in a situation where someone was yelling at you so forcefully that you felt intimidated and yet you don't remember a single word? You may have blocked out the words and the grammar, but the intent of the other person's message came through loudly and clearly.

The expressive-affective component of communication has not received much attention in the deaf education literature. Maybe this is because affect is difficult to capture and convey to a child with a hearing loss. Prosodic features of speech carry affect and expression. Nonmanual markers do the same in ASL; however, there is no such vehicle when English-based signs are used. Further, because few states require that Teachers of the Deaf pass minimum standards in the use of American Sign Language and because affect is often lost in a spoken message, many deaf students do not have appropriate models of linguistic expression and affect.

Relationship of Theories to Philosophies and Approaches

We know from the theories above that there is a complex set of thinking skills associated with learning in general and language learning in particular. We know that there is a symbiotic relationship between language and thinking; the development of one influences the development of the other. The contribution of the information processing theory is that it describes the possible avenues by which one might take in, process, and use language. If one avenue does not work, we can try another. The contribution of the neurolinguistic theory is that we now know that the brain doesn't care what language it uses in order to think, just as long as it has an accessible, complete language. The contribution of the cognitive-socialization theory is that the purpose for using language takes precedence. Once students understand the purpose behind a segment of language, it is irrelevant whether a child codes that through an auditory pathway or through a visual pathway. The CCCE model provides a new way of looking at languages and modalities.

Additional Perspectives on Appropriate Pathways

The research on hearing children points out additional factors we should consider when determining the child/code (pathway) match. These might provide additional insights with children who are deaf and hard of hearing.

Teaching/Learning Style.   Bates, Dale, and Thal (1995) reviewed the literature on individual differences in language learning and stated that "[m]ost cognitive variables correlate with what the child *knows* about language (indexed by comprehension), as opposed to what the child *does* (indexed by production)" (p. 113). In other words, cognitive skills correlate more with language understanding than language use. This means that good language instruction should promote understanding before application. They further indicated that grammatical development "depends on the establishment of a critical lexical base" (p. 119). This means that we must not rush into instruction in grammar until the student can spontaneously communicate thought and can express his basic intentions. Word combinations emerge in the hearing child when his vocabulary is in the fifty-to-one-hundred-word range, and the use of verb morphology emerges when the child is in the four hundred-to-six-hundred-word range. After the child's vocabulary is within this range, he begins to develop more and more complex grammatical use by leaps and bounds. In deaf education, both natural and structural approaches encourage the development of connected language, or grammar. Stress on the development of grammar may have caused us to overlook the importance of the sufficient development of a lexicon capable of supporting grammar and expressing intent.

Bates, Dale, and Thal (1995) also pointed out differences between an *analytic style* and a *holistic style*. They see this as an issue of speed and accuracy of processing stating that "[a] holistic strategy corresponds to emphasizing speed by selecting a larger unit for processing; an analytic strategy corresponds to emphasizing accuracy, by selecting a smaller unit" (p. 132). Traditionally, development of English has been thought of as a sequential process of increasing unit length and ASL has been likened to a more holistic, visuo-spatial process. Suppose you are developing language strategies analytically with a child whose brain thinks holistically, or vice versa. Problems might then be related more to the child's innate learning style, memory constraints, and attending skills rather than instructional mode. The need for memory capacity varies within language levels. Lack of sufficient memory to handle the perceptual load may interfere with language acquisition. Easterbrooks and O'Rourke (in press) found that parental report of a child's attending skills correlated with success in a particular language instructional approach. The relationship between attention and language development is only recently being examined in hearing students and has potential for providing insights into the language instruction of students who are deaf and hard of hearing.

General Intelligence. There is much confusion about the relationship between intelligence and language development when English is signed or when the language is ASL. The layman often confuses the ability to speak with intelligence. Although lack of speech does not mean lack of intelligence, if one's capacity is diminished, the ability to acquire language at the same pace as others will also be diminished. Another factor to consider is that language is most often thought to relate to verbal intelligence rather than nonverbal, or performance, intelligence. Watson, Sullivan, Moeller, and Jensen (1982) looked at the nonverbal intelligence of a sample of deaf students and found that nonverbal intelligence, as measured by the Wechsler Intelligence Scale for Children-Revised (Wechsler, 1974) and the Hiskey-Nebraska Test of Learning Aptitude (Hiskey, 1966), was a predictor of English language ability. Visual memory was highly related to language skills, and memory plays an important role in language learning. Teachers must understand the memory limitations of their students so that they may present language in accessible, "rememberable" segments. In addition, we must be aware that some students with diminished capacity will be at risk for developing a language system unless they receive additional support.

Child Temperament.   A growing body of literature suggests that one's basic temperament may be related to language acquisition. For example, in a study of several hundred infants from different cultures, Martin, Wisenbaker, Baker, and Huttunen (1997) found that during infancy, girls showed more distress at novel stimuli than boys. This might indicate that infant girls' greater physiological maturation allows them to attend to the world better than boys. Children who showed distress and were difficult in infancy (identified as fussy/demandingness in infancy) adapted poorly to stimuli at age five. Bornstein and Ruddy (1984) found that four-month-old infants who habituated more rapidly to novel stimuli have larger vocabularies at twelve months. The willingness to adapt to novel situations requires that children first attend to differences, and attention to stimuli in infancy is a predictor of later language development (Dixon & Shore, 1997). Therefore, nonadaptability and poor habituation in infancy might be seen as a risk factor for language development.

Likelihood of Family Follow-Up.   The veracity and tenacity with which families follow up recommendations for language intervention with their children correlates highly with language success (Bornstein, 1989; Easterbrooks, O'Rourke, & Todd, 2000). When families defer their children's development to the schools, the outcomes are poorer. We have no literature to advise us if there is a breaking point at which schools can compensate for lack of parental involvement or not. We know that the earlier intervention occurs, the better. It is the quality of the intent that matters, without which the likelihood that communication will develop becomes nil. We do know that if families are not involved actively in fostering and using a communication system with youngsters, then no matter what approach we take, that child is at risk for failure to learn to communicate.

Where Students Are Taught

The education of students who are deaf and hard of hearing occurs in a variety of settings from residential schools to local school systems to private schools and clinics. The diversity of our world is reflected in all these settings. Below we introduce you to two teachers and twelve students to whom we will refer throughout the remainder of the first part of this book. As you read through their descriptions, try to think about how all the theories we described might apply to these students, especially as regards the multiple pathways by which humans can learn to communicate.

Imagine that we are on a field trip. On the first day of the trip we are going to the School for the Deaf to visit Mr. Wilson's classroom. Mr. Wilson teaches in the middle school and has a caseload of six students who range in ages from ten to thirteen years. Two are cousins whose families have other deaf members. These students have strong ASL skills. One student has a severe hearing loss, suspected learning disabilities, and Attention Deficit/Hyperactivity Disorder (ADHD). He does not have a good grasp of either ASL or English signs. One has a severe hearing loss and comes from a home where the language spoken is Spanish. One has a moderate loss, has been from foster home to foster home, and has experienced great physical, emotional, and language neglect during his first four years of life. He detects sounds well, including spoken input but shows numerous traits associated with a language processing problem. One student received a cochlear implant at age seven and has made little or no progress in spoken production, although he does demonstrate awareness of the presence of speech and recognition of some highly stereotypic phrases. The spoken languages of his home are Hindi and English. During our visit we see Mr. Wilson carefully managing a wide range of language and reading levels, even though there are only six students in the class.

Back on the road, we head out of town to a rural school system an hour and a half away. There we meet Mrs. Troutman, whose caseload includes six students from four to fifteen years of age. Three students are from ethnic backgrounds not native to the area. The preschooler has a cochlear implant. One student is profoundly deaf. One has significant learning challenges above and beyond those imposed by the hearing loss. During our visit we follow Mrs. Troutman to three different buildings and are amazed at the complexity of her schedule.

Each of these teachers is charged with the responsibility of making the regular education curriculum accessible to the students. Simultaneously they must understand each child's communication style and address through-the-air and written-language development. While this task may seem daunting, it is not unlike the responsibility many teachers of children with hearing losses face. The teacher must manage his or her group from the perspective that there are multiple pathways to learn language and to impart information and there are multiple factors that influence learning. Some perspectives work well with one child while some work well with others. The teacher cannot pick or choose the communication philosophy he or she champions. First, one never knows what skills or communication system a child will bring to the classroom, and secondly, in the typical everyday classroom of deaf children, teachers have a responsibility to select strategies that will take each child from his present level of performance forward. School-age students use a variety of pathways to learn in general and to learn language in particular, and the teacher must be able to meet each child at his or her own level, no matter the communication mode or learning style, in order to advance that child's skills. Multiple pathways to learning exist within each classroom, and the teacher's sensitive response is necessary.

Characteristics of the child should determine the pathway through which learning occurs most rapidly, and the philosophies and prejudices of the adult should not. This requires us to rethink the importance of the brain in language learning. It also requires us to rethink how we assess children in terms of the pathway that is most appropriate for each child.

Kevin is an example of a student who learns through a visual pathway. This is evidenced by the rate at which he has picked up the ability to read through print exposure. Mercedes is an example of a student who learns through the auditory pathway. Their teachers must understand both pathways and must respect their differences.

Heterogeneity of the Population

Students who are deaf and hard of hearing form a widely heterogeneous group (Bowe, 1988; Easterbrooks, 1999). Unless a teacher works in a large residential

Meet Kevin

Kevin is an eight-year-old male who has been profoundly deaf since birth. He wears bilateral hearing aids but makes very little use of them. His loss is of unknown origin. He lives in a rural area. Kevin's loss was diagnosed when he was two years of age. Kevin has no additional disabilities. He lives with his mother, who is divorced. She is an intelligent young woman who is still exploring available options for her son. One of these options is the possibility of moving to a larger school system with more services. His mother is very active in the local parents' support group. Initially she chose an oral option for early intervention because the interventionist told her that she could always sign later to Kevin if oral instruction proved unsuccessful. She participated in a correspondence course that assisted her in teaching her son. Kevin's mother started signing in English word order to him when he was five years old as she was dissatisfied with his progress under oral instruction. He does not have access to ASL. A look into the crystal ball shows that he will not have access to ASL until adulthood. But for now, both the teachers and his mother are committed to English development. Kevin's mother is a voracious reader who has read with him and modeled good reading habits since infancy. While Kevin seems to have a knack for reading, which he is able to do on an early second-grade level, he shows little progress with written skills. Kevin is in a self-contained classroom for the whole day with the Teacher of the Deaf, who uses a signed form of English.

Meet Mercedes

Mercedes is a thirteen-year-old female of Hispanic descent. She has a moderate-to-severe loss in one ear and a mild-to-severe loss in the other. The etiology is of unknown origin. Her parents suspect that an older family member had a hearing loss, but there are no records to confirm this. They did not suspect the hearing loss until Mercedes was two years old because she jabbered incessantly as a toddler. However, at two years of age, very few of these chatterings had formed into actual words. Both parents are educated and jointly run a successful business. They have been in the U.S. for fifteen years and speak English well when talking with the teacher. At home they speak Spanish. Mercedes attended a private oral preschool, where she made good progress with spoken English. She uses her hearing aids well. At home the parents encourage her development of spoken Spanish. There is no evidence of additional learning challenges other than the fact that she enjoys interacting with her peers more than with the school task at hand. Mercedes remained in the private oral school until she was eight years old, then was mainstreamed for most of the day into a regular third-grade class. Her reading comprehension scores on the Woodcock Reading Mastery Test-Revised place her at a 6.8 grade reading level, however, everyone fully expects that with continued support, her reading skills will catch up to grade level. Although she does not use ASL, she sometimes signs in English to the teacher. She enjoys watching others sign but is not interested in learning more than a basic sign lexicon. She is cognitively bright and socially popular. Academically she has the potential to do better if she were less preoccupied with the social environment around her. She is mainstreamed into regular education eighth grade classes without an interpreter. She sees the Teacher of the Deaf for an hour and a half daily for reading, language arts, study skills instruction, and to monitor her academic studies.

school in a large city, it is highly unlikely that the students with whom he works will all be on the same language level or have the same instructional needs. An itinerant teacher in a rural county may be the only one serving seven or eight different students at seven or eight different grade levels in multiple school buildings. In addition to this, these students are probably very different. One might be profoundly deaf and have parents who refuse to allow the school to use sign language. Another might have a moderate-to-severe hearing loss but also have mild retardation. Still another might have a mild-to-moderate loss along with a significant medical challenge such as cerebral palsy, which would impact his ability to speak, write, and navigate around the school. Even in those few classrooms that have several children at the same grade level, the teacher can expect variety. One student might have a learning disability that requires the teacher to use alternative instructional techniques while another child might have ADHD, requiring the teacher to spend extra time refocusing that student's attention. Yet another student might be a recent immigrant from a foreign country, who rarely attended school in the past due to the impact of a long-standing war in that country. It is also likely that this child never wore a hearing aid before, and that his family's adjustment to the new culture results in his missing a lot of school.

Not only will teachers have caseloads that are heterogeneous, but also the problems, life situations, and communication needs of students will change over time. For example, one youngster might understand his teacher well through the oral channel when he and the teacher are in the resource room face-to-face, but when he is in a mainstream classroom, the demands of the situation might warrant the use of an interpreter. Thus, he would need to know sign language. Another student whose additional mild learning disorder was negligible during her younger years might need additional support to compensate for her different learning style now that she is in higher grades. There are no easy caseloads of students who are deaf and hard of hearing.

According to the U.S. Department of Education (DOE) (1999), 5,388,483 students with disabilities ages 6 through 21 were identified under IDEA in the public schools during the 1997–1998 academic year. Of those, 1.2% were categorized as "hearing impaired." Trends reveal that there is an increase in the 6-to-17-year age group. Placements revealed that 82.52 percent were educated in their local school systems (regular education, 37.57 percent; resource environments, 18.33 percent; separate classes, 26.62 percent) and 17.48 percent in separate facilities (public day, 4.96 percent; private day, 2.61 percent; public residential, 8.64 percent; private residential, 0.86 percent; hospital-homebound, 0.41 percent). A tally of the numbers of students attending local schools listed in the 1998 reference edition of the *American Annals of the Deaf* revealed that 34 percent served seven or fewer children who were deaf or hard of hearing. These students received a variety of services and had a variety of needs. In order to understand the demands that the teacher of students who are deaf and hard of hearing faces on a daily basis, we must take a closer look at the heterogeneity within the population.

Deaf Students with Deaf Parents

In an extensive study of the literature regarding the impact that deaf parents have on their deaf children's communication development, Spencer and Lederberg (1997) clearly pointed out the benefits to language development that come with having parents who are themselves deaf. Deaf children of deaf parents acquire communication skills ranging from communicative turn-taking to early gestures to later vocabulary and grammar development at the same ages and through the same stages as hearing children of hearing parents. This is because deaf children of deaf parents are surrounded by a rich linguistic environment that is quantitatively and qualitatively appropriate. Deaf children of deaf parents have also been reported to engage in early literacy activities including reading and writing. As a result deaf children of deaf parents come to school with a language base upon which they may develop skills in ESL, reading, writing, and knowledge across academic and curricular areas. On average, Deaf children of Deaf parents perform better on reading comprehension tasks (Padden & Ramsey, 2000) than their peers with hearing parents.

Jonathan is a deaf child from a culturally Deaf family who is progressing well. He is an example of a child whose language pathway is visual. However, his cousin Ashley is struggling in school, and we can only speculate about the cause. Perhaps a dual language code confused her. Perhaps her mother had an undetected learning disability or was cognitively less able, resulting in her early departure from school, and perhaps Ashley inherited the propensity to struggle academically from her mother. Perhaps she is not motivated to do her school work. No matter the reason, even in a seemingly homogeneous group such as Deaf children of Deaf parents, individual differences emerge.

Deaf Students with Hearing Parents

The path to language learning is often very different for deaf students with hearing parents. Most hearing parents who have deaf children are taken by sur-

Meet Jonathan

Jonathan is a ten-year-old Deaf male growing up in a family with Deaf-World orientation. Both of his parents are Deaf. His parents attended their state's school for the deaf, which is located in the neighborhood in which they live. Jonathan has had a severe-to-profound bilateral hearing loss due to heredity since birth. His parents began signing ASL with him immediately, as did a Deaf uncle, a hard-of-hearing aunt, and his Deaf grandfather. Jonathan and his family were seen routinely by an early interventionist, who supported their choice of ASL. His parents read to him routinely. The family is very active in the Deaf Community, and they travel frequently. Jonathan has attended the school for the deaf since preschool. Jonathan's school followed a bilingual-bicultural philosophy of interaction, involvement, and instruction with the students. He progressed rapidly with English development. At ten years of age, he is capable of being mainstreamed into a general education fifth-grade classroom with an interpreter; however, he and his parents agree that his overall needs would be better met in the environment provided by his current school. His Teacher of the Deaf follows the school's block schedule for language and literacy development, focusing at least two hours on English and reading and a third hour on ASL literacy. He is reading at a 4.2 grade equivalent level, based on recent scores on the Woodcock Reading Mastery Test-Revised. Jonathan does not vocalize. His cousin, who also has a hearing loss, is in his class. All of his classmates use ASL. Jonathan is happy, well liked, and appears to be comfortable in the school environment.

Meet Ashley

Ashley is an eleven-year-old Deaf female. Her father is Deaf. Her mother is hard of hearing. Her father attended his state's school for the deaf, along with his brother. His mother attended her local school system until the age of 16, when she left school to take a job. Ashley has had a severe bilateral hearing loss due to heredity since birth. Her father began signing ASL with her immediately, as did a Deaf uncle (Jonathan's dad), a Deaf aunt, and her Deaf grandfather. Ashley's mother, who has usable oral speech and language skills, uses ASL for routine conversations and also encourages her daughter to develop oral English ability. Ashley and her family were seen routinely by an early interventionist, who supported the father's choice of ASL and gave the mother information on developing her residual hearing and speech. Her parents read to her routinely. The family is very active in the Deaf Community. At the mother's wishes, Ashley attended preschool at an oral program then transferred to the school for the deaf in kindergarten. From that point on she made slow but steady progress with English development. However, she struggled academically, and both the school and the parents agreed that it was in her best interest to repeat the second grade. At eleven years of age, she is partially mainstreamed into a regular fourth-grade classroom located in a school two blocks from the school for the deaf. She is accompanied by an interpreter, who also provides tutorial assistance in her science, health, and social studies classes. She sees the Teacher of the Deaf half of the day to work on English, reading, and math. She sees the Speech-Language Pathologist in the local school for half an hour twice weekly for auditory training, speech, and language support. She is reading on a 3.6 grade equivalent level based on recent scores on the Woodcock Reading Mastery Test-Revised. Ashley has understandable speech, reads well, and converses well with her peers at the local school in speech and at the school for the deaf in sign. However, she is still struggling with school subjects, and she will continue to need a lot of encouragement and academic assistance.

prise. They have never considered the possibility of having a deaf child much less their role in that child's communication development. The reality, however, is that ninety percent of children who are born deaf and hard of hearing are born to parents who themselves can hear (Moores, 2000). In addition to dealing with grief over and adjustment to a hearing loss, hearing parents are faced with the task of sorting through medical, communication, and educational options. Never having considered that they will need to learn to be their child's instructor in communication, many parents are overwhelmed with the responsibility. It is no wonder that many parents have difficulty instilling a native, or first, language system in their children. Musselman and Kircaali-Iftar (1996) pointed out that deaf children who are most successful have parents who are highly committed to their communication development. As challenging as this is, it is essential for parents to take an aggressive approach to helping their children learn to communicate. Jahan is an example of a youngster whose family struggled with a variety of communication options and technologies before finding the appropriate pathway through which he could learn.

Deaf Students with Cochlear Implants

Carney and Moeller (1998) provided a comprehensive review of the literature on cochlear implants. A cochlear implant is a device that, when implanted into a child's cochlea, provides stimulation to the auditory nerve, thus giving the

Meet Jahan

Jahan is a thirteen-year-old male who was born with no hearing. Although there is no confirmation of the etiology, his mother was hospitalized several times during her pregnancy for various viral and/or bacterial related illnesses, some of which required high doses of antibiotics. The family moved from India to the U.S. after Jahan's fourth birthday in search of appropriate services for their son. His father is in the medical field. His mother is a homemaker. The languages of the home are Hindi and heavily accented English. Jahan's mother read to him extensively as a youngster. He demonstrated a knack for lipreading his mother and relating this to the printed word. Jahan entered a private preschool where he made slow but steady progress in understanding communication but not in speech for several years. At seven years of age, he received a cochlear implant and entered intensive follow-up therapy. After a year of therapy, he made little or no progress with spoken communication, although he demonstrated awareness of the presence of speech, recognition of some highly stereotypic phrases, and understood basic requests and instructions. During his eighth year, Jahan's parents agreed to the addition of sign language to his communication system. They were very firm in their conviction that during instruction signs should be used in English word order, although they had no objections to allowing Jahan to use ASL with other deaf students. At nine years of age, he stopped wearing his implant. Jahan possesses high average intelligence and began to use signs rapidly once in a signing environment. After five years of such exposure, he has made great language strides in English and understands most compound sentence forms as well as some complex forms, especially adverbials. He is reading at the 5.7 grade equivalent level. He has a passion for reading, enjoys learning, and is masterful with the computer. Jahan is partially mainstreamed for math, science, and social studies in a sixth-grade classroom in a school nearby. He uses the services of a transliterator. He sees the Teacher of the Deaf daily for English, reading, and study skills associated with his academic subjects. There is a general consensus among all parties that he is ready to transfer full-time to the regular education program to complete his schooling. He has high aspirations, and his teacher is convinced that he will achieve these.

child an awareness of sound. Cochlear implants have both their supporters and their detractors. Supporters point out the benefits to various aspects of communication development (Geers & Moog, 1994; O'Donoghue, Nikolopoulos, Archbold, & Tait, 1999; Tomblin, Spencer, Flock, & Gantz, 1999). Detractors express their concerns over the impact of this technology upon Deaf Culture and point to the fact that the success rate of the implant is variable (Lane, 1993; Tucker, 1998). In fact, the picture is still unclear. Data regarding the influence of placement, whether in total communication or oral programs, suggest some accelerated performance of children in auditory-oral programs (Osberger et al., 1991; Tyler, 1990). Easterbrooks and Mordica (2000) studied all of the fifty-one implant users in a population of nearly three hundred students who were deaf and hard of hearing. Of these, 74 percent of the females but only 50 percent of the males were rated by their teachers as using the implant as a tool for communication. It is probable that the Teacher of Deaf students will have children with implants on her caseload. Some may be successful users, and some not. The student may be a long-time user or may be a new implantee. If the student

Meet Sissy

Sissy is a four-year-old female whose hearing loss is of unknown origin. The pediatrician's audiology consultant identified Sissy's hearing loss when she was fifteen months of age after much urging and, finally, insistence from her mother. Because Sissy has twin sisters who are a year older than she, the mother was concerned when her response to sounds and communication were delayed relative to her older sisters. Sissy received a cochlear implant when she was nineteen months old. The family lives in a rural community and did not have access to therapy locally, so the mother drove her an hour and a half each way three times weekly to attend therapy sessions in the city. The mother is a freelance reporter for the local newspaper, whose schedule could accommodate therapy. The father works in an administrative position with the postal service and is on a ten-hour-day work plan, so he was also able to attend therapy on occasion. The older girls attended therapy sessions at least once a week and became avid supporters of their little sister's communication development. When Sissy turned three, she became eligible for her school system's early intervention services. An Individualized Family Services Plan (IFSP) was written to include twice-weekly visits to the Speech–Language Pathologist (SLP) for continued speech and language support, although her skills are nearly age-appropriate. She is eligible to attend the school's special-needs play group but the mother prefers to have her attend a small preschool program conducted by her local church. The Teacher of the Deaf in the local school system attends the same church and offered advice to the preschool teachers. Recently the family has asked that the Teacher of the Deaf spend some time with Sissy as they are trying to decide the most appropriate placement for her when she starts kindergarten. This was an unusual request, but the school willingly complied.

---

is a new implantee, then the teacher will not only be responsible for the child's linguistic and academic development, but will also be expected to assist the child in developing appropriate listening and auditory language skills. Sissy and LaShawndra are students for whom an implant was successful—for them, technology made an auditory code accessible. Jahan is a student for whom it did not. Apparently he is one of those youngsters who was gifted in lipreading, who developed a visual base for language through lipreading and print, and whose visually functioning brain did not benefit from auditory stimulation.

Compare LaShawndra's experiences with a cochlear implant to Jahan's experiences. Teachers of children who have cochlear implants may expect to see a variety of uses of the technology, from no use to use for environmental awareness to use as a primary means of understanding communication.

Hard of Hearing Students

Students who are hard of hearing are among the most misunderstood and underserved (Bowe, 1988; Davis, 1990) of this population. Precisely because hard of hearing children have some usable, obvious hearing, they are often overlooked and underidentified. This results in their being identified late, often

Meet LaShawndra

LaShawndra is a nine-year-old female of African-American descent. She was born with a profound bilateral hearing loss of unknown etiology. Her hearing loss was identified in the neonatal unit of her birth hospital and confirmed by a pediatric audiologist at six months. The audiologist recommended that the parents receive counseling and begin learning about cochlear implants. Her father, an attorney, searched the Internet and found a wealth of information about the procedure. LaShawndra received a cochlear implant at twenty months of age and intensive auditory, speech, and language therapy until the age of five, when she was placed in a regular kindergarten. Both parents were involved with her therapy, although the mother more so, especially since she negotiated flex-hours on her job so that she could transport LaShawndra to her therapy sessions. The home language is English. LaShawndra had some difficulty adjusting to group instruction after such intensive one-to-one treatment, but with time and encouragement she adjusted well. She remains in speech therapy, where they continue to work on articulation of the more difficult sounds. Sometimes the vocabulary demands of the school day seem to overwhelm her, but she easily catches on with support from the SLP. The Teacher of the Deaf sees her monthly for consultation with the classroom teacher, to monitor her grades, and to advise her on any listening-related problems she may be having. Other than these services, she is doing well in the regular fourth-grade classroom, is reading on grade level, and is included in all aspects of school life.

long after they have begun to experience language and academic problems (Meadow-Orlans, Sass-Lehrer, Scott-Olson, & Mertens, 1998). A student who has a mild hearing loss may hear the teacher but may not understand the message clearly. You may get a glimpse into this situation by imagining yourself at a family gathering. You are upstairs. The rest of the family is downstairs. You think you hear them say your name. You hear them talking and laughing, you understand a word every now and then, but you cannot hear them clearly. This is what it is like for the hard of hearing child, and it puts him at risk for academic failure and retention. The child who hears only a partial message will require extra time to process auditory information (Pillai, 1997), but this is not a trait of most fast-paced classrooms. Consequently, the child cannot follow extended conversations, and he will miss out on a considerable amount of vocabulary and grammar such as verb tense. Because language can be affected, there are some who recommend the use of sign language, even with hard of hearing students. The place, amount, and type of signs that are appropriate for hard of hearing students are under debate (Preisler, 1997).

The accumulated effects of years of misunderstanding and half-messages are usually felt around the third or fourth grade, along with jeopardized self-esteem. By this time, the reading demands are great. Now the child who was shut out of instruction earlier because he could not understand the teacher's speech is shut out of instruction because his reading level is not adequate for instructional purposes.

Even a very slight amount of hearing loss can have an effect on a child's achievement. Davis, Elfenbein, Schum, and Bentler (1986) studied 112 children with moderate sensorineural hearing losses. They grouped the subjects by degree of loss (Group A = <41 dB better ear average, Group B = 45–60 dB, and Group C = >61 dB) to determine the effects of degree of hearing impairment on intellect, social, academic, and language behavior. Their results showed that the degree of a hearing loss in the moderate range did not predict language or educational performance. No matter how moderate the loss was, the subjects had problems. Reich, Hambleton, and Houldin (1977) also studied this phenomenon and found similar results. Davis et al. (1986) found that hard of hearing children had delays in verbal skills, academic achievement, and social development. Antia and Dittillo (1998) studied a group of children who had hearing losses both in hard of hearing and deaf ranges and found that no matter what degree loss the children had, they displayed similar patterns of initiation and response to their hearing peers.

Many students with mild hearing losses do not define themselves as having a loss (Albertson, 1996). These students may suffer academically and experience rejection, insensitivity, lack of understanding of what is happening around them, and the need for assistive devices. Their ability to use good speech fools the hearing individuals around them into assuming that they hear equally as well. This is not the case. Good speech can mask poor comprehension. These students still need academic and counseling support. Trisha is an example of such a student.

Students Who Are Hard of Hearing Due to a Unilateral Loss. A student with a unilateral hearing loss, or loss in one ear, is also at educational risk (Oyler & Matkin, 1988). Children with unilateral losses are often undetected in the schools and suffer the consequences (Mauk, Barringer, & Mauk, 1995). Because the child hears well in one ear, she usually has good speech and an adequate vocabulary, but many times subtle language problems exist. In addition, the child is often accused of "hearing what she wants to hear" when, in fact, she hears those things directed at her good ear and misses those things directed at her bad ear. Like the mildly hard of hearing child, the child with a unilateral loss will not hear the teacher clearly, especially when that teacher is at a distance. In trying to locate the source of a sound or the teacher's voice, the child may turn around in her seat a lot. Often this is seen as a behavior problem, not a problem in trying to access information and communication. The child with a unilateral

Meet Trisha

Trisha is a fifteen-year-old female whose moderate-to-severe hearing loss was identified after a bout of meningitis when she was three years of age. Both her parents are fully hearing. Trisha was placed in the special-needs preschool and kindergarten classes as a youngster. She adjusted immediately to her hearing aids and depends upon them as a primary source of information. Hearing aids bring her hearing into the mild-to-moderate range. She also received daily speech, auditory, and language instruction from an SLP. She was placed full-time with the Teacher of the Deaf for first and second grade after which time she began to participate in mainstream classes. She was fully mainstreamed by fourth grade, using an auditory trainer in the classroom. This period of her life was very stressful as she was dealing with the demands of the regular classroom while also struggling with her parents' divorce, which occurred the previous year. Trisha lives with her mother. The father moved to a different state, where he started a new family. Trisha sees him rarely and is in conflict over this aspect of her life. While Trisha is an academically capable student in English and content area subjects, she has been identified as having a learning disability in the area of mathematics. Trisha is a large, mature young woman who is in the tenth grade. She attends the school's resource class for students who have difficulty with math and sees the Teacher of the Deaf for one period each day for study skills, which primarily includes assistance in managing her schedule of assignments as well as some academic tutoring. She wants to work in a child care center when she graduates because she has enjoyed helping to raise her younger siblings.

loss will need speech and language support, especially as they relate to phonics instruction.

Students Who Are Hard of Hearing Due to a Fluctuating Loss.   The child with a fluctuating loss due to otitis media, or middle ear infection, is also at risk for early language and learning delays (Roberts, 1997). When he reaches school, more often than not, neither the teacher nor the child may be aware that there is now or was in the past a temporary hearing loss. When the teacher reports a concern to the parent, it is usually that the child appears to be having good days and bad days. Actually, he is having hearing days and deaf days. Children with severe allergies can have fluctuating hearing losses. Recurring otitis media can impact language and cognitive development, leaving gaps in information and communication skills that are difficult to detect. These are especially difficult to detect once the middle ear infection is gone. However, if left untreated a middle ear infection can develop into a permanent hearing loss.

The lack of consistent auditory input that children with fluctuating losses experience may result in their not learning to pay attention to sounds. Children with fluctuating losses are often called inattentive, distractible, and immature, when in fact they hear some things well some days but not others. In addition, fluctuating hearing loss can impair classroom participation.

A higher degree of fluctuating hearing loss due to otitis media exists among the Native American population (Gregg, Roberts, & Colleran, 1983). In addition, the hearing losses of Native American children tend not to be identified until school age (Baker, 1996). Poor identification coupled with increased encounters with hearing loss places these children at great risk academically.

Students with Central Auditory Processing Disorders

A central auditory processing disorder (CAPD) is a disorder in the ability to understand what one hears in the face of intact peripheral hearing (Cacase & McFarland, 1998). Although the outer, middle, and inner ear mechanisms are intact, the individual is unable to process incoming auditory messages because of problems associated with the brain stem, ascending auditory pathway, or auditory cortex. CAPD has a significant impact on the ability to pay attention and to process language receptively (Chermak, Hall, & Musiek, 1999) and is often associated with other learning and behavioral problems. Children with CAPD have problems listening both in stressful and ideal listening situations (Smoski, Brunt, & Tannahil, 1992). Central auditory processing disorders are challenging to identify, and there is controversy over who is responsible for the CAPD child. No matter which category he falls into among the special education array of terminology associated with disorders, this child will have difficulty listening, and this will cause problems in developing and using language. Children with CAPD have characteristics similar to children who are hard of hearing, and they will benefit from speech and language intervention.

Hearing Students from Culturally Deaf Families

Very little research is available regarding the needs of hearing children from culturally Deaf families (CODAs, or children of deaf adults), and these children's needs are poorly understood. The child of Deaf parents has a very different experience with English than other children who hear. Many of these children learn ASL as their first language and English as a second language, so English is not seen as a primary source of nurturing and support. Because hearing is not a component of that family's experience, the child may mistakenly learn that sound is not important. This is especially problematic if the child does not learn to pay attention to sound. A child who grows up ignoring sounds will continue to do so in the classroom, with disastrous effects. For example, teachers often use variations in the tone of their voices to get children's attention, to signal important information, and to add emotion and excitement to their message. The hearing child who has grown up in a Deaf family may be unaware that the teacher is conveying important information with her voice. The cultural, linguistic, and experiential differences that CODAs bring with them when they come to school often cause cultural tensions, unnecessary misunderstandings, reduced participation in class, and great frustration (Singleton & Tittle, 2000). These students may need speech and language services to catch up to their hearing peers who grew up in hearing homes because their native language, even though they can hear, is different from that language used at school.

Deaf and Hard of Hearing Students Who Have Not Had Early Intervention

The evidence that early intervention is an important component in communication development in deaf and hard of hearing children is incontrovertible (Calderon & Greenberg, 1997). Unfortunately, fewer than 50 percent of students with hearing losses are identified in the years most critical for impacting communication development, even though the benefits are clear (Carney & Moeller, 1998). Children who have had the benefit of early language instruction are more likely to begin their formal school years with a functional communication system upon which teachers may base additional instruction in communication. Similarly, these students may come to school without a sufficient foundation for instruction in reading, writing, math, and other academic subjects. While early onset of hearing loss has increased slightly due to increased occurrences of otitis media and cytomegalovirus etiologies, early identification has not.

As more and more states develop early screening and identification programs (Arehart, Yoshinaga-Itano, Thomson, Gabbard, & Stredler-Brown, 1998), the likelihood that all children with hearing losses will have early access to communication increases. While this is a necessary first step, it must be followed by diligent efforts to prepare an early intervention force that understands that there are multiple pathways to language learning. Early interventionists in only a handful of states have sufficient knowledge of the heterogeneity of the population. In addition they tend to lack sufficient skills in both auditory development and ASL to allow them to assist families in learning how to provide their children with a complete and consistent language code. This is another crisis in the education of students who are deaf and hard of hearing. Martin is an example of a youngster who did not receive appropriate early intervention services because his home life was so complicated. This is even more tragic because he had so many needs in so many areas.

Deaf and Hard of Hearing Students with Secondary Disorders

Sabatino (1983) pointed out that the federal definition of a learning disability results in a conundrum; by nature of the definition, "there are no . . . hearing . . . impaired learning disabled children in the world—the idiocy of such a rule denies the evidence" (p. 26). National data (Holden-Pitt & Diaz, 1998) sug-

Meet Martin

Martin is a twelve-year-old male with a moderate bilateral hearing loss. His birth mother was of African-American descent, as was his birth father. Martin showed signs of Fetal Alcohol Syndrome and was hospitalized during his first few years of life for various reasons including mild encephalitis. There is no indication in the school records as to whether he received early intervention. Martin has been in foster care since he was an infant and has had many different placements. He experienced physical, emotional, and linguistic neglect during the first four years of his life, at which time an African-American family of modest income adopted him. He is the only child in his new home and has attended the school for the deaf since he was five years old. His adoptive parents have worked long and hard with him, learning ASL at the suggestion of the school. He detects sounds well, including speech sounds; however, his vocabulary is deficient and his grammar has traits similar to those of hearing children who have language processing problems. He falls in the borderline-average range of intelligence and has notable memory problems. He is reading on a late-first-to-early-second-grade level based on his response to questions asked informally after reading leveled story books. He becomes frustrated and distracted during formal assessments. Martin attends homeroom and PE with his near-aged peers but is in the lower sections for academic instruction. He is seen by an Occupational Therapist weekly, by the Speech-Language Pathologist for half an hour three times weekly, and spends the remainder of his school day with the Teacher of the Deaf.

gest that about 8 percent of students with hearing losses have some degree of mental retardation and about 9 percent have some type of learning disability. Taking into consideration all the different categories of disability, an estimated 25 to 33 percent of deaf and hard of hearing students have some kind of additional disability (Schildroth & Hotto, 1996). Because schools tend to provide services based on the primary disability (e.g., a child whose deafness is his

Meet Colton

Colton is an eleven-year-old male. Both of his parents are fully hearing, and there is no evidence of hearing loss in any other family member. Colton's father struggled in school and is very concerned because his son is doing the same. Colton has a severe bilateral hearing loss of unknown etiology, probably since birth; however, it remained undetected until he was two and a half years old. Colton and his family were seen by an early interventionist, but the visits were sporadic as his mother often forgot the appointments. While the family was not opposed to the use of ASL, neither did they make anything other than half-hearted attempts to learn the language. Colton's mother had a difficult time accepting his hearing loss, but with support, and after seeing some development, she now attempts to assist him with his schoolwork and occasionally reads to him. His father was a poor reader in school and does not read to any of his children. Colton has had exposure to the Deaf Community because of his involvement with his schoolmates, but the family chooses not to participate in Deaf Community activities. Several years ago, they experienced family conflict due to the father's work-related issues. In addition, the mother had some personal problems of long standing with which she was still dealing, and there is a nonsupportive extended family. Colton attended the special-needs kindergarten for children with developmental delays in the local school system. The teacher in this program signed in English word order, but her skills were minimal. This school system was in a moderately sized suburban area where there were several other students with hearing losses, but none who signed, and none who was in Colton's school building. At this time, family pressures came to a head, the parents divorced, and the mother moved several times in one year before settling down. Colton was placed at the school for the deaf in a nongraded classroom, and the mother agreed to start learning sign language. Today, Colton exhibits behavior and attending problems that make it difficult for him to participate in class. He is making poor progress both in English development and ASL, and he struggles academically. He is reading on a 2.5 grade equivalent level, based on recent scores on the Woodcock Reading Mastery Test-Revised. Colton attempts to use speech but is understood only by those closest to him. He was evaluated by the Diagnostics and Evaluation team and was found to have evidence of a learning disability. In addition, the family physician and school psychologist have determined that he has ADHD. Colton appears frustrated, and his moods vacillate between agitated excitement and mild depression.

primary disability might also have tunnel vision, which would be his secondary disability), little effort has gone into determining profiles of behaviors associated with additional learning disorders. Without available profiles to validate the existence of secondary learning problems, researchers have difficulty identifying appropriate educational interventions, and teachers are left to their own devices to infer the best approach (Powers, Elliott, Fairbank, & Monaghon, 1988). This means that teachers must understand two sets of information: the impact that a hearing loss has on language development, and the impact that learning disabilities, retardation, attention problems, central auditory processing disorders, behavior problems, and visual problems, among others, have on language development as well. Colton and Montel are students whose additional learning problems pose significant challenges in addition to those imposed by the hearing loss. These problems include attention and memory to different degrees for each boy.

Deaf and Hard of Hearing Students Whose Home Language Is Not English

About 40 percent of students who are deaf and hard of hearing come from homes either where English is not the primary language or where the family

Meet Montel

Montel is a six-year-old male of mixed race. His mother is a first-generation Jamaican-American and his father first-generation Laotian-American. The parents are in their early twenties. They never married. Montel lives with his father and maternal grandmother, although his mother lives in the same apartment complex and sees him routinely. Montel has a severe-to-profound hearing loss, which was identified at birth by the neonatalogy staff when they noted complications associated with cytomegalovirus. Montel was a small baby who had difficulty eating. He has allergies, mild motor delays, and appears to catch every virus that goes through the school. This results in his missing school frequently. Developmental testing estimates his intellectual ability to be in the low-average-to-borderline range. However, he does well in pre-mathematics skills. He is a friendly, happy fellow who loves everyone he meets. He is placed for the first half of the day with the Teacher of the Deaf, who works on language, concept development, early literacy, and math concepts. She uses sign-supported speech as her communication approach. Montel goes to the special-needs kindergarten in the afternoon for socialization with his hearing peers. In an unusual twist of fate, the special-needs kindergarten teacher had a deaf friend during high school and knows sign language adequately to keep Montel informed of the goings-on in the classroom. Montel is a favorite among the school staff, and he loves to go to school.

uses a dialect of English. In many instances students are in trilingual or multilingual environments (Walker-Vann, 1998). MacLeod-Gallinger (1993) studied deaf persons from ethnic minorities and found that deafness and ethnicity posed a dual restriction on academic and employment outcomes. Students who are deaf or hard of hearing and whose families do not speak English (Christensen & Delgado, 1993; Cohen, Fischgrund, & Redding, 1990) or whose families are African-American (Moores & Oden, 1977) are at greater risk academically. Primarily they are at greater risk for acquiring adequate communication skills, either in English or ASL. Jorge is an example of a young man whose bilingual status is complicated by extreme language deprivation. Information regarding critical periods for language acquisition suggests the likelihood that Jorge will make only minimal progress with ASL.

Meet Jorge

Jorge is a thirteen-year-old Mexican-American male who has a severe hearing loss caused by meningitis when he was three years of age. His family entered the United States two years ago and moved periodically during the first year. His family is from a small town where there are no services, so Jorge's first educational experiences occurred when he entered the school system in the U.S. Jorge was never seen by an early interventionist. The home language is the dialect of Spanish used in the parents' home town. Jorge communicates with his parents and siblings through a system of home signs, gestures, and situationally based vocalizations that are primarily unintelligible. His mother reads to all his siblings, so he is growing up exposed to print in Spanish. The family has had no contact with the Deaf Community, but they are very active in the local Hispanic Community. Jorge has a large extended family and is an active member of the social culture of the family. During his first year of school he moved several times as the father was employed as a migrant farm worker. Recently his father has secured a more stable job, so Jorge has attended the school for the deaf for the better part of the academic year. Jorge's signs are composed primarily of one- and two-word utterances. His mother reports that he understands most basic instructions and directions that she gives him and that he recognizes several words in Spanish print. He has a sight-word vocabulary in English of around fifty to seventy words. Jorge does not enjoy taking reading tests in English, consequently the D&E team is still gathering checklist and anecdotal records on both his reading and language development. He is well aware that he is behind the other students. Recently there has been some discussion about allowing Jorge to live in the residential facility at the school for the deaf, where he would be immersed in an ASL environment, but his parents remain concerned about this option. Jorge is athletic and skilled mechanically. He enjoys sports activities with friends and family members after school but as yet is not in any organized sport. Jorge spends his day in a classroom with a Teacher of the Deaf, where they work on ASL, print recognition, math, and general science and social studies concepts.

Because communication develops through interaction with others (Haydon, Mann, & Fugate 1995), difficulty in establishing and maintaining communication can have a devastating impact. In other words, children who have mild and moderate hearing losses are at great risk for academic failure, along with their peers whose hearing losses are more severe. The need for services to children in the severe-to-profound range is obvious. No matter what the degree of hearing loss, student support teams should consider the impact of that loss on communication development and must make every attempt to see that the loss does not diminish academic progress.

Summary

In this chapter we proposed that there are multiple pathways by which children learn to communicate. We built the case that the human brain works in mysterious ways, and that the different styles by which humans think may have direct influence on how they learn language. We demonstrated that the population of students we serve is heterogeneous, with vastly differing needs. Based on research and the heterogeneity of the population, teachers of students who are deaf and hard of hearing have many challenges. They must develop better strategies to address the diverse linguistic needs of students. Some students are analytic learners, others are holistic learners. Issues such as maternal input, the child's temperament, global IQ, style of information processing, basic neurological functioning, and completeness of language code are absolute outcome-determining preconditions to success.

Questions for Critical Thinking

1. What does it mean to encode information, and what options do children who are deaf and hard of hearing have?

2. What are the implications of brain research?

3. What language pathway is each student presented in the chapter using?

4. In addition to the pathway, what cognitive factors influence language learning?

5. What contribution does the CCCE model make to our understanding of language learning?

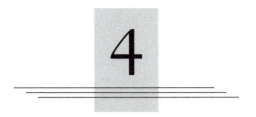

Assessment of Language

What to Expect in This Chapter

In this chapter you will learn about the complex nature of evaluation, the particular challenges we face when assessing students who are deaf and hard of hearing, and the assessment options available. You will see that a collaborative approach to assessment is essential.

Assessment is a process requiring time and effort. Assessment is meaningless unless we use the information to impact educational outcomes. Unfortunately, the tools at our disposal and the time frame within which we must complete the task usually mold what and how we assess. The purpose of this chapter is to provide the reader with an overview of formal language evaluations as well as classroom-based assessment practices. Although we will describe the formal assessment process, our main purpose is to provide an overview of the issues that make assessment of students with hearing losses different from assessment of other students. In the previous chapter you met several students who represent those found in schools and programs around the nation. You will read about language assessments that are appropriate for these students. First, however, we present a discussion of assessment standards and an overview of formal assessment.

Standards for Assessment

In 1994, the International Reading Association and the National Council of Teachers of English published joint recommendations for standards that should be applied to the assessment of children's language and literacy skills. Although referring primarily to reading, they have application to our students because facility with language undergirds literacy.

The standards are:

1. *The interests of the student are paramount in assessment.* (p. 13) The assessment process is often perplexing and intimidating to a student. When we invade the student's privacy in this way we must be sure we are doing it to obtain useful information.

2. *The primary purpose of assessment is to improve teaching and learning.* (p. 15) Sometimes we get so wrapped up with issues of eligibility and standards that we forget to spend sufficient time relating the process of assessment to the process of teaching and learning.

3. *Assessment must reflect and allow for critical inquiry into curriculum and instruction.* (p. 17) It is important that assessment reflect the complexity of the curriculum that we are expecting the child to master.

4. *Assessments must recognize and reflect the intellectually and socially complex nature of reading and writing and the important roles of school, home, and society in literacy development.* (p. 19) For assessment purposes, we must recognize the intricate relationships between reading, writing, and language. This means that assessments must take multiple forms because a "one-size-fits-all" approach does not work with this diverse population.

5. *Assessment must be fair and equitable.* (p. 21) Not only is this a legal requirement, but also it is a challenge to the assessor in providing unbiased, factual, and thoughtful documentation.

6. *The consequences of an assessment procedure are the first, and most important, consideration in establishing the validity of the assessment.* (p. 25) The more an assessment directly serves the needs of the student in the classroom, the more valid is that test.

7. *The teacher is the most important agent of assessment.* (p. 27) In other words, the more the teacher is involved in the assessment process, the more directly that assessment will influence instruction. This places a clear preference on the use of informal, classroom-based assessments over formal, normed assessments.

8. *The assessment process should involve multiple perspectives and sources of data.* (p. 29) If it is true that language and literacy are intertwined in complex ways, then it will require multiple perspectives and sources of data to tease out this complexity.

9. *Assessment must be based in the school community.* (p. 33) Diversity of perspective surrounding a classroom-based issue promotes the use of assessment for progress rather than blame.

10. *All members of the educational community—students, parents, teachers, administrators, policymakers, and the public—must have a voice in the development, inter-*

pretation, and reporting of assessment. (p. 35) Because different stakeholders have different concerns, a collaborative effort has the best chance of bringing about results that can satisfy everyone.

11. *Parents must be involved as active, essential participants in the assessment process.* (p. 37) Productive schools have active, participating parents. That participation must include participation in the assessment process. Parents have a unique perspective not only on their child's language development but also on their aspirations for their child's future. Any given teacher has a fleeting impact on development. The parents' impact is pervasive.

Why Do We Assess?

There are a number of purposes for testing students, and each of these purposes leads to a different choice of test products or processes. For example, if you want to see if a student can maintain a conversation regarding a specific topic, you would not give that student a formalized test. Conversely, if you were considering placing the student in a regular education class, you would give her a test that compared her with other individuals in the class. Some purposes of testing require numerical results. Some purposes require results based upon a previously set criterion. Some purposes of testing require observation and documentation of a specific skill. Knowing one's purpose for evaluation will help narrow the range of possible test products and processes to use. We evaluate students after initial referral or for screening purposes to determine appropriate placements and teaching approaches, to determine present levels of functioning and instructional need for the IEP, and to document our success (Taylor, 1997).

New Referrals

The first reason we evaluate a student's language is to document that student's eligibility and need for special instructional services. This happens when a student is new to the school or program. Perhaps the student recently has been diagnosed with a hearing loss, or maybe she just moved into the school or system from elsewhere. For example, Mrs. Troutman, whom you met in Chapter 3, is interested in the kinds of assessments that will help her decide if Sissy is eligible for her services as well as decide what instructional services Sissy will need.

In deciding what tests to give, consult the requirements of your own state's department of education. IDEA requires that students receive assessments but it does not specify the actual tests you must give. If you do not know your state's requirements for assessment, contact your special education director.

Planning Instruction

The most important reason for testing is to decide what to teach. Mr. Wilson, whom you met in Chapter 3, is very interested in arranging a comprehensive evaluation for Colton, who is struggling in his class. When beginning an evaluation on a student with whom you are not familiar, gather as much information as you can to narrow the range of skills you will assess. Use information from the following sources:

- Previous testing by another school or clinic
- Audiograms
- Parents' reports and perceptions
- Conversations with other individuals who have knowledge of the student
- Observations of the student that you have made
- Screening tools such as the Kendall Communication Proficiency Rating (French, 1999), the Teacher Assessment of Grammatical Structures (Moog & Kozak, 1983), or the Teacher Assessment of Spoken Language (Moog & Biedenstein, 1998).

After gathering the information listed here, narrow the range of language skills to evaluate. Table 4.1 provides a thumbnail sketch of language and thinking skills at five different levels. Use this information to help you decide what to investigate. This is an important step because we want to evaluate only those areas where the student has demonstrated a weakness (Schirmer, 1984). For example, Jorge is at the pre-grammatical level. We would choose early language inventories. Montel is also at this level, although he does use some simple sentence grammar. He might benefit from early grammar screening tools as well as a language inventory. Martin understands simple sentences and in production applies conjoining, negation and questions to three and four word utterances. His evaluation should focus on the morphological features that would improve his production. Kevin does well in the simple-sentence stage and is starting to move into compound sentences but does not understand sentences with multiple verbs. The teacher would want to focus on what types of multiverb sentences he misses. He would also benefit from the ASL checklist. Jonathan exhibits good thought processes associated with compound sentence structure and knows early clauses but is unable to understand or use later clauses, especially those involving time concepts. The Speech-Language Pathologist might be able to recommend a more traditional language assessment. Colton appears to have strengths and weaknesses all across the simple-to-compound range. He will require some diagnostic teaching to narrow his needs. Ashley's skills range across the compound and complex levels. She has more problems in English than appear on the surface. She would benefit from a primary-level language test. The rest of the students understand and use skills associated with the

TABLE 4.1 *Selected Language and Thinking Skills Associated with Major Developmental Stages of English*

Major Stages of English Grammar	Key Traits and Examples	Associated Thinking Skills
Pre-grammatical forms One and two word utterances	Nouns, action words, modifiers, personal-social and functional words; primacy of nouns ~50–100 words	Discrimination, matching, imitation, making simple choices
Non-inflected three and four word utterances	~200+ words e.g., *Daddy go work?* Simple conjunction, possession, entity, attributes, action, existence, recurrence	Sequencing 2–3 items/objects Organizing in space
Simple sentence forms and traits	**Basic sentence patterns** Subj. + intransitive verb Subj. + transitive verb + object Subj. + linking verb + adjective Subj. + linking verb + subject renamed Subj. + linking verb + prep. phrase Conjoining sentence parts and whole sentences, negation, simple question forms	Sequencing 4+ objects Seriation of events Simple coding Cause-effect awareness Categorization hierarchically
Compound sentence forms	More than two verbs not related as auxiliary (helping) and main verb Coordinating conjunction (for, nor, but, yet, so) Complements (know that ..., think that ..., hope that ..., feel that ...)	Seriation of thoughts Categorize serially and hierarchically Organize events Advanced symbolic thought
Complex sentence forms Early clauses Later clauses	**Subordinating conjunction** Because, before, after, until, when, while Although, as long as, even if, as if, whenever Wh- infinitives clauses know how to, show me what to	Sequencing time and thought Organizing in time Analysis and synthesis Problem-solving Abstract coding Creative
Compound-complex forms and traits	Can use with dependent clause first, second, or third in sequence	Advance reasoning Mental hypothesis testing

Sources: Moog, 1999; Nelson, 1998; Owens, 1996; Schumaker & Sheldon, 1999.

complex level, so they could be given tests for hearing students that are age-appropriate.

Once you have a general sense of the level on which the student is communicating, choose tests that focus on language within that level. The thought process you will go through in deciding what to test is like a series of gradient filters. You start with the entire realm of possible languages, language components, and language modes. Next, you narrow these down with one filter (i.e., which languages to assess) then with a finer filter (i.e., which stage within that language to assess), and ultimately you are left with a manageable amount of information to assess. Table 4.2 summarizes these steps.

Documenting Progress

IDEA requires that teachers document a student's progress toward his goals and objectives at regular intervals, which often coincide with the grading period of the school that the student is attending. This is sometimes called "benchmark testing" and is related directly to the language goals and objectives identified in the student's IEP. For example, one student might have the objective "____ will choose the correct picture in an array of pictures when given a stimulus sentence in passive voice." This does not require a formal test; however, it does require that you have a well thought out format for documenting actual use. Checklists, tallies, assessment rubrics, artifacts from a portfolio of products, interviews, and analysis of language samples are all examples of informal ways that you might accomplish this. Mr. Wilson sends a checklist weekly to Ashley's mainstream teacher so that the teacher can check whether she has seen evidence of specific pragmatic language objectives in classroom context on which Mr. Wilson and Ashley have been working.

End-of-Year Evaluation

Like a benchmark evaluation, the end-of-year evaluation looks at the progress a student has made relative to his goals and objectives. At the end of each school

---

TABLE 4.2 *Steps in Planning a Language Assessment of Students Who Are Deaf and Hard of Hearing*

Step 1	Narrow down concerns within the range of possibilities (i.e., English or ASL; simple language or complex language; visual or oral presentation mode).
Step 2	Identify a section of the language realm that applies to the students (i.e., phonology, morphology, syntax, semantics, or pragmatics).
Step 3	Choose tools that evaluate the appropriate components of that section.

year you will evaluate what the student has learned, how well he has learned it, and what he needs to learn next. Everyone is very excited about gathering end-of-year evaluations on Jahan in anticipation of his move to a local school program.

End-of-year evaluations generally include a combination of formal and informal testing. You will assess the student using norm-referenced or criterion-referenced measures to document on his IEP that he is making progress relative to other students, and you will assess using language samples, checklists, rubrics, and the like to document that he is making progress relative to himself. Progress relative to oneself is an important part of assessment in that this is how we make decisions concerning the language instructional practices we are using. For example, we might not expect a profoundly deaf second-grader who received no preschool services to improve one grade level in vocabulary in one academic year, but we would expect her to meet the goals and objectives we set. It is reasonable to expect students to make progress. If progress is not made, then it is time to question whether our instructional practices represent the best match between the teacher's teaching style and communication mode and the learner's learning style and communication mode. If progress is not made, it may be time for the IEP team to:

1. recommend more comprehensive testing to determine if there are other learning problems involved,
2. consult individuals with additional expertise in how students who are deaf and hard of hearing learn language best, and
3. reconsider placement and instructional practices.

Legal Mandates

According to the 1997 revisions of IDEA, IEPs must now contain a written statement of how teams have considered a deaf child's communication needs. This is a necessary addition to the requirements for appropriately serving students with hearing losses, but unless done well, it will miss the mark of its intention. In many instances, individuals making decisions do not have the necessary background in deaf education to ask all the right questions (Commission on Education of the Deaf, 1988; Easterbrooks, 1999; Gutierrez, 1994), so the potential exists that this requirement will be glossed over. In addition, it may first appear that this is a question about the appropriate philosophy under which a child should be educated. We contend that the question should not be about which philosophy to use but about a particular student's style for coding and mediating information and the system that will best match that style. Not only must we abide by the letter of the law and consider the student's communication needs, but we must also abide by the intent of the law and act on those needs.

Types of Tests and Test Scores

Tests are described based on the way scores are organized and reported. Formal tests are described by the technical nature that makes scores meaningful and are reported in a number of manners.

Norm-Referenced Tests

"A norm-referenced test is one in which a person's score is compared to a specific reference group. The reference group is also called the normative or standardization sample and provides the norms on which to base the comparison" (Taylor, 1997, p. 28). We use norm-referenced tests when we are trying to compare an individual student to a group of students. Most available language tests are normed on students with normal hearing. This poses a problem for deaf educators. We already know that most of the students we teach will score lower than hearing students on most norm-referenced tests. If they didn't, then they would not need our services. Few language tests exist that have been normed on the deaf and hard of hearing population. It is very difficult to norm tests on such students. First, it is difficult to find enough students at any given age to determine norms. Second, norms may differ depending upon degree of hearing loss. Finally, norms will be influenced when students have secondary learning disorders. It would not be helpful to compare Mercedes and Martin to the same set of deaf norms, for although they are close in age, they have very different communication needs.

Criterion-Referenced Tests

A criterion-referenced test "does not specifically compare an individual's score to other people's scores. Rather, it measures an individual's mastery of content" (Taylor, 1997, p. 32). For example, the Brigance Inventory of Early Development-Revised (1991) is a criterion-referenced test that looks at eleven content areas, including speech and language. In a criterion-referenced test, the student must get a pre-specified number of answers right in order to get credit for success in at a certain level of skill. There is a cut-off point below which the student is not rated as successful and above which the student is rated as successful. Criterion-referenced tests give us a better understanding of what a student knows relative to himself rather than how much he knows compared to others. Mrs. Troutman would find this kind of test very helpful in Sissy's case.

Standard Scores

When a test is normed on a group of individuals, that group is called the *standardization* group. In other words, their scores are the standard by which other students' performances are judged. Another term for a standard score is a *de-*

rived score. Results are not reported as raw scores but as adjusted scores that reflect the standard deviation within the group. Taylor (1997) defined standard scores as:

> transformed raw scores with the same mean and standard deviation. The *mean* represents the average score, and the *standard deviation* reflects the variability of a set of scores. In the standardization of a test, approximately 34 percent of the subjects score within one standard deviation of the mean; approximately 14 percent score between one and two standard deviations; only about 2 percent score between two and three standard deviations. Thus, approximately 68 percent of the subjects score between +/–1 standard deviations, and approximately 96 percent score between +/–2 standard deviations. (p. 30)

There are many kinds of standard scores (see Lyman, 1998), but the one most commonly reported are those with a mean of 100 and a standard deviation of 10. The reason we use standard scores is so we can compare scores from one test to another. For example, most IQ tests have a mean of 100 and a standard deviation of 15. Certain subtests of the Oral and Written Language Scales have a mean of 10 and a standard deviation of 3, so if a child had an IQ of 115, we would expect him to get a 13 on this test. Mrs. Troutman might give Trisha a standardized test to compare her spoken language skills with her written language skills.

Percentile Rank

A percentile score is a score that tells us the student's position relative to the norm group (Lyman, 1998). For example, if a student's score is at the 50th percentile, then we know that he has scored as high as 50 percent of the students in the norming group. Percentile ranks are widely used in high-stakes testing. High-stakes testing is that testing which schools use to label, place, promote, graduate, or somehow give designation to students. An example of a high-stakes test is the Iowa Test of Basic Skills (ITBS). When you took the Scholastic Aptitude Test or the Graduate Record Examination, your acceptance into college was at stake. For students in school, their acceptance into special education or their promotion to the next grade may be at stake. LaShawndra's teachers might look very carefully at her language arts scores on the ITBS, especially because she has a tendency to become overwhelmed with classroom vocabulary.

Age-Equivalent Scores

According to Lyman (1998), "age scores can be developed for any human characteristic that changes with age; however, they are used most frequently with intelligence and achievement tests of children of school-age or below" (p. 113). If you were to give a test to 1,000 randomly selected children from ages 6 to 10, you would expect roughly an equal number of children who were 8 years old, 8 years 1 month old, 8 years 2 months old, and on, up to 10 years old. Suppose you took the scores of all the children who were a specific age, say 9 years 3 months, and found that the average or median of their scores was 72. That raw score would become the expected score for other children who are 9 years 3 months old. You would expect a child that age to get a raw score equivalent to 72. The problem with using age-equivalent scores is that they are often overinterpreted. For example, if a child who is 6-years 9-months-old were to get a raw score of 72 on a test, we would say his age-equivalent score was 9 years 3 months. This might lead us to believe that the child was gifted. However, this depends on what is being tested. Suppose the test looked at the ability to name letters of the alphabet. We would expect the average 6-year 9-month-old to score about the same as a 9-year 3-month-old, so this information would be meaningless. As another example, suppose a 10-year-old were to receive a 9-year 3-month age-equivalent score on a test. One might be concerned that the child was falling below expectations on that test. This too would be useless information. For one reason, we don't know if the correct raw score for a 10-year-old is 72 or 73 or 88. We don't know how far away from expectation he is. Nor do we know anything about the actual skills he missed. What reading skills, for example, does a 10-year-old have that a 9-year 3-month-old does not? Further, language develops in spurts (Muma, 1998). A child may be making great strides in one area but slow strides in another. This does not necessarily mean that the second area is delayed. The age-equivalent score gives us no information to help us decide what the student needs to learn. It does not mean that a student is slow or advanced. All it means is that student was able to accrue a particular raw score.

Grade-Equivalent Scores

Lyman (1998) stated that "the basic rationale for grade-placement scores is similar to that for age scores, for their values are set to equal the average score of school pupils at the corresponding grade placement" (p. 115). Grade-equivalent scores have the same basic flaw as age-equivalent scores. Suppose we used the same test results from the preceding example, but this time we averaged the raw scores based on the grade the child was in (e.g., 2.1, 2.1, 2.3, etc.). Our first-grader who achieved a third-grade equivalent score might be considered gifted, and our fifth-grader who achieved a third-grade equivalent score might cause his teacher concern. However, information is not this discrete. We don't all learn the exact same thing at the exact same point in time. One child halfway through the third grade in School A might have been exposed to different things than was another child halfway through third grade in School B. Grade- and age-equivalent scores give us ballpark guesses about a student's performance. They are not absolutes. You probably noticed that grade-equivalent reading scores were given for most of the students in Chapter 3. This allowed you to get a general sense of whether the students were performing below, at, or above expectations, but it did not tell you what to teach.

Issues in Assessment of Deaf and Hard of Hearing Students

The main problems associated with the assessment of language of children with hearing losses have always been and still remain:

- the lack of skilled examiners,
- confusion over the use of deaf norms or hearing norms, and
- the lack of easily administered materials (NASDSE, 1995).

Language in and of itself is extremely complex, and a firm grasp of language does not come with just one or two courses. If you are going to assess the language of deaf and hard of hearing children, then you need an extensive knowledge base in the following general areas:

- developmental and language issues specific to students who are deaf or hard of hearing,
- the variety of languages and language modes which students who are deaf and hard of hearing may use,
- the ability to communicate in the language or mode of the student, and
- the impact of additional disorders on deaf students' language acquisition.

Such knowledge does not come quickly, and those with only a passing understanding of the issues in deaf education do not possess the skills needed to look in depth at a deaf or hard of hearing student's communication needs. At minimum, the evaluator's knowledge base must include specific information related to the issues described in Table 4.3. Without a firm understanding of how children who are deaf and hard of hearing perform or of the languages and modes they might use, examiners may misunderstand the student. Common misunderstandings include:

- The student may attempt to imitate your question, leading you to think he understood the answer (e.g., Examiner: "Is this a cat or a dog?" Student imitates last word seen or heard, *dog*, and accidentally gets it correct.).
- The student may watch your facial expression very carefully and catch that, unbeknownst to you, you always look at the correct answer after asking the question.
- The student may fake her way through the answer by responding to your facial expression (e.g., You ask "Which does not belong: dog, cat, bug?" Student answers "dog," eliciting a raised eyebrow from you, then says, "I mean bug.")

Poorly skilled evaluators produce poor evaluations.

TABLE 4.3 *Skills Needed By Language Evaluators of Children Who Are Deaf and Hard of Hearing*

Skill	Description
Knowledge of the forms, functions, and uses of English	The phonology, morphology, syntax, semantics, and pragmatics of English are very complex. Evaluators must be able to identify the stage at which a child is communicating. Refer to later chapters to learn about this aspect of language.
Knowledge of the forms, functions, and uses of American Sign Language	ASL has distinct systems of phonology, morphology, syntax, semantics, and pragmatics that are also complex. Gaining a metalinguistic understanding of English and ASL is a challenge. Do not expect to understand everything about how to teach both languages all at once. If you follow a process and apply it with each student, then you will learn the complexities of these languages over time as you need them and in relation to a specific student.
Knowledge of the forms, functions, and uses of other languages	The home language of many students is something other than English or ASL. Lane, Hoffmeister, & Bahan (1996) identified the six most common languages founds in schools today in the following order: English, Spanish, Italian, German, French, and ASL. As the Hispanic population increases in this country, you will be faced with more and more students who use Spanish. You will also need to learn this language so that you can determine its influence on your students' English and/or ASL development. If you do not, then you need to consult an outside expert who can identify for you those language skills that the student may already possess in his home language.
Ability to communicate in the student's preferred language or mode of communication	Someone who is just learning English can not rate your ability with your own language because he or she misses a lot of what it is you are capable of doing. The same holds true for ASL. One who does not know ASL should not be assessing a child who uses ASL. One who does not know how to sign English should not be assessing the English of a child who signs it. One who is not familiar with the speech patterns of an oral deaf or hard of hearing child should not be assessing that child's oral communication. This will lead to misinformation. Those new to the field tend to overestimate their own skills and to underestimate the skills of the student. Under- or overestimation leads to the development of inappropriate goals and objectives and wasted instructional time. Use of an interpreter can invalidate test results and should be done with caution. Locating appropriate evaluators often requires seeking outside resources.

Ability to determine the stage of language at which a child is functioning	You will need to determine the stage at which a student is functioning as a first step in the process of examining what your student can do and what he or she needs to learn. There are both formal and informal means of doing this.
Ability to judge the rate at which a child is making progress in a language or mode	Two errors occur frequently: (1) the approach a child needs is often made based on what is available; and (2) progress through a program, or lack thereof, is never questioned relative to the skills of the teacher. Most parents send their children to school where schooling is available. Seventy-five to 80% of students who are deaf and hard of hearing attend their local school systems (Holden-Pitt & Diaz, 1998; U.S. Department of Education, 1999). Approximately 34% of them attend schools where there are seven or fewer deaf and hard of hearing students (Easterbrooks, 1999) limiting access to a variety of teachers of the deaf with a variety of skills across modalities and approaches. The result is that the student is not matched to the teacher based upon his or her needs but based upon the luck of the draw. Further, there are few attempts made to look at the influence of the instructional mode on the student's progress. We rarely consider the rate at which a child is progressing. This practice contributes to the low educational outcomes.
Knowledge of indicators suggesting that a student may not be progressing sufficiently	This is a corollary to the issue above. In order to judge the rate of a particular student's language relative to the mode by which he is learning or the language he is being taught, we need to know what to look for. In addition to proposing a standard for rate of development later in this chapter, we propose a set of questions that you should ask to determine if your student is making sufficient progress in communication.
Collaborating on all available tools	No single individual can be an expert in all languages and modes of instruction, therefore, it is essential that evaluators and teachers communicate well with one another. The problem is this: How do you know that a child is not making progress in ASL if you don't know what ASL is? How do you know whether a child may or may not benefit from a different style or mode of input if you do not know that style or mode? Keeping a child in a program where there is a mismatch between the language needs of the child and the skills of the teacher will result in language delay. An alert teacher must seek outside help. Some possibilities that you may want to pursue are:

(continued)

TABLE 4.3 *Continued*

Skill	*Description*
	• forming a language-learning community with two or three other teachers from around your state who have different skills than you have and engaging in routine e-mail dialogues regarding the students each of you is serving, • utilizing the diagnostic services available from your state's school for the deaf, • contracting for services from others who can evaluate a child relative to a different perspective, • contracting with consultants who are experts in a particular mode of language who can evaluate a child relative to their perspective, • regionalizing services so that schools in a particular geographic area can share access to individuals who are educated in a variety of perspectives, and • sharing your knowledge, and sharing the responsibility. Collaboration is essential during the assessment process.
An understanding of the language demands of the curriculum	An often overlooked area of evaluation is the academic context within which the student is using language. This includes the language the teacher will use, the language the teacher will teach, and the language in the textbooks. While we want to provide our students with a sound, developmentally based language instructional program, it is also necessary to consider the demands of the real world the child faces.
An understanding of the interrelationship of the communication systems used at home and in school	When the language at home differs from the language at school, students do not have after-hours access to models of the school language. Parental involvement in language development is crucial for students who are deaf and hard of hearing. In addition, if a student already has a linguistic skill in his home language, then it is easier to use this language to teach the new language. The knowledge that a child has about his home language has implications for how a teacher will instruct a child when learning English or ASL. If you do not know the language used in a student's home, then at minimum you will need to consult an individual who does.

| An awareness of the relationship between the language of test administration and the language being tested | Some tests that seem to be assessing comprehension contain a production component that may obscure what the student knows, and some tests that seem to be assessing an earlier stage of language pose their questions in language more difficult than the target. Evaluators must consider the language of instructions and indicators of comprehension. By "comprehension" we mean this: what does the student understand when the examiner presents a language stimulus? The examiner can present a stimulus through gesture and pantomime, voice, signs presented in English structure, signs presented in ASL, Cued Speech, or print. First, if you present a language stimulus to a child via speech and he communicates in ASL, then you are assessing his ability to lipread, not his ability to understand the language stimulus. Likewise, if you present a grammar construction in ASL to a child who uses Cued Speech, you are assessing his ability to understand ASL, not his ability to understand the language stimulus. Second, it is important to know if the language of the instructions is within the child's repertoire. Third, it is important to know if the student understands how he is supposed to respond. All these issues can obscure what the student can and can't do. |
| An awareness of the differences between communication through-the-air and language in print form | It is very difficult to separate language in and of itself from language in the printed form because so much of what goes on in language lessons involves the use of print either directly or indirectly. You must be careful in assessing language through print. If a student missed an answer, did he miss it because he didn't understand the underlying language or because he couldn't read? |

Formal and Informal Measures of Language

In designing a language assessment protocol, you will choose a combination of formal and informal assessment packages and procedures. The choices you make will depend on the age of the student, the reason for your assessment, and the student's present levels of performance. In general, you have formal options and informal options.

Formal Tests of Language

The market today has numerous test options. Some are helpful with deaf and hard of hearing students and some are not. When reviewing this smorgasbord of possibilities, keep in mind the kind of test you are looking for. A description of the kinds of tests that are available follows. We present only a few here as examples of possibilities. Additional tests are reviewed in Appendix A of this chapter. For a more comprehensive examination of published test materials, see American Speech-Language-Hearing Association (ASAH) (1998), Bradley-Johnson and Evans (1991), Nelson (1998), and Zieziula (1982).

Tests of English Grammar.   Tests of English grammar are commonly used with students who are deaf and hard of hearing. This is one of the few areas of assessment where we have several options developed specifically for students with hearing losses. Some of these tests require students to point to a picture given a language stimulus, such as The Rhode Island Test of Language Structures (Engen & Engen,1983); some require them to manipulate materials, such as the Grammatical Analysis of Elicited Language sets (Moog & Geers, 1979). Others require the teacher to observe each student and chart when a specific structure has been elicited or used spontaneously, such as the Teacher Assessment of Grammatical Structures (Moog & Kozak, 1983) or the Teacher Assessment of Spoken Language (Moog & Biedenstein, 1998). Some are useful as screening devices, such as The Kendall Language Proficiency Scale (French, 1999). All of these tests provide a look at one specific aspect of language; that is, grammar.

Other tests of grammar that were designed for use with hearing students have found their way onto the shelves of many examiners because they have proved themselves to be useful. While some of these mainly evaluate grammar (The Test of Auditory Comprehension of Language-Revised, Carrow-Woolfolk, 1985), others take a broader look at language (The Test of Language Development series by PRO-ED). These tests are helpful in that they are more likely to be normed on hearing children but not on children with hearing losses. If you are looking for a numerical rating to put on a some form, these tests are useful. Be advised, however, that you might not find specific direction for choosing goals and objectives from these kinds of tests.

Tests of ASL Grammar. Unfortunately there are relatively few tests available that evaluate the ASL grammar of students with hearing losses. Most available tests were designed either for interpreters or to assess the communication proficiency of those who can hear. However, with the increased awareness of the need to evaluate deaf students' ASL skills and with continued research into the nature of ASL grammar, actual test materials are surely on the horizon. Until such time as these become readily available, we suggest several sources. First is the checklist in Table 4.4. To use this test, choose a language skill that you want to evaluate, then observe your student in both natural conversation and prompted activities to determine if it is currently in the student's repertoire. A second checklist by Evans, Zimmer, and Murray (1994) is presented in Table 4.5. You will find another source of information on ASL goals and objectives by going to http://www.doe.k12.ga.us/qcc/asl. This is the website for the Quality Core Curriculum of the Department of Education of the State of Georgia. This state permits students to take ASL as one of their foreign language objectives. Three levels of objectives are available. Use this as you would any other checklist.

Tests of English Word Meaning. Tests of English word meaning are abundant; however, there are only a couple that were designed specifically for students who are deaf and hard of hearing. Typically, vocabulary tests use a picture-pointing format. Most available tests of vocabulary were developed for hearing students, but these are useful in that they give a general assessment of where a student's vocabulary skills lie relative to his hearing peers. Most look strictly at vocabulary understanding or use (e.g., The Receptive One Word Picture Vocabulary Test, Gardner, 1985 (ROWPVT); The Expressive One Word Picture Vocabulary Test, Gardner, 1981 (EOWPVT); The Peabody Picture Vocabulary Test-R (PPVT-R), Dunn & Dunn, 1981), but some look at advance applications such as multiple meanings of words or the ability to categorize (e.g., The Test of Adolescent and Adult Language-3, Hammill, Brown, Larson, & Wiederholt, 1994). When choosing a test, you will need to decide whether you want a test that looks at language per se, a test that uses a student's ability to write to assess language, or a test that does both (e.g., The Oral and Written Language Scales (OWLS), Carrow-Wollfolk, 1994).

Tests of ASL Word Meaning. As with ASL grammar, very few tests are available that look at a student's ASL vocabulary. One exception is the Semantic Awareness Test Kit (1991) by Sign Media, Inc. This test evaluates the deaf student's understanding of words with multiple meanings both in ASL and English.

Tests of Spoken English versus Signed English. Although there are no tests that are developed specifically to compare spoken English to signed English,

TABLE 4.4 *Checklist of Emerging ASL Skills**

Language Skill	Indicator	Not Observed	Emerging Immature	Functional Use	Age-Appropriate
Nonlinguistic markers	1. Engages in communicative pointing.	1	1	1	1
	2. Allows self to be tapped on shoulder to view mutually an object, action, or event that is being labeled.	2	2	2	2
	3. Watches faces for communication.	3	3	3	3
	4. Engages in mutual gazing.	4	4	4	4
	5. Early gestures are context appropriate.	5	5	5	5
	6. Communicates well by showing.	6	6	6	6
Phonology	1. Uses various *distinctive features* of handshapes, or cheremes. Circle those observed: compact, concave, index, touch, broad, full, radial, ulnar, dual.	1	1	1	1
	2. Emerging handshapes fall into one of the categories below: Stage 1 A S L bO[1] 5 C G Stage 2 B F O Stage 3 I D Y P 3 V H W Stage 4 8 7 X R T M N	2	2	2	2
Morphology	1. Uses classifiers. Circle those observed: General person (index) Vehicle (thumb up, middle & index pointing in direction of movement) Stationary object wider than tall/movable (closed fist/thumb up) Stationary object taller than wide/fixed (arms extend up elbow to fingertip) Flat object/portable (flat hand/palm up) Flat object/fixed (flat hand/palm down)	1	1	1	1
	2. Uses facial expression to modify the meaning of a specific sign (e.g., widening eyes to indicate emphasis).	2	2	2	2

3. Uses eyebrow movement to indicate change in question forms.	3	3	3	3
4. Uses other nonmanual markers such as leaning forward or holding the last sign of a sentence to convey meaning.	4	4	4	4
5. Uses directionality of signs to change the meaning of sentences.	5	5	5	5
6. Uses the following mouthing forms meaningfully: tongue slightly forward (e.g., lazy) cha (e.g., large)	6	6	6	6
7. Uses reduplication of signs to form plurals.	7	7	7	7
8. Locates object of conversation "in space" and later refers to object by pointing to or moving a sign toward that space in a meaningful fashion.	8	8	8	8
9. Incorporates negation into signs to create the following: want, don't want (one sign) like, don't like (with headshake) know, don't know (one sign) care, don't care (one sign)	9	9	9	9
10. Used deictic pointing (to self, others, third person, single nonperson locus, multiple loci).	10	10	10	10
Syntax				
1. Uses "topic, comment" structures.	1	1	1	1
2. Produces two signs per communication act.	2	2	2	2
3. Produces three signs per communication act.	3	3	3	3
4. Produces multiple signs per act	4	4	4	4
5. Indicates "wh" questions by signing the indicator both at the beginning and at the end of the sentence.	5	5	5	5
6. Uses time and location indicators in the beginning of a sentence to set the frame of reference.	6	6	6	6
7. Uses rhetorical questions (ME WORK WHERE? School).	7	7	7	7
8. Produces simple sentence where there is one subject and one verb action.	8	8	8	8
9. Produces complex sentence forms where there may be embedding of one idea into another to expand or explain.	9	9	9	9
10. Produces specific grammatical structures such as conditionals (e.g., suppose if) and relatives (e.g, You know, boy tall? He. . . .)	10	10	10	10

(continued)

TABLE 4.4 *Continued*

Language Skill	Indicator	Not Observed	Emerging Immature	Functional Use	Age-Appropriate
Semantics	1. Uses gestures symbolically.	1	1	1	1
	2. Can illustrate the shape of objects.	2	2	2	2
	3. Can spell/sign own name.	3	3	3	3
	4. Has a recognizable lexicon of signs (e.g., numbers/colors). List several:	4	4	4	4
	5. Illustrates another person's features (e.g., face, clothes).	5	5	5	5
	6. Uses different signs to indicate negation *(no)*, nonexistence *(no, none, nothing)*, and denial *(not, don't, didn't)*.	6	6	6	6
	7. Can present synonyms and antonyms in ASL.	7	7	7	7
	8. Given a category, can sign examples.	8	8	8	8
	9. Given enough examples, can sign the label of the category.	9	9	9	9
	10. Can summarize and comment on a short story presented in ASL.	10	10	10	10
Pragmatics	1. Can style shift to accommodate communication with adults versus peers.	1	1	1	1
	2. Expresses appropriate facial affect associated with context.	2	2	2	2
	3. Provides information concerned culturally important (e.g., DEAF IX (V/N) INSTITUTION, GROW UP, IX (wh-q) MOTHER FATHER DEAF (V/N)	3	3	3	3
	4. If child signs English, do signs nativize in presence of other deaf individuals ?	4	4	4	4
	5. Maintains eye contact through conversation.	5	5	5	5
	6. Allows self to be touched for attention or emphasis.	6	6	6	6

*See Appendix B for instructions.
[1]bO = baby O

Sources: McIntire, 1994; Valli & Lucas, 1995; Wix & Supalla, undated.

TABLE 4.5 *ASL Development Checklist*

Stage 1

- Begin to use simple handshapes (e.g., B, C, O, A, S, 1, 5).
- Begins to use simple movements (e.g., straight forward, up, down).
- Begins to use simple single-sign vocabulary.
- Begins to combine signs into simple two-sign sentences.
- Uses classifiers (Object) (e.g., 2h CL: O—pole).
- Negation—headshake alone or headshake with negative sign

    headshake   headshake
       NO   CAN'T

- Questions used include Yes/No and What, Where

    wh—q (frown)   Yes/No—q (eyebrows raised)
      WHERE   MINE

- Indexes (points to) present objects and people.
- Storytelling is not always clear—copying actions and facial expressions.

Stage 2

- Tries to use complex handshapes, but often simplifies (substitutes simple handshapes) (e.g., WATER with 5 handshape replacing the W handshape). Uses simple movement (straight forward, up down).
- Use of verb modification
  WALK—stroll; WALK—quickly; WALK—for a long time.
- Three- or four-sign sentences.
- Classifiers: Object + Movement (e.g., CL: 3—car driving forward).
- Negation—headshake with non-negative sign

    headshake
    ME WANT MILK

- Questions used include Yes/No and What, Where, Why

    whq (frown)
    GO HOME WHY

- Storytelling (different roles, body shift, facial expression)
  - Substitutes present objects to talk about objects and people not present.
  - Character identification and shifts not always clear.

Stage 3

- Begins to use complex handshapes (e.g., X, Y, T, R, 3)
- Begins to use complex movements (e.g., wiggly movement)

(continued)

TABLE 4.5   *Continued*

- Begins to use verb modification to indicate number and distribution (e.g., FALL, singular; FALL, plural; FALL, random)
- Begins to use noun modification to indicate intensity, size, and quality of objects. (e.g., bowl—big)
- Questions used include Yes/No and What, Where, Why, For-For, Who

Sentence structures:

$$\underline{\quad\quad}^{t}$$

- Begins to use topicalization IX (*my*) ROOM, PAINT TOMORROW

$$\underline{\quad\quad\quad\quad}^{rhet}\text{ (raised eyebrow)}$$

- Begins to use rhetorical questions (e.g., TURTLE RUN, WHO WIN, TURTLE)

Storytelling:

- Inconsistent use of points in space to represent nonpresent objects/people.
- Role-play through body shifts, eye gaze, and facial expression.

Stage 4

- Consistent use of complex handshapes and movements (e.g., fingerspelling short words and names).
- Use of noun modification to indicate the spatial arrangement of objects (e.g., TREE++ in a row; TREE++ in a cluster).
- Use of bracketing to indicate "wh" questions

$$\underline{\quad\quad\quad\quad}\text{wh (frown)}$$
WHERE GO WHERE

Sentence structures:

- Topicalization (topic continuation)
- Rhetorical questions
- Conditionals (IF or SUPPOSE)

$$\underline{\quad\quad\quad\quad}\text{cond. (brow raised)}$$
IF—SUPPOSE RAIN, GAME CANCEL

- Appropriate use of full abstract referencing for objects/people not present.
- Storytelling (character identification, role-play, role shifts) is clear and consistent.

Reprinted with permission from Evans, Zimmer, and Murray (1994). *Discovering With Words and Signs* (p. 42–44).

this is a relatively easy comparison to make. Several tests have two different forms that have been designed to yield comparable results (e.g., Boehm Test of Basic Concepts, Boehm, 1986; the Northwestern Syntax Screening Test (NSST), Lee, 1971). If a comparison is needed to document that a particular student is progressing more rapidly in one mode than another, or if documentation is needed to measure comparative progress of one mode to another, then give one of the test forms in spoken English and the other in signed English.

Tests of the Vocabulary of Instruction and Test-Taking. A frequently overlooked component of vocabulary instruction is the body of vocabulary that a student must know in order to take tests. We assume that students understand the language that we are using to provide test directions, but often they make errors because they do not understand the directions. These include simple vocabulary at younger ages (e.g., Circle the picture that does not belong with the one on the left.) to those with more complex cognitive and grammatical demands (e.g., Was the Marshall Plan enacted before or after World War I?). While there are few actual tests that measure these skills, one source developed to teach these skills (The Language of Directions) contains several test options. In fact, there are many curriculum guides and instructional manuals available that contain checklists and rubrics for assessment in many areas of language. Contact schools for the deaf to locate these.

Tests of English Pragmatic Skills. Pragmatic language is very difficult to assess. We know of no tests that have been designed specifically for students who are deaf and hard of hearing. Several are available that a skilled evaluator could use (e.g., The Test of Problem Solving (TOPS), Zachman, Jorgensen, Huisingh, Barrett, 1984; The Test of Pragmatic Language (TOPL), Phelps-Terasaki & Phelps-Gunn, 1992).

Tests of ASL Pragmatic Skills. As with grammar and vocabulary, the field lacks options for assessing pragmatics. However, numerous checklists are available that can be adapted for this purpose such as those found in Tables 4.4 and 4.5.

Tests of Classroom Discourse Rules. We want to know about a student's knowledge of the rules of classroom discourse because language is more than just words and sentences. Language is a tool to help us engage in learning and to share this learning experience with others. Available formal tests (e.g., Interpersonal Language Skills Assessment (ILSA), Blagden & McConnell, 1985) are normed on hearing students but might be adapted by a skilled examiner for students who are deaf and hard of hearing. This is another area where checklists or rubric assessments are appropriate.

Tests of Figurative Language.   Few tests are available that evaluate figurative language use in students who are deaf and hard of hearing. Most tests described in the literature were designed for use in research. For example Rittenhouse and Kenyon (1991) designed a multiple choice test of vignettes and pictures to examine a student's understanding of sentences as metaphors. Easterbrooks (1983) designed a forced-choice test where students applied physical properties (e.g., warm/cold) to psychological traits (e.g., smiling woman/stern man) to examine a student's understanding of words as metaphors. She found that the deaf subjects in her study were able to apply adjectives metaphorically but at a much delayed age compared to their hearing peers. We need tests of figurative language in English and ASL because nonliteral language forms are found pervasively throughout all forms of the printed word. They occur as early as the primer level and increase in complexity and amount rapidly. They account for some of the problems that deaf and hard of hearing students have in learning to read.

Informal Procedures for Language Assessment

In the preceding section you learned that in addition to formal evaluations, we participate in informal ways of gathering information about a student's language understanding and use. The following describes a variety of informal procedures by which we gather information, including a key feature of language assessment, the language sample analysis.

Curriculum-Based Assessment.   *Curriculum-based assessment* involves measuring expected curriculum outcomes (Taylor, 1997; Tucker, 1985). Curriculum-based assessment uses as its frame of reference the curriculum standards of the school or school district. *Language-based curriculum analysis* (Prelock, 1998; Prelock, Miller, & Reed, 1993) is similar to curriculum-based assessment in that it is based on the needs of the general education curriculum and provides a "process for systematically reviewing the curriculum and evaluating curriculum demand, predicting breakdowns for students with communication impairments, and brainstorming modifications" (Prelock, 1998, p. 35). Table 4.6 provides a format you can use to examine the language needs of deaf and hard of hearing students' language skills relative to a specific instructional segment in the general education classroom.

Performance-Based Assessment.   Tests must measure what they say they measure (i.e., they must be valid), and tests are more valid when the assessment is attached to real-world uses of language and literacy (International Reading Association and National Council of Teachers of English, 1994). *Performance-based assessment* uses as its frame of reference how that skill or knowledge appears in the real world. This means that assessments must include real, authentic appli-

TABLE 4.6   *Questions to Ask in a Language-Based Curriculum Analysis for Students Who Are Deaf and Hard of Hearing*

1. What are the curriculum objectives?
2. What language objectives are emphasized?
3. What classroom communication objectives are emphasized?
4. What prerequisite vocabulary is necessary for achieving stated objectives?
5. What new vocabulary is to be introduced?
6. What are the allowable options the student may use to indicate comprehension: (Please check all that apply.)

__ pointing/showing   __ circling/drawing/ringing   __ answering questions

__ ordering/sequencing __ role-playing   __ following oral directions

__ pictures/words   __ manipulating objects   __ solving problems at chalkboard

__ sentences/numbers   __ following written directions __ other (please specify)

7. What are the allowable options of expression that the student may use? (Please check all that apply.)

__ defining vocabulary   __ storytelling

__ using complete oral utterances   __ reading to class

__ using complete signed utterances __ clarifying response

__ asking and answering questions   __ demonstrating

__ explaining answers   __ acting out

8. What are the allowable options for written expression?

__ tracing number/letters   __ copying numbers/letters/words

__ writing numbers/letters   __ filling in sentences

__ spelling words   __ writing complete sentences

__ making outlines   __ writing stories

__ writing book report   __ writing research reports

__ writing an explanation   __ reading word problems

__ writing equations/formulas   __ other (please specify)

9. Do/Does student(s) have the prerequisite vocabulary?
10. What semantic confusions are likely with the new vocabulary to be introduced?
11. What syntactic confusions are likely?
12. Does the class, overall, have the prerequisite knowledge?
13. What semantic, syntactic, and/or phonological confusions are likely to be experienced by the class, which were not mentioned for the identified student(s)?

Semantic:
Syntactic:
Phonological:

(continued)

TABLE 4.6 *Continued*

14. Which of the requirements identified above is/are likely to be difficult for

Identified student(s)?
Whole class?

15. How will you modify prerequisite vocabulary for the identified student(s)?

16. How will you modify prerequisite vocabulary for the whole class?

17. How will you introduce new vocabulary for

Identified student(s)?
Whole class?

18. How will you make modifications to meet language comprehension requirements for

Identified student(s)?
Whole class?

19. How will you make modifications to meet expressive language requirements for

Identified student(s)?
Whole class?

20. How will you make modifications to meet written language requirements for

Identified student(s)
Whole class?

Adapted with permission from Prelock (1999). *Journal of Children's Communication Development.*

cations of language. Paper-and-pencil tasks or pointing to the correct answer in an array do not show what the child can do with real language in real situations. According to Taylor, performance assessment is "an alternative assessment that requires the student to *do* (produce, demonstrate, perform, create, construct, apply, build, solve, plan, show, illustrate, convince, persuade, or explain) some task" (p. 143). Performance-based assessments are absolutely appropriate for students who are deaf and hard of hearing. They allow us to avoid problems of confusion between speech and language, reading and language, and comprehension and production. For example, if Mr. Wilson wants to see whether Kevin understands the use of *where* as a relative pronoun, he can tell him to go to a location when the direction contained the relative pronoun (e.g., Your science paper is in the room where Mrs. Plimpton works.). Performance assessments require the student to show us a correct action that corresponds to the intent of the sentence, allowing us to be confident that the student does in fact understand the language construction that we used. *Authentic assessment* is a form of performance assessment "that requires the *application* of knowledge to real-life, real-world settings, or a simulation of such a setting using real-life, real-world activities" (Taylor, 1997, p. 143). Real-life and real-world assessments should be a mainstay of your ongoing monitoring and assessment process.

Observational Assessment and Diagnostic Teaching. Observational assessment uses as its frame of reference the point of view of the individual doing the observation. That may be the point of view of a parent comparing the child to his siblings. It may be that of the teacher comparing the child to other students with whom he or she has worked. Teachers routinely observe children, and when they notice a problem, a more organized approach to the assessment can begin.

Diagnostic teaching is a process of field-testing instructional strategies that involves observation of a student's performance under specifically designed conditions. To set up a data collection system for your observation, follow the procedures outlined in Table 4.7.

Portfolio Assessment. Portfolio assessment is a performance assessment that uses "observable evidence or products completed by the student over time" (Taylor, 1997, p. 143). A portfolio contains educational artifacts that a student has actually made or used. Examples that apply to the area of language include but are not limited to:

- videotapes and audiotapes of conversations
- logs and journals
- representative classwork and assignments

TABLE 4.7 *Procedures for Designing an Observation Form for Use during Diagnostic Teaching*

1. Identify the instructional objectives targeted and gather baseline performance data.
2. Determine the current conditions (baseline conditions) under which instruction is taking place.
3. Choose or develop an informal assessment tool (e.g., rubric, observation form) to monitor student performance.
4. Gather data on the student's performance under the baseline instructional condition for at least one week to get an adequate picture of performance.
5. Choose or design a new instructional strategy or condition to use diagnostically with student.
6. Implement the new instructional strategy for a period of at least one week. The period of time chosen should correspond to the period of time during which baseline data were gathered.
7. Note if progress has been made.
8. Continue for at least one more week, gathering data daily.
9. Compare progress over the three-week segments.

- reports
- scrapbooks of activities demonstrating performance associated with the language objective
- illustrations and diagrams
- evaluations and checklists
- observation reports from others
- tests and quizzes
- teacher's notes and anecdotal observations
- photographs and projects

Rubrics. A rubric is a specific form of observation that uses a set of criteria to evaluate a student's performance on predetermined objectives. Rubrics are constructed by determining a fixed measurement scale, of usually four or five points, and a list of criteria that describe the characteristics of products or performances needed to score a particular point. These are plotted down the columns of the rubric (or across the top) while the skill to be examined is across the top (or down the side). Rubrics differ from *checklists* in that each rubric defines the quality of a skill of one individual while a checklist may be used to identify quantity of performance. Schirmer, Bailey, and Fitzgerald (1999) found that rubrics are also a useful instructional tool. When students understand the quality of work expected of them and the way their work will be evaluated, they

TABLE 4.8 Rubric to Evaluate Pragmatic Language Skills: Manners

Student: Montel

Asks for help appropriately (e.g., raises hand, uses "please," explains self)	Interrupts conversations appropriately (e.g., "Excuse me," raises hand, waits turn).	Responds to communication from others with acknowledgment, answer, or request for clarification.	Says "Thank you" after receiving something (e.g., object, compliment, etc.).
4 Uses clearly and consistently.	4 Uses clearly and consistently.	4 Uses clearly and consistently.	4 Uses clearly and consistently.
3 Uses spontaneously in some situations.	3 Uses spontaneously in some situations.	3 Uses spontaneously in some situations.	3 Uses spontaneously in some situations.
2 Uses with prompts.	2 Uses with prompts.	2 Uses with prompts.	2 Uses with prompts.
1 Does not use.	1 Does not use.	1 Does not use.	1 Does not use.

have a clearer picture of what they must do. Table 4.8 is an example of a rubric assessment of pragmatic language associated with manners that might be used with a child like Montel.

Inventories.   Inventories use as their frame of reference a previously determined set of indicators to which a particular group, organization, or agency has ascribed importance. There are two types of these: hierarchies and formal inventories. You will find many different hierarchies of language in the second half of this book. To use these, determine the general stage at which your student is functioning, transfer the skills just before and just after this level to an inventory sheet, then use this to check off whether or not the student has mastered the skill. You will find several language inventories listed in Appendix A of this chapter.

Language Sample Analysis.   *Language sampling and analysis* procedures have been used in assessment for many years (Miller, 1981; Tyack & Gottsleben, 1977). It is the key pin around which you will base the rest of your assessment. The language sample helps you determine where the student is functioning so you may choose appropriate formal tests. It gives you an authentic look at what the student is actually doing, and it provides you with a wealth of information about the student's language competence. Both language sampling and language analysis are time-consuming tasks; there is no easy or quick way to do them. However, the effort expended is well worth the time because it provides a rich source of information about a student.

There are many ways to gather a language sample. Videotaping is essential when sampling the language of students who are deaf and hard of hearing in order to gather both nonlinguistic cues to meaning and visual language skills associated with ASL. Gather samples from multiple sources such as:

- student-to-student interactions in the classroom
- student-to-student interactions during noninstructional time
- student-to-teacher formal classroom interactions
- student-to-teacher informal, noninstructional interactions

Gather language samples from multiple situations such as:

- the classroom
- the lunchroom
- the playground or school hallways
- one-on-one
- in groups
- at home

Typically students are told to gather approximately one hundred utterances (Schirmer, 1989) over a period of time in order to get a representative sample of the student's true language capabilities. Muma (1998) studied the language samples of ten subjects and found that much larger samples of utterances were needed depending upon the error rate you are willing to accept and the language being evaluated. For an error rate of 25 percent, from 113 to 119 utterances might be needed. For an error rate of 15 percent, from 167 to 266 utterances might be needed. For an error rate of 5 percent, from 244 to 334 utterances might be needed, the range determined by the language being assessed. Clearly the larger the sample, the better. Once you have collected a sufficient body of utterances, transcribe these onto a form such as the one found in Table 4.9. There are several formats available for purchase (Long & Fey, 1991; Miller & Chapman, 1991; Stickler, 1987; Tyack & Gottsleben, 1977). Some schools for the deaf have designed their own formats, but you must always start by gathering a sufficient body of utterances. An utterance is defined as one unit of thought or one unit of communication. For example, if a little child says or signs "Doggie jump," that represents one thought or one unit of communication. However, if an older student says or signs "I do that when I finish," that is one thought or communication unit and is considered a single utterance. If a student makes a sentence break as in "My brother went to store late last night. Buy ice cream," we consider that to be two thought units. Luetke-Stahlman (1988) recommended Bloom and Lahey's (1978) taxonomy of semantic categories as another tool to assess language samples. An additional category that you must apply to a language sample of deaf students is ASL signs, classifiers, facial information, and other nonmanual markers of the language. We suggest that you use two colored pens, one to indicate the English components of the utterance and one to indicate the ASL components of the utterance. Table 4.9 gives an example of how we might complete a language sample on Ashley. Recall that Ashley's skills range across the compound and complex levels. We consulted the charts in Chapters 6 and 7 to complete the form.

After transcribing your student's language sample, you will begin the analysis. You may use one of the systems identified above, or you may examine the utterances from the perspective of available language hierarchies in the areas of morphology and syntax (grammar), vocabulary and semantic cases (meaning), and pragmatics (social application). Determine the stage the student is in (see Table 4.1). Search for examples of language skills within that stage. If you use the form included in this chapter, you need to identify a skill only once. For example, although you may see several subordinate clauses beginning with *until*, you need to identify it only once. Use the hierarchies in later chapters of this book to identify that section of the language maze where the student is beginning to miss skills. These skills will become your IEP objectives. If your student uses ASL, we suggest that you evaluate the sample twice, once to record English skills and once to record ASL skills.

TABLE 4.9 *Language Sampling and Analysis Form*

Child's Name: Ashley
Date:
Transcriber/Evaluator:

CA:

Context	Utterance	Morpho-syntactic forms observed	Categories of semantic meaning observed	Pragmatic category used
Narrating story from picture of boy looking at dog in front of school building.	1. OK. There is a boy name Jack and he have a dog name Jane. 2. and he have a dog name Jane. 3. When he have to go to school, then the dog was following and then 4. when the boy turned (signed LOOK-AT) the dog was moving (CL:3 bent). 5. And he saw the dog (FS-barked). 6. He was so mad because the dog didn't respect the boy.	Articles, t-there, linking verb, attempted passive, SP2, when-clause, quasimodal have-to, if/then clause, attempts at double-verb sentences, classifiers, because clauses, negative contraction, intensifiers	Limited use of descriptive terminology, no derived adjectives, uses basic noun categories and action, stative and process verbs	Micropragmatic rules, narration, third person (dog) perspective

128

Evaluators and Students

Language assessment is conducted in a variety of manners depending upon what school a student is attending. Different people are given the responsibility for this kind of assessment at different times and in different places.

Types of Evaluators

Students are educated and evaluated in many different locations and by a variety of individuals. Schools for the deaf may have a Speech-Language Pathologist (SLP) with a background in deaf education as well as speech/language pathology and who is simultaneously skilled in ASL. This person may do all the speech and language evaluations. Realistically, however, individuals with this level of skill are very rare. More commonly a team of specialists works together to determine the needs of students with special problems; the Teacher of the Deaf serves on the team. Many schools for the deaf have a Diagnostics & Evaluation Team (D & E) whose function it is to do in-depth, diagnostic testing on students referred both from within the school and outside of the school in the case where a local school system lacks expertise. In addition to having the necessary communication skills, D & E team members have expertise and experience in testing this population. D & E team members generally have advanced degrees and advanced assessment skills.

Some larger local school systems have a sufficient number of students to warrant hiring an individual skilled in evaluating the deaf and hard of hearing students. This person may have a background as an SLP, a Teacher of the Deaf, or an Audiologist. Depending upon the job description from the system's central office, she may do all of the evaluations, including academic evaluations, may specialize in one area of evaluation such as language or reading, or may assist the teachers where needed. Quite often, the Teacher of the Deaf evaluates students.

Larger cities may have private clinics and centers that do testing on a contractual or fee-for-services basis. Sometimes these assessment centers are affiliated with private schools for deaf and hard of hearing students, with university programs training Speech-Language Pathologists and Teachers of the Deaf, or are part of a larger diagnostic program.

When deciding who will do an evaluation, consider the different skill levels required. Some tasks might be accomplished by a trained technician such as the paraprofessional or by a parent volunteer. These individuals might be involved, for example, in observing a child for the purpose of filling out an assessment rubric or a checklist. They may help gather language samples, or they may engage the child in an activity while the teacher gathers a language sample. Some tasks might require a teacher or other professional with specific skills. For example, you may need an oral teacher to assess the communication skills of an oral child; a teacher who is skilled in the understanding and use of English-based signs to assess signed English skills; a teacher who is an expert in ASL to assess the communication skills of a child who uses ASL; or a teacher who is an expert in Cued Speech to assess the skills of a child who cues. In some instances it may be appropriate to include the services of an interpreter or transliterator during your evaluation, especially if you are not skilled in the use of signs or cues. You may need to ask a native speaker of Spanish or another foreign language to participate in the evaluation.

There are often times when we must consult individuals with special credentials to conduct parts of the evaluation. These certified examiners have special expertise and credentials that allow them to perform certain tests. For example, the SLP has in-depth knowledge of the kinds of language disorders that may occur in addition to those imposed by the hearing loss. The School Psychologist is trained and credentialed to give certain protected tests such as IQ tests and neuropsychological tests. Although few and far between, there are individuals who have specialized skills in assessing difficult-to-test deaf and hard of hearing children. Given the severity of the language problems involved, their services may be warranted.

We invite you now to meet some real people whose job it is to do real language evaluations on students who are deaf and hard of hearing. We asked them to read the case histories from the previous chapter and to tell you how they would approach an assessment of these students. Meet the evaluators below.

Case Study #1 Laura's Perspective

Laura is a Teacher of the Deaf in her local school system's high school located in a rural area a considerable distance from the nearest city. Laura serves five students, as a resource teacher, interpreter, and on a half-day self-contained service plan. Laura has a B.S. in deaf education, ten years' experience, and intermediate signing skills. Among her duties, Laura evaluates the language of her students. Here are Laura's answers to her interview:

Q: When and for what purpose do you evaluate your students' language skills?

A: There are two of us in my building. I am responsible for all the three-year re-evaluations on the deaf and hard of hearing students. If they are with me, I do some sort of evaluation at the end of each semester. For new students, the deaf and hard of hearing teachers do all the evaluations since the state doesn't require them to have psychologicals.

Q: With whom do you collaborate on the evaluations?

A: I collaborate with the other teacher of the deaf. If possible we get writing samples from the regular education teachers, but the rest is up to us. If a student were to come in whom I couldn't evaluate, I would refer that student to the school psychologist. We would probably consider sending the student up to the school for the deaf for an evaluation by the D & E team.

Q: *About how much of your time is devoted to language assessments?*

A: Usually a lot of time is spent in testing at the beginning of the year, at the end of the semester, and at the end of the year.

Q: *How do you decide on appropriate language objectives for your students' IEPs?*

A: I use their existing IEP, the results of the language testing, and my personal observations from working with them.

Q: *What are some formal language assessment tools that you use routinely?*

A: That depends on the student's age, what language they already have, and whether they will be pulled out or mainstreamed for English. I like the old Test of Syntactic Abilities because it breaks down language into small parts and you can really see what is going on. I use the EOWPVT and the ROW-PVT so I can compare the vocabulary they know with what they might need in the mainstream.

Q: *What is your favorite informal means of gathering and recording information about your students' language needs?*

A: I read their book reports. We have a graded reading bank, so I get them to pick a book then tell me the story in their own words. I also use other books that they are able to read. I ask them to define a word and use it in a sentence. This gives me information about the vocabulary, grammar, and concept awareness as well.

Q: *You read the case of Sissy. If Sissy were to enter your school system tomorrow, what would your assessment plan include?*

A: As far as communication goes, since she's just a little behind normally hearing children, I would want to go into the preschool during center time. I'd do a language-building activity, then see how she compares to her hearing peers. I would also use some basic checklists to gather observational information.

Q: *You also read the case of Kevin. If Kevin were to enter your school system tomorrow, what would your assessment plan include?*

A: I would compare what he can do with English signs and with ASL. I would be most concerned about improving his grammar base, any grammar base. I would try to start using ASL to teach him ESL, but I would also need to work on his basic ASL skills too. I would use the Woodcock-Johnson subtests for writing to see how well he is expressing English since he is such a good reader.

Case Study #2 *Abby's Perspective*

Abby is a Speech-Language Pathologist at a public day school for the deaf located in a large metropolitan area. She has a B.S. in Speech-Language Pathology and an M.S. in Deaf Education. This is her second year in the profession. Here are Abby's answers to her interview:

Q: *When and for what purpose do you evaluate the language skills of students who are deaf and hard of hearing?*

A: I serve about sixty students, maintaining ongoing speech and language records on a daily basis. In addition I do the intake speech and language evaluations and three-year re-evaluations on all students (approximately one hundred seventy). I also assist the classroom teachers in completing their annual evaluations.

Q: *With whom do you collaborate on the evaluations?*

A: I work on a daily basis with a lot of people at the school for the deaf. I collaborate with the D & E team, with other SLPs in the school, and with the classroom teachers.

Q: *About how much of your time is devoted to language assessments?*

A: Approximately twenty percent.

Q: *How do you decide on appropriate language objectives for each student's IEP?*

A: If they have a recent RITLS, I use that. We do language sampling annually and use the information we gather extensively. Sometimes I use information from their written assessments.

Q: *What are some formal language assessment tools that you use routinely?*

A: The RITLS, EOWPVT, ROWPVT, and a language sampling analysis process developed at our school.

Q: *What is your favorite informal means of gathering and recording information about your students' language needs?*

A: I engage students in conversations to get an understanding of what they can convey and understand. I also like to watch their interactions with their peers, record evidence of their developing skills, and compare this to formal measures.

Q: *You read the case of Ashley. If Ashley were to enter your school tomorrow, what would your assessment plan include?*

A: Our assessment plan is pretty standard. We give a pragmatic checklist to the teachers who fill them out as soon as they are comfortable with the student's language. We use the Ling Phonologic and Phonetic assessment, and I give the Mono-syllable Spondee Trochee test—once for speech reading and once for audition. I help the classroom teachers begin gathering a language sample.

Q: *You read the case of Jorge. If Jorge were to enter your school system tomorrow, what would your assessment plan include?*

A: He would be a real challenge because there is no speech to evaluate, and there aren't that many tools available in Spanish that also work for deaf kids. Mostly we would use observations and early language checklists. I had four years of Spanish in high school, so when I recognized a word I would write it down. We had several students like Jorge this past year, and I consulted a lot with our teacher's aide who is Hispanic when communication was questionable.

Q: *You also read the case of Jahan. If Jahan were to enter your school tomorrow, what would your assessment plan include?*

A: I would use the RITLS to see what he does and doesn't have. I would do a written sample because of his age and an oral-versus-signed sample to see what challenges he'd have in the regular classroom. Mostly I would use language sampling because of his advanced grammar. I might want to consider a more advanced standardized test such as the TOAL since he is going to go into the mainstream. I would want to know what he is up against so we could inform his new teachers.

Case Study #3   BJ's Perspective

BJ is an Educational Diagnostician at a school for the deaf. She has a B.S. and M.S. in Deaf Education, an M.S. in School Counseling, and a Ph.D. in special education/learning disabilities. She has thirty-three years of experience as a teacher, university instructor, and diagnostician. The school, where she has worked for the last eighteen years, is located in a large metropolitan area. BJ's primary role is to evaluate students, including language testing, to make recommendations for IEPs and instructional objectives, and to consult with teachers on appropriate ways to meet these objectives. She evaluates students across all academic areas, including language. Here are BJ's answers to her interview:

Q: *When and for what purpose do you evaluate students' language skills?*

A: Whenever a student is referred for any reason we begin with a language assessment.

Q: *With whom do you collaborate on the evaluations?*

A: I collaborate with the classroom teacher on in-house students. When we have an outpatient evaluation we collaborate with the parents, but we can't always observe interactions with the parents of in-house students. We also look at peer-to-peer interactions.

Q: *About how much of your time is devoted to language assessments?*

A: At least seventy to eighty percent of my time is spent in evaluations, and about fifty percent of that is on language per se. If you look at language-related tasks like reading, it is a higher percentage than that. Really, everything is related to language, even math. The only time we are not looking at language is when the school psychologist evaluates nonverbal skills.

Q: *How do you decide on appropriate language objectives for a student's IEPs?*

A: I don't get to do that specifically. The input I give is in designating a level of vocabulary and connected language. The teachers then consult the school's curriculum to decide on specifics.

Q: *What are some formal language assessment tools that you use routinely?*

A: For the deafer students whose language is more limited, we use the RITLS, Assessment of Children's Language Comprehension (ACLC), and Carolina Picture Vocabulary Test (CPVT). We use other tests for students with more English, such as EOWPVT, ROWPVT, and the PPVT. We may also use these with the deafer students if we are trying to make a point of how far below a child is for his age. The language test of choice for us is the Clinical Evaluation of Language Functions-III (CELF-III) when we want to assess the skills required in the mainstream. Unfortunately there are no tests of ASL that I know of.

Q: *What is your favorite informal means of gathering and recording information about your students' language needs?*

A: I get the most from observing them in their own classroom when there is an activity involving teacher and student interactions. That's when they are communicating the most naturally. That's when I see things I never see in the testing situation, both good and bad.

Q: *You read the case of Jonathan. If he were to enter your school tomorrow, what would your assessment plan include?*

A: I would try to use standardized tests comparing him to hearing kids. The tests for the less capable kids wouldn't give me enough specific information. I would look at his connected language and vocabulary and how his understanding of language relates to reading. I would need to collaborate with somebody who knows ASL so I wouldn't miss anything. I assume that ASL is his normal, natural language. I would expect that language to be comparable to the language of the same-aged hearing peers. I would expect his reading of English might be better than his through-the-air language. He'd be fun!

Q: *You also read the case of Colton. If Colton were to enter your school system tomorrow, what would your assessment plan include?*

A: Colton is more like the students I usually see. I would probably start by comparing his English to other hearing impaired children his age. I would try to get an informal assessment of his developing ASL skills. It would be very important to look at the relationship between language and literature. I would include observations and a written and oral language sample. Unfortunately there are no tests to evaluate language learning disabilities in these students. I would have to get some basic information and that would help me decide what to do next, which usually would be to formulate an informal task. Half the time we are inventing tasks to look at specific language issues.

Q: *You also read the case of Martin. If you were asked to assess Martin's communication skills, what would your plan be?*

A: I think it would look a lot like the one for Colton. You start out with the basics for all kids then modify for their individual needs. Since he has problems with testing we might watch carefully the length of each session. We might also try to test him in ways that he would be unaware of within the limits of the test. Martin by far has the most significant problems. He lost so much prime time. With him particularly I would try to consult with the SLP. He might require the use of a lot of informal measures.

Case Study #4   Susan's Perspective

Susan is an elementary teacher in her local school system. The school system is located in a rapidly growing rural area outside a large city. She has an M.S. in Deaf Education and has taught for many years. Her signing skills are rated as advanced. Her job involves a combination of self-contained and resource students. She spends about 10 percent of her time evaluating the language of students who are deaf and hard of hearing in addition to the running records she keeps on a daily basis. Susan evaluates, makes recommendations for services to the IEP committees, and collaborates with the classroom teachers. Here are Susan's answers to her interview:

Q: *When and for what purpose do you evaluate the language skills of the students in your school who are deaf or hard of hearing?*

A: I evaluate the language of my students all the time. There isn't much time that goes by that I'm not thinking what they are doing, what I am doing, and whether we have a good mix. Formally, however, I am responsible for new students entering the school, for three-year re-evaluations of my students, for benchmark assessments at the end of the grading period, and for end-of-the-year documentation of their successes.

Q: *With whom do you collaborate on the evaluations?*

A: I collaborate with the other Teacher of the Deaf in my building, with my principal, with the parents of my students. I work routinely with the regular education teachers and the hearing students in the classes where my students are mainstreamed.

Q: *How do you decide on appropriate language objectives for student recommendations?*

A: The decision is made by the IEP committee based on lots of input from multiple individuals, including the parents, and on tons and tons of data and records. I am a firm believer in ongoing assessment.

Q: *What are some formal language assessment tools that you use routinely?*

A: That depends on the child. I have been known to use the Sequenced Inventory of Communication Development (SICD), Preschool Language Assessment Inventory (PLAI), CELF-R, RITLS, OWLS, PPVT-R, and just about anything I can get my hands on if it works with a particular student. For the cochlear implant kids I use checklists from some of the books on Auditory-Verbal therapy. For the hard of hearing kids or other kids who are using sign-supported speech and are primarily English users, I use all the above. For my ASL users, a Deaf friend comes in once a month to read to all my students. I have her spend extra time with the Deaf student. She tells me if she thinks the student is more like her own Deaf three-year-old or her five-year-old or better or worse. I do a lot of PR with my school regarding the importance of ASL.

Q: *What is your favorite informal means of gathering and recording information about the students' language needs?*

A: I love to read to kids. I act the story out, read it, sign it. We dress up and act it out. Then I get the students on videotape telling the story to someone else. It is a real eye-opener to see how much they have grasped, even with limited communication skills. They almost always get the gist of the story, and I can use what they give me on the tape to compare it to developmental checklists. I have made up some of my own checklists for basic skills in ASL. I wish someone would publish a really good ASL test.

Q: *You read the case of Mercedes. If she were to enter your school system tomorrow, what would your assessment plan include?*

A: With an eighth-grade reading level, I would use all the tests that the regular education folks use. I might use the OWLS or the CELF-R, but I wouldn't really need that much of a diagnostic nature since she is doing so well. Mostly I would be concerned with her written language and would use my state's assessment rubric for the eighth-grade assessment to see how she was doing.

Q: *You also read the case of LaShawndra. If LaShawndra were to enter your school system tomorrow, what would your assessment plan include?*

A: Since I would only see her for consultation, I would develop my assessment around what is happening in the regular classroom. I would use standardized language tests and I would do some curriculum-based assessments. I would need to work with the teacher so she or he was aware of any problems with some of the more difficult language that LaShawndra might face.

Q: *You also read the case of Montel. If Montel were to enter your school system tomorrow, what would your assessment plan include?*

A: I would use the Kaufmann Scales of Early Development, the kindergarten skills checklist from my school, the Boehm, etc., but those are where I would start with language. I would use my ASL checklist and would also probably try to work with the parent to move toward the use of ASL.

Choosing a Battery of Tests and Other Assessment Procedures

The first step in an evaluation is to narrow down the areas of language that you want to evaluate. Next, you will choose a battery of tests and testing procedures to meet your particular needs based on your reason for testing, what you are testing, and the functional age of the child. The functional age is the age at which a child is performing, not his or her chronological age (Thompson, Biro, Vethivelu, Pious, & Hatfield, 1987, p. 52). It is very important to keep this notion of functional age in mind with students who are deaf and hard of hearing because their current levels of performance are often well below that of children with normal hearing. A battery may contain formal and/or informal measures. Consider all of a test or parts of a test.

Designing an Assessment Plan

Table 4.10 provides an Assessment Planning Form with which to organize assessment. As you read through this next section, follow along on the table. If you are a new teacher or parent, or if you are uncomfortable with the assessment process, you will need to collaborate with one or more individuals who can help you work through this plan. A collaborative team might include such individuals as the parents, the teacher of the deaf and hard of hearing, the SLP, the ASL linguistic specialist, and the teacher of students with learning disabilities.

The first decision the team should make is the reason for assessment. Is the evaluee a new student, are you evaluating to develop or change the IEP, are you evaluating to monitor benchmarks, or are you doing end-of-year assessment? Sometimes we suspect an additional language disorder and need to develop a diagnostic assessment plan. Other times we are looking at the mismatch between the student's present linguistic skills and the linguistic demands of the classroom or lesson. Next, determine which skills are the target of study. Are you looking at English, ASL, Spanish, another language, or a combination thereof? Determine whether or not you have sufficient expertise on your team to choose and perform the assessments.

Next, decide who should be involved in the assessment process. Consider

TABLE 4.10 *Assessment Planning Form*

Student's Name:
Date of Birth:
Date of Test:

Languages to be Assessed: English, ASL, Other

Examiner(s):

Circle Reason for Assessment	*Circle Evaluator Skills*	*Circle Grammatical Stage*	*Circle Meaning Stage*	*Circle Stage of Intention*
New student	Technician	Pre-grammatical One- and two-word utterances	Simple word meanings and lexical tallies	Performatives
Program decisions/IEP	Skilled teacher: Oral skills English sign skills	Noninflected three- to four-word utterances	Multiple meanings and simple idiomatic expressions	Pragmatic intentions and purposes Social uses
Re-evaluation: Benchmarks End of year	American Sign Language	Simple sentence forms and traits Compound sentence forms and traits	Verb idioms and figurative expressions	Discourse and later purposes
Diagnostic	Interpreter	Complex sentence forms and traits Early clauses Later clauses	Metalinguistic skills Giving definitions Categorization Word analysis	
Classroom/lesson analysis	Other (specify)_____ Certified examiner: SLP School psychologist	Compound-complex sentences		

List Tests you Will Use:

using a technician such as a paraprofessional or a parent volunteer. Decide if your teachers have the necessary skills to evaluate spoken English, signed English, ASL, Cued Speech, or another foreign language. Decide if an interpreter or transliterator should assist you or if you need an evaluator who is skilled with the languages and modes above. If you do not have the necessary expertise or if you are considering the use of protected tests, call upon the services of other individuals in the system with special expertise and certification. If you need outside assistance, contact the appropriate administrator to locate and contract with an outside expert. The school for the deaf is usually a valuable resource. This is most important when doing an initial evaluation on a new student or when evaluating a student who is not making sufficient progress.

Finally, decide what stage of language a child is in, what aspects of that stage need to be evaluated, and what tests and procedures would be most helpful in gathering the kind of information you need. Consider evaluating the areas of grammar (morphology and syntax), meaning (semantics), and intent or purpose (pragmatics).

A Closer Look at Services and Placement

Earlier in this chapter we expressed concern over the lack of care with which we monitor a student's rate of progress. This results in poor outcomes. For example, over 500 students who are deaf and hard of hearing and were 14 years of age or older dropped out of U.S. schools during the 1996–97 school year (U.S. Department of Education, 1999). In regular education, as a rule of thumb, we do not worry about hearing children if they are satisfactorily passing (i.e., with C averages) from one grade to another. However, many students with hearing losses are socially promoted or are promoted based on "passing" the objectives in their IEPs. These are often written to ensure success, so a measuring stick by which we determine adequate progress does not exist. In its place we deferred to the wishes of the IEP team. Some sort of standard needs to be applied rigorously and routinely with all children who have hearing losses. We challenge researchers to identify an appropriate standard for communication and academic progress. Nelson (1998) stated that we should accept no less than the same degree of progress we expect in hearing children. In the absence of research and theory, we propose that educators reevaluate teaching/learning interactions when students' profiles contain the indicators listed in Table 4.11. Schirmer (1985) demonstrated that the language of children who are deaf and hard of hearing is delayed, not deviant. This being the case, then all children should make *some* progress, and that progress should follow the normal developmental sequence. Normally developing hearing children exhibit as much as a six-month gap among various language processes (Muma, 1998), so gaps greater than these among any given student's language processes should give us concern. In the absence or serious delay of progress, or if areas of language show unusual developmental patterns, we need to be concerned.

TABLE 4.11 *Evaluation of Present Placement and Mode*

Name: CA:
Current Placement: IQ:
                           MA:

Check each item that applies to student being evaluated.

1. Current placement or reading comprehension scores are greater   1 pt _____
   than one year below MA.
2. Current placement or reading comprehension scores are greater   1 pt _____
   than two years below MA.
   (Earns point in addition to point for #1.)
3. Did not meet reading IEP objectives first time around.   1 pt _____
4. Did not meet overall IEP objectives first time around.   1 pt _____
5. Additional learning problems suspected or documented.   1 pt _____
6. Age/grade equivalent remained the same or standard score went   1 pt _____
   down on standardized test after a year of instruction.
7. Age/grade equivalent and standard scores went down after a year   1 pt _____
   of instruction. (Earns point in addition to point for #6.)
8. Did not receive intervention services prior to age three.   1 pt _____
9. Is not developing language skills over time as indicated by   1 pt _____
   progress through various linguistic sequences (e.g., negation
   sequence, question sequence).
10. Is not forming social groups or is not communicating with peers.   1 pt _____

                                                      Total:

Total equals 1 to 3 points: Increase services in current placement.
Total equals 4 to 6 points: Consider other placement/communication mode options.
Total equals 7 or greater points: Unlikely that student will make reasonable progress in
     present placement and communication mode. Seek other options.

Language Development versus Language Disorders

Little is known about the interactions between the language problems imposed by a hearing loss and the problems related to additional language disorders a child might have even in the presence of normal hearing. One is an issue of development, the other an issue of disability. We can document language disorders in hearing children, and just about everyone can point to a deaf or hard of hearing child whom he or she "just knows for sure" has a language problem. However, there is little to guide us in making a clear diagnosis. This kind of evaluation requires a highly skilled examiner who is experienced with the deaf and hard of hearing population, with appropriate modifications to tests, and with hypothesis testing.

Many hearing students with additional learning disorders exhibit problems with thinking and reasoning that interfere with the ability to learn and use language. In particular, students with language disorders have difficulty on tests that assess memory, attention, word retrieval (a memory function), and sequencing. If a hearing student's cognitive processes are associated with language and learning disorders, then the thought processes of a deaf or hard of hearing student must be similarly influenced. In order to understand the nature of language disorders not associated with a hearing loss, we need to understand the fundamental interactions between cognition (thinking) and language. Various syndromes, acquired brain injuries, aphasia-like symptoms, and illnesses influencing the brain such as encephalitis and meningitis can cause language impairments in children with normal hearing, so we must consider them as possible causes of language impairments in children who are deaf and hard of hearing. Language disorder traits can occur across the categories of phonology, morphology, syntax, semantics, and pragmatics. Collaboration is essential in learning how to handle these kinds of problems.

Summary

The purpose of this chapter was to provide an overview of why we test, what we test, how we test, and who does the testing. A daunting task to begin with, language assessment is even more challenging when a student has a hearing loss. The communication skills of children who are deaf and hard of hearing are perhaps the most difficult of all areas to evaluate. On the one hand, many students have trouble with everything. On the other hand, we cannot teach everything in one year. We need to narrow down the areas upon which we should focus. This chapter provided a format for organizing assessment as well as several tools to apply in the classroom. Collaboration with others is an essential component to a successful language evaluation.

Questions For Critical Thinking _____

1. Compare and contrast the assessment process you would follow for Jahan and Sissy, for Colton and Kevin, or for Ashley and Montel. What are the similarities and differences?

2. When completing a language analysis sample, what are the benefits of identifying present skills versus identifying errors?

3. How would you establish a collaborative community of support both inside and outside your particular school system? What are the benefits of such a support group? How would this impact assessment?

Appendix A
Available Tests

Title, Author, Publisher	Type/Scores	Norms/Target Population	Description
Assessing Semantics Skills Through Everyday Themes (ASSET) Barrett, Zachman, Huisingh 1988 LinguiSystems East Moline, IL	Norm-referenced Age equivalents Standard scores Percentiles	Norms: hearing Population: hearing Target: 3:0 to 9:11	Semantics; vocabulary Responses are elicited by questions or directions from the examiner, referring to illustrations in the picture stimuli book. Receptive tasks require the subject to make picture-pointing responses. Expressive tasks require a verbal response using language to include labeling, making comparisons, describing, and defining.
Assessment of Children's Language Comprehension Foster, Gidden, and Stark 1972 Consulting Psych. Press, Inc. 577 College Avenue Palo Alto, CA 94306	Norm-referenced Percentiles	Norms: hearing Population: hearing Target: 3 to 6:6	Vocabulary The test stimuli are arranged on a series of 40 plates with each plate containing 4 or 5 picture stimuli. The child "points to" or "shows" the picture corresponding to the verbal stimulus.
Bilingual Syntax Measure I and II (BSM) Burt, Dudley, and Chavez—I Above with Taleporos—II 1978—I/1980—II The Psychological Corp. San Antonio, TX	Criterion-referenced	Norms: hearing Population: hearing Target: K–12 (I); 3–12 (II)	Measures oral language proficiency; oral syntax in Spanish and English Proficiency level: (1) responds to minimum number of questions, (2) number of grammatically correct responses, (3) number of correct responses to specific questions. Series of multicolored, cartoon-like pictures. Twenty-five test questions that correspond to specific pictures. Some questions require examiner to point to specific aspects of the pictures as questions are asked. Examiner writes the student's responses verbatim.

Test	Type	Norms/Population/Target	Description
Boehm Test of Basic Concepts-Revised (BTBC-R) Boehm, A. The Psychological Corp. San Antonio, TX	Norm-referenced Percentiles	Norms: hearing Population: hearing Target: K, 1, 2	Concepts Students mark an "X" on the test booklet in response to the instructions of the examiner, such as, "Look at the toys. Mark the toy that is next to the truck." Test may also be used with older hearing-impaired children as a criterion-referenced instrument.
Boehm Test of Basic Concepts-Preschool Version Boehm, A. 1986 The Psychological Corp. San Antonio, TX	Norm-referenced Percentiles, t-scores	Norms: hearing Population: hearing Target: 3:0 to 5:11	Relational concepts The child is presented a picture paired with the verbal stimulus and required to point to the correct concept target.
Bracken Basic Concept Scale Bracken, A. 1984 Charles E. Merrill Pub. Co. 1300 Alum Creek Drive Columbus, OH 43216	Norm-referenced Age equivalents Percentiles	Norms: hearing Population: hearing Target: 2:6 to 8 years	Color, letter identification, numbers/counting, comparisons, shapes, etc. The child is shown a plate with four stimulus pictures and is instructed to "show me _____" or "point to _____."
Brigance Inventory of Early Development-Revised Albert H. Brigance 1991	Criterion-referenced raw scores	Norms: none Population: hearing Target: birth to 7	Perambulatory-motor, gross-motor, fine-motor, self-help, speech and language, general knowledge and comprehension, social and emotional development, readiness, basic reading, manuscript writing, basic math Easily administered by aides, volunteers, or tutors. Record book profiles assessments administered, responses, skills recently mastered, and objectives; record books help monitor classes; response formats vary: on the phonics portion the student is given a letter (written) and

(continued)

APPENDIX A *Continued*

Title, Author, Publisher	Type/Scores	Norms/Target Population	Description
			is told to find a picture of an object that starts with the sound the letter makes.
Carolina Picture Vocabulary Test (CPVT) Layton, T.L. and Holmes, D.W. 1985 Pro-Ed Austin, TX	Norm-referenced Age equivalents Percentiles	Norms: deaf Population: deaf Target: 4:0 to 11:6	Receptive sign vocabulary Picture book contains 130 numbered test plates with four black-and-white line-drawn pictures per plate. The examiner signs stimuli to the child. The child points to the corresponding line drawing.
Comprehensive Receptive and Expressive Vocabulary Test (CREVT) Gerald Wallace and Donald Hammill 1994	Norm-referenced Age equivalents Standard scores Percentiles	Norms: hearing Population: hearing Target: Receptive: 4:0 to 17:11 Expressive: 5:0 to 17:11	Oral vocabulary Picture identification and word definition
Expressive One Word Picture Vocabulary Test Gardner, M.F. 1981 Academic Therapy Pub. 20 Commercial Boulevard Novato, CA 94947	Norm-referenced Age equivalents Percentiles	Norms: hearing Population: hearing Target: 2 to 12½	Vocabulary The child looks at a series of pictures, one per plate, and is asked to tell the examiner the "names of things" in the pictures. The test ends on six consecutive incorrect responses.

Test	Type	Norms	Description
Grammatical Analysis of Elicited Language Moog, J.S. and Geers, A.E. 1979 Central Institute for the Deaf 818 So. Euclid St. Louis, MO 63110	Norm-referenced Percentiles	Norms: hearing/oral hearing-impaired Population: deaf and hard of hearing Target: three language ranges	Syntax The examiner models specified sentence structures and the child is prompted to produce the same structured utterances.
Interpersonal Language Skills Assessment Blagden and McConnell 1985 LinguiSystems, Inc. Moline, IL	Norm-referenced Standard scores Percentiles	Norms: hearing Population: hearing Target: 8 to 14	Use of social language skills The examiner obtains an expressive language sample while observing 3–4 students playing a table game for approx. 15–30 min.
Language Processing Test-Revised (LPT-R) Richard, G.J. and Haner, M.A. 1995 Pro-Ed Austin, TX	Norm-referenced Age equivalents Standard scores Percentiles, raw score	Norms: hearing Population: hearing Target: 5 to 11	Language processing deficits Verbal responses to questions such as "What do you do with _____?" The child must also verbalize the likeness and differences among specific stimuli.
Maryland Syntax Evaluation Instrument White, A.E. 1981 Support System for the Deaf Box 428 Sanger, TX 76266	Norm-referenced	Norms: deaf Population: deaf Target: 6 to 11:11	Syntax Scoring is complicated; instead of scoring errors, the examiner gives credit for what the child knows about syntax. Children are given a colored filmstrip with ten pictures. They write one sentence per picture. Young children may respond using speech or signs.

(continued)

Title, Author, Publisher	Type/Scores	Norms/Target Population	Description
Northwestern Syntax Screening Test Lee, L.L. 1971 Northwestern University Press 1831 Hinman Ave. Evanston, IL 60201	Norm-referenced Percentiles	Norms: hearing Population: hearing Target: 3 to 8	Syntax The child is given two to four pictures, and after the examiner reads a sentence, the child points (receptive). For expressive, the child produces a sentence for two pictures after the examiner first produces the sentence.
Oral and Written Language Scales (OWLS): Listening Comp and Oral Exp. Carrow-Woolfolk, E. 1994 AGS Circle Pines, MN	Norm-referenced Percentiles Test-age equivalent, stanine, normal curve equivalent	Norms: hearing Population: hearing Target: 3 to 21:11	Higher order thinking, semantics, syntax, vocabulary, pragmatics Picture pointing (listening comp. scale), answering questions, and sentence completion (oral exp. scale)
Peabody Picture Vocabulary Test-Revised Dunn 1981 American Guidance Service Publisher's Building Circle Pines, NM 55014	Norm-referenced Age equivalents Standard scores Percentiles	Norms: hearing Population: hearing Target: $2^1/_2$ to 40	Receptive vocabulary The subject's task is to select the picture which best illustrates the meaning of the stimulus word presented by the examiner.

Test	Type / Scores	Norms / Population / Target	Skills
Preschool Language Assessment Instrument (PLAI) Blank, Rose, and Berlin, 1978 Grune and Stratton, Inc. Orlando, FL	Norm-referenced Age equivalents Percentiles	Norms: hearing Population: hearing Target: 3 to 6	Discourse skills The examiner shows the child one test plate at a time and asks questions related to the picture stimulus. Verbal responses are usually required.
Rhode Island Test of Language Structures Engen, E. and Engen T. 1983 Pro-Ed Austin, TX	Norm-referenced Percentiles	Norms: deaf and hearing Population: deaf and hearing Target: 5 to 17+	Morphology, syntax The child selects the picture which describes the sentence the examiner read, given three pictures from which to choose.
Ski-HI Receptive Language Test Longhurst, Briery, and Emery 1975 Project SKI-HI, Dept. of Communication Disorders Utah State University Logan, UT 84322	Criterion-referenced Percentiles Percent correct	Norms: none Population: deaf Target: 3 to 6½	Vocabulary The child is required to point to the picture corresponding to the word, phrase, or sentence read by the examiner.
Ski-HI Language Development Scale Tonelson and Watkins 1979 Project SKI-HI, Dept. of Communication Disorders Utah State University	Criterion-referenced Age equivalents Checklist	Norms: none Population: deaf Target: 0 to 5	Communication behaviors The LDS is developmentally ordered and contains a list of communication and language skills in varying intervals for different ages. Each age interval is represented by enough observable receptive and expressive language skills to obtain a good profile of a child's language ability.

(continued)

Title, Author, Publisher	Type/Scores	Norms/Target Population	Description
Test of Auditory Compre-hension of Language-Revised Carrow-Woolfolk 1985 DLM Teaching Resources P.O. Box 4000, 1 DLM Park Allen, TX 75002	Norm-referenced Age equivalents Standard scores Percentiles (by age group)	Norms: hearing Population: hearing Target: 3 to 10	Morphology, syntax The child points to the correct picture in the test booklet in response to the examiner's verbal stimuli.
The Word Test-Revised (Elementary) Huisingh, Barrett, Zackman, Blagden, and Orman 1990 LinguiSystems East Moline, IL	Norm-referenced Age equivalents Standard scores Percentiles	Norms: hearing Population: hearing Target: 7 to 12	Semantics, vocabulary Procedures vary based on which subtest is being evaluated.
Receptive One Word Pic-ture Vocabulary Test Gardner 1985 Academic Therapy Pub. 20 Commercial Boulevard, Navato, CA 94947	Norm-referenced Age equivalents Language standard scores Percentiles	Norms: hearing Population: hearing Target: 2 to 12	Vocabulary The examiner provides a stimulus word that depicts one of four pictures the child sees on a page. The child is re-quired to identify the picture that illustrates the stimulus word.

Receptive-Expressive Emergent Language Test (REEL-2) Bzoch and League 1991 Pro-Ed Austin, TX	Criterion-referenced Age equivalents	Criterion: hearing Population: hearing Target: up to 3	Receptive and expressive language Uses observable information reported by parents or guardians to identify major receptive and expressive language problems in young children. The examiner's manual provides examples of questions to elicit information about each item on the scale.
Teacher Assessment of Grammatical Structures *Moog and Kozak* 1983 Central Institute for the Deaf 818 So. Euclid St. Louis, MO 63110	Criterion-referenced Checklist Age equivalents	Norms: none Population: hearing-impaired children who use spoken and/or signed English Target: 0 to 9	Morphology, syntax, semantics Teacher observes students in natural situations and notes various language skills as they emerge and/or are mastered.
Teacher Assessment of Spoken Language (TASL) Moog and Biedenstein 1998 The Moog Oral School St. Louis, MO	Criterion-referenced	Target: all ages Norms: none Population: hearing and deaf	Syntax Based on teacher's experience with the particular child or that child compared with other children in the teacher's experience. Children are observed by their teacher over a period of several days or weeks. The teacher focuses on sentence structure and syntactic elements. Ratings are based on actual observation of the child while he/she is communicating.

(continued)

Title, Author, Publisher	Type/Scores	Norms/Target Population	Description
Test for Examining Expressive Morphology Shipley, Stone, and Sue 1983 Communication Skill Builders 3130 N. Dodge Blvd., P.O. Box 42050 Tucson, AZ 85733	Norm-referenced Age equivalents	Norms: hearing Population: hearing Target: 3 to 8	Morphology The examiner shows the child a picture(s) and provides partial information about it. The child is then required to complete a sentence about the picture(s).
Test of Adolescent and Adult Language–Third Edition (TOAL-3) Hammill, Brown, Larson, and Wiederhold 1994	Norm-referenced Standard scores Percentiles, raw scores, composite scores	Norms: hearing Population: hearing Target: 12:0 to 24:11	Syntax, vocabulary Pointing, speaking, reading, and writing
Test of Early Language Development (TELD-2) Hresko, Reid, and Hammill 1991 Pro-Ed Austin, TX	Norm-referenced Percentiles Language age Language quotient Normal curve equivalents	Norms: hearing Population: hearing Target: 2:0 to 7:11	Syntax, semantics Naming responses, picture pointing, gestures, following directions, and conversational speech.

Test of Expressive Language Ability (TEXLA) Bunch 1981 G.B. Services, Ltd. 100 Waterton Rd, Weston Ontario, Canada M9P2R3	Norm-referenced Age equivalent Standard scores Percentiles	Norms: deaf Population: deaf Target: 7 to 12	Morphology, syntax An illustration is presented with one or two written sentences describing it. One sentence is incomplete. The student must complete the sentences by writing an appropriate response.
Test of Language Development PI—Second Edition (TOLD-P:2) Newcomer, and Hammill 1988 Pro-Ed Austin, TX	Norm-referenced Standard scores Percentiles	Norms: hearing Population: hearing Target: 4:0 to 8:11	Morphology, semantics, syntax, vocabulary Picture pointing, word definition, sentence repetition, sentence completion, discriminating two words as "same" or "different," and picture naming.
Test of Pragmatic Skills-Revised Shulman 1986 Communication Skill Builders/ The Psychological Corp. San Antonio, TX	Norm-referenced Percentiles Mean composite score, raw score	Norms: hearing Population: hearing Target: 3:0 to 8:11	Use of language to signify conversational intent Conversation/role-playing in each of four context: (1) playing with puppets; (2) playing with pencil and sheet of paper; (3) playing with telephones; and (4) playing with blocks. Each task is presented in numerical sequence.

(continued)

APPENDIX A *Continued*

Title, Author, Publisher	Type/Scores	Norms/Target Population	Description
Test of Problem Solving-Elementary-Revised Zachman, Huisingh, Barrett, J. Orman, and LoGiudice 1994 LinguiSystems East Moline, IL	Norm-referenced Age equivalents Standard scores Percentiles	Norms: hearing Population: hearing Target: 6 to 12 years	Critical thinking ability The student responds verbally to spoken questions from the examiner dealing with common occurrences depicted in fourteen illustrations.
Test of Receptive Language Ability (TERLA) Bunch 1981 G.B. Services 10 Pinehill Cresent, Toronto Ontario MGM 2B6, Canada	Norm-referenced Criterion-referenced Age equivalents Standard scores Percentiles	Norms: deaf Population: deaf Target: 7 to 12	Morphology, syntax The test administrator reads a single printed word or verb phrase for each item; each item is accompanied by the written word or phrase and three illustrations. The child selects the illustration that best represents the printed word or phrase.
Test of Syntactic Abilities Quigley, Steinkampf, Power, and Jones 1982 Pro-Ed Austin, TX	Norm-referenced Age equivalents Percentiles	Norms: deaf Population: deaf Target: 10 to 18:11	Syntax Tests items are written in a multiple-choice format; the student marks his/her choice in a test booklet.

Test			
Test of Word Finding (TWF) German 1986 Pro-Ed Austin, TX	Norm-referenced Standard scores Percentiles Comprehensive score, range of confidence	Norms: hearing Population: hearing Target: 6:6 to 12:11	Word finding skills, semantics Picture naming, sentence completion, and description naming
Test of Word Finding in Discourse (TWFD) German 1991 Pro-Ed Austin, TX	Norm-referenced Standard scores Percentiles	Norms: hearing Population: hearing Target: 6:6 to 12:11	Word finding skills in discourse Picture description and storytelling
Test of Word Knowledge (TOWK) Wiig and Secord 1992 The Psychological Corp. San Antonio, TX	Norm-referenced Criterion-referenced Age equivalents Standard scores Percentiles Stanines	Norms: hearing Population: hearing Target: 5:0 to 17:11	Semantics Picture naming, picture describing, picture pointing, word finding, using synonyms and multiple meanings, describing use of idioms, conjunctions, and transition words
Total Communication Receptive Vocabulary Test Scherer 1981 Mental Health and Deafness Resources, Inc. P.O. Box 1083 Northbrook, IL 60006	Norm-referenced Age equivalents	Norms: deaf and hearing Population: deaf Target: 3 to 6	Vocabulary The student indicates the correct picture after being given the directions, "show me _____." Test consists of seventy-five test plates (four pictures per plate).

(continued)

Title, Author, Publisher	Type/Scores	Norms/Target Population	Description
Word Finding Referral Checklist (WFRC) German and German 1993 Pro-Ed Austin, TX	Checklist	Population: hearing Target: elementary, middle, and secondary students	General understanding of language, word finding skills in single-word retrieval contexts, and word-finding skills in discourse. Provides specific language behaviors that screen for word finding difficulties in single-word retrieval contexts and in discourse. Doubles as a guide to inservice classroom teachers in the area of child word finding.
Wiig Criterion-Referenced Inventory of Language (Wiig CRIL) Wiig 1990 The Psychological Corp. San Antonio, TX	Criterion-referenced Percentiles	Population: children with language impairments	Morphology, semantics, syntax, pragmatics The examiner administers probes only for structures/concepts thought to be in question following in-depth language testing. Response: picture naming, sentence completion, parallel production, and elicitation.
Woodcock Language Proficiency Battery-Revised (WLPB-R) Woodcock 1991 Riverside Publishing Company Itasca, IL	Norm-referenced Raw scores Age equivalents Grade-equivalents Standard scores Percentiles Relative mastery indexes	Norms: hearing Population: hearing Target: 2 to 90+	Reading comp, language comp, cipher knowledge, morphology, semantics, vocabulary Test procedures vary depending on which subtest is being administered.

Appendix B

Instructions for Using Checklist of Emerging ASL Skills

The *Checklist of Emerging ASL Skills* (see p. 114) provides a series of indicators to judge whether a deaf child has components of ASL in his or her communication system. Do not attempt to judge skills based on student's English ability. Focus only on ASL. This list should be filled out by at least three different evaluators. Evaluators should be familiar with the child and should themselves have skill in American Sign Language.

Read each indicator, then check the category that best describes this student's ASL skills *relative to other students you know who have the same degree of hearing loss and are of the same age.* This requires that the evaluator have experience both with ASL and with students in the same age group as those being evaluated.

Rate all Items

Rate each item.

"Not observed/Immature" means that you have not seen the student use this skill or that the student confuses this skill with another most of the time.

"Emerging" means that you have seen the student attempt this skill, but the attempt is erroneous at least 50 percent of the time.

"Functional Use" means that you have seen this skill used correctly better than 50 percent of the time, and the student is able to use it to meet his needs.

"Mature Use" means that you have seen this skill used correctly most of the time in at least two different environments.

Provide Descriptions and Ratings

Some questions in the checklist ask you to give examples. Please give as many as possible. Always give at least one example. Where an example is given, provide a rating of that language skill as well. Rate all skills.

Rating the Phonology Section

Use the descriptors below to determine which handshapes the student uses meaningfully in appropriate contexts.

"Compact" refers to signs made with no fingers extended.

"Concave" refers to signs made with at least two bent fingers.

"Index" refers to signs made with all fingers except the index closed.

"Touch" refers to signs made with one or more fingertips contacting the thumb.

"Broad" refers to signs made with three or more fingers extended.

"Full" refers to signs made with all four fingers extended.

"Radial" refers to signs made with at least the thumb extended.

"Ulnar" refers to signs made with at least the pinky extended.

"Dual" refers to signs made with only two fingers extended.

Stage 1: A S L BO 5 C G*

The student in this stage substitutes these handshapes for those required in later stages, for example, substitutes 5-handshape for F-handshape to make sign for *cat*. *BO refers to the baby form of O.

Stage 2: B F O

The student in this stage substitutes these or earlier handshapes for those in stage three and four, for example, substitutes B- or A-handshape for 3-handshape of classifiers for vehicles.

Stage 3: I D Y P 3 V H W

The student in this stage substitutes these or earlier handshapes for those in stage four, for example, substitutes H-handshape for R-handshape in sign for *restaurant*.

Stage 4: *8 7 X R T M N* ———————————————————

The student in this stage uses all handshapes appropriately.

Note ————————————————————————————

It is not sufficient to have the child imitate your production of the alphabet and the numbers. You must observe these handshapes appropriately used in specific signs.

5

From Theory to Practice

What to Expect in This Chapter _____

In this chapter you will read about the methods, approaches, and practices that are used to teach students who are deaf and hard of hearing to communicate. You will see that there are many different ways to teach the same skill.

Throughout this book we have built the case that there are multiple languages to learn, multiple ways to learn and use them, and multiple factors that can confound the language-learning process. We begin this chapter with a discussion of pragmatic intent, which is the reason why we communicate in the first place. Everything that we say or sign has an inherent motivation behind it. That motivation is either to understand another's intention or to make our own intentions understood. Muma (1998) refers to this as the *centrality of intent;* it is at the core of why we communicate. In this chapter we show you how to present language skills from various perspectives, but these should always be couched within pragmatics. We describe three instructional contact points where the teacher or parent might work with children: *learning a first language, learning about language, and learning via language.* We also present a variety of approaches, practices, and techniques that facilitate language learning. Remember as you read this chapter that there are many ways to teach the same skill, so any examples discussed here are not necessarily definitive.

Pragmatic Intent: The Heart and Soul of Language Learning

The study of pragmatic intent is a relatively new field that places linguistics within a social context (Mey, 1998a). Little research has been conducted relative to deaf and hard of hearing students and pragmatic intent, but pragmatic

158

intent in spoken languages has common features that cut across all languages, whether signed or spoken. In addition there is some variation from language to language because pragmatics is greatly influenced by culture. Mey defines pragmatics as the "study of language in a human context" (p. 724) and "from the user point of view, where the individual components of such a study are joined in a common, societal perspective" (p. 725). Early pragmaticians (Austin, 1962; Grice, 1975) talked about "the speech act" and its social implications. More recently, theorists have recognized that communication is not limited to speech and are using instead the terms *language act* or *communication act* to refer to an act of communication that occurs between communicators (interlocution) or within a communicator (intralocution) for some social purpose. Communication occurs in manners other than spoken or signed languages. We communicate through gestures, body language, vocalizations, looks, signs, symbols, and other codes (e.g, Morse Code). These acts of communication are all used to serve pragmatic intent. Figure 5.1 demonstrates the relationship of communication, language, speech, sign, and other means of expression.

FRAME OF REFERENCE: THE COMMUNICATOR

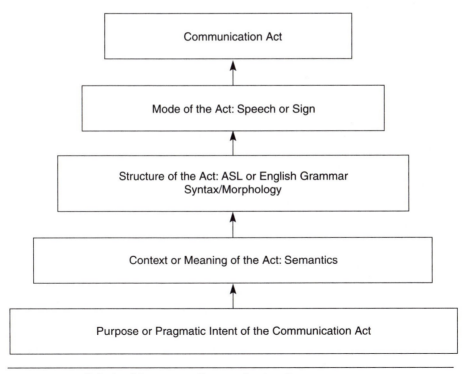

FIGURE 5.1 *Relationships among Communication Components*

Pragmatic skills ensure common understanding of a language act. Mey (1998b) stated that "in daily life, the usual, unfortunate situation is that one person does not understand what the other is saying, not because the words are unclear or the phrasing ambiguous, but simply because the one interlocutor does not grasp what the other is talking about, or because she or he interprets that which the other is talking about as something entirely different" (pp. 701–702). A successful communicator measures the situation and speaks accordingly, situating his or her language act within the appropriate social context. The process of *situating language acts* involves many pragmatic skills.

The ideal language situation (called ideal speech situation by Togeby, 1998) occurs when interlocutors have a common set of knowledge, symmetrical status, and are in agreement about the sincerity of the communication act. Our common set of knowledge comes from a shared culture and shared experiences. A symmetrical status occurs when the balance of power between communicators is the same (e.g., adult to adult, child to child). Asymmetrical status occurs when there is an imbalance of power between communicators (e.g., teacher to student, governor to governed). Agreement on sincerity occurs when both interlocutors maintain the same degree of openness with one another rather than one intentionally or subconsciously obscuring the message. Asymmetrical communications often occur between hearing and deaf communicators for a variety of reasons. First, students with hearing losses may miscommunicate or misperceive a message. Second, they do not always share a set of experiences with hearing communicators. Third, Deaf cultural experiences differ from the majority culture. In this situation hearing culture may perceive Deaf culture as having lesser status due to communication differences.

Pragmatics is the practical use of all language acts based upon contextual need. For example, we expect people to speak (phonology) in certain ways. If they do not, then we assume they are less capable, causing a mismatch between interlocutors. Pragmatic requirements have an impact on grammar (Dahl, 1998; Carston, 1998a, 1998b; deVilliers, 1982). We expect people to use standard grammar (morphology and syntax). If they do not, we make assumptions about their level of intelligence and experience. We expect people to talk about certain topics at certain times and places (semantics). If they do not, we perceive them negatively and wonder about their manners, upbringing, and education. In other words, a person may use perfectly good grammar and speech, but we still judge them as communicatively competent or incompetent based on whether they appropriately situate the language act within the expected social context.

There are three broad divisions of pragmatics: *micropragmatics, macropragmatics,* and *metapragmatics* (Mey, 1998a). Micropragmatics is the study of intention, especially at the word and sentence level. Macropragmatics looks beyond the purpose of a language act to the social context or setting of the conversation. Speakers have different expectations in different environments. For example, the medical environment (e.g., doctor to patient), the educational environment (e.g., student to teacher), the workplace, generation-specific environments (e.g., adolescent to adolescent, child to adult), gender-related environments (e.g., boy to boy, boy to girl), and environments based on social privilege all carry certain expectations. We use the term *discourse* to describe conversation as opposed to single words or sentences. Discourse processes are related both to conversation and to text. Classroom and conversational discourse rules are especially important to address because the school environment is one in which we spend most of our time with students. The most obvious pragmatic intentions of language in the classroom are to inform, to instruct, to control structure of the exchange of information, to control behavior, to elicit information, and to change the awareness of others (Mercer, 1998). Classroom discourse is based on an understanding of the role of the teacher and the role of the students. This includes knowledge of the organization of information-sharing, the rules for participation, the procedures for asking questions as well as the kinds of questions that are allowable, all of which surround the topic of instruction (Merritt, Barton, & Culatta, 1998). Metapragmatics refers to one's social awareness of what one is saying. For example, if I were to say "I agree with you one hundred percent and I'm not just saying that because you are my boss" I am engaging in metapragmatics. I have recognized that the situation in which I am communicating could have two pragmatic intentions: to agree or to flatter. I realize that my communication partner is aware of these two possibilities. I look at the social context I am in related to these two possibilities and realize that it is in my best interest socially to appear genuine rather than disingenuous, so I add a qualifying statement to my basic proposition. Metapragmatics involves understanding micro- and macropragmatic issues and manipulating them appropriately.

In summary, pragmatics requires that we take the communicator seriously: his needs, wants, and social situation. Table 5.1 outlines pragmatic content. Any time you design a language lesson, you must consider the user of the language. Simply attempting to impart a set of rules is not sufficient. The lesson must take into consideration when, where, and why the student would want to use a linguistic rule.

Language Instruction in Students Who Are Deaf and Hard of Hearing

There are many different contact points where teachers and parents engage students in language activities. Table 5.2 outlines the primary ways that we ask children to interact with language. We ask them: (1) to learn a language for communication purposes; (2) to learn about their language; and (3) to learn other information using their language as a tool.

First and foremost, students who are deaf must learn a primary or native language. For this to happen, we must make sure that the child's primary

TABLE 5.1 *Micro-, Macro-, and Metapragmatic Skills*

Category	Description	Components
Micropragmatic performatives	Babies express intentions through *performatives* or actions. Performatives are what the child does.	Pointing (deixis)—use of the index finger to show intention related to person, time, and space Gesturing—moving hands in a meaningful manner Gazing—early eye-contact and shifting of focus to call adult's attention to something Shouting/babbling/crying—using pre-linguistic vocalizations to express intent Posturing—turning head and body toward or away from adult to express intent Using facial expression—expressing emotions Touching/holding/tugging—communicating through physical contact Joint reference—the ability to garner another person's attention with regard to an object of mutual attention
Micropragmatic intentions: early	Intent refers to why a child communicates. The prelinguistic baby is able to express a variety of intentions.	Labeling—asking for an object to be named Repeating—asking for a label to be given again Answering—responding to the communication partner Requesting and action—trying to get someone to do something Requesting an answer—trying to get someone to respond to an utterance Calling—trying to get someone's attention Greeting—acknowledging another's presence Protesting—not wanting to do something Practicing—rehearsing Directing—ordering another's action Complaining—expressing affect relative to an action Questioning—asking for information

Micropragmatic intentions: later	Children begin to understand that conversation is a two-way street, and develop conversational skills.	Conversational turn-taking—conversation is a two-way street with specific rules of conduct • Selecting and initiating topics—the rules for getting conversation started • Maintaining topics—the rules for maintaining topics • Using appropriate pause time—too long or too short provides inappropriate cues to listener • Commenting on topics—the rules for commenting on the speaker's utterances • Giving feedback—the rules for interrupting the speaker's utterance and giving one's perspective • Seeking clarification/contingent queries—the use of questions to initiate, clarify, or continue an exchange • Appropriate interrupting or overlapping another's conversation • Quantity—too much or too little information • Changing topics • Topic closure—the rules for ending a conversation Register—the ability to assume various roles when speaking Types of intent—to explain, express, describe, direct, report, reason, imagine, hypothesize, persuade, infer cause, and predict outcomes
Macropragmatics: early	Discourse rules within a social context occurring at the suprasentential level; apply to conversations and text. Each two-way interaction is called an *adjacency pair.*	Directive/compliance—speaker/signer states personal need, asks permission, asks question, gives hint, and listener/watcher complies Query/response—speaker/signer requests information, confirmation, for repetition, and listener/watcher provides appropriate response Request/response—speaker/signer makes direct request, inferred request, request for acknowledgment and listener/watcher responds Comment/acknowledgment—speaker/signer describes activity, state or condition, names, and makes acknowledgments that are positive, negative, expletive, or indicative and listener/watcher acknowledges comment

(continued)

TABLE 5.1 *Continued*

Category	*Description*	*Components*
Macropragmatics: later	Additional skills occur after conversational turn-taking.	Presuppositions—the degree to which the speaker is aware of the listener's prior experiences with the topic Turn-taking—advanced use of earlier turn-taking to include stylistic language demanded by the communication environment, such as teenaged slang Code-switching—more sophisticated ability to switch register as well as the ability to switch from one language to another in a bi- or multilingual situation Conversational style changes—changes demanded by the subculture, such as the use of adolescent language versus the use of language for a formal presentation Social deixis—where the speaker acknowledges social status Requests for clarification—where the listener or responder recognizes the presence of miscommunication Nonegocentrism—the ability to take the perspective of another person Decentration—the process of moving from rigid descriptions of objects to smooth, flexible, and multidimensional descriptions
Macropragmatic: spoken or written text		Use of narratives—to tell a story, recount an event, or explain a situation Discourse deixis—where the writer/speaker points out what is upcoming Rules associated with speaking and writing for the following purposes: descriptive, narrative, persuasive, expository, explanatory, and for the purpose of giving directions Text grammar—the organized, predictable, rule-governed organization of narratives

Metapragmatics	A language user's ability to judge the adequacy of his choice of language acts	Thinkability—thinking about and choosing the best match between form and social intent Feasibility—using strategies to match language form and social intent Recognizability—narrowing down a partner's information and focusing on informative clues such as context, facial expression, or emphasis Reflexivity—reflecting on shared knowledge and editing impressions during conversation Monitoring—editing impressions based on micro- and macropragmatic skills assumed in a conversation as the conversation proceeds

Sources: Anderson, 1992; Bates, Camaioni, & Volterra, 1975; Caffi, 1998; Dore, 1975; Levinson, 1998; Owens, 1996; Shatz, 1987; Stephens, 1988; Tough, 1977.

TABLE 5.2   *Contact Points in Language Instruction*

Language Learning

Learning a first language before school
- Spoken English
- English-based signs/cues
- ASL

Learning a first language at school
- Spoken English
- English-based signs/cues
- ASL

Learning about language (metalinguistic instruction)
- Simultaneously with first language learning
- Through print

Learning via language
- Bridging the communication gap

---

language-learning pathway is used and that the child is receiving a complete language code. In the past a child had to mold to the method or service available regardless of the way he learned best. We need to take a different approach, looking at the child's best pathway for language acquisition and then determining the appropriate methods or approaches. For example, Kevin would probably benefit from a strong bilingual program. Ashley would probably benefit from a primarily English-based program supplemented with ASL when appropriate. Trisha, on the other hand, is learning very well through the auditory pathway and would benefit from print support for language.

At some point, learning to use language becomes learning about language arts, which forms the traditional language instruction that occurs in elementary and middle schools across the nation. Teachers instruct students in how to use their language as a tool, both to read and to learn new information. After students have a foundation in reading and writing they begin learning about their language and identifying such components as compound and complex sentences. This can be a daunting task (and quite counterproductive) for a child without a native or first language.

The final language task students must master is that of using language as a tool to learn other information. Sometimes that other information is math, science, or history. Sometimes that other information is another language. This is the case when students are learning English as a new language based on their knowledge of ASL (as in the case of Jonathan) or English as a new language, despite previous partial awareness of some other spoken language (e.g., Spanish, as in the case of Jorge). Unfortunately, many deaf and hard of hearing students are put into situations that assume an available language base that is not there. For example, an elementary-age deaf student (such as Martin) having little prior experience with sign language is mainstreamed into a regular classroom with an interpreter. This puts the child in a difficult situation. First he doesn't know enough sign language to access the interpreted message. Second, he doesn't have sufficient knowledge of English to understand the written text. Finally, he does not have prior information necessary to understand the subject matter. This may seem like an unbelievable situation, but it commonly occurs in school districts throughout the country. We describe each of these three contact points for language below.

Learning a First Language at School

The best place to learn a first language is at home from your parents. When that doesn't happen, then teachers must take on the task. The process of learning a first language differs if a child is learning it at home during normal developmental stages or if he is learning it as an older child at school. When a child arrives at school we may not know his primary language learning pathway, and he will not show us this until he has had sufficient opportunities to experience a variety of language-learning options. During this investigation we need to provide complete language codes while exploring different options thus allowing the child to show us the pathway with which his brain learns most efficiently. Table 5.3 lists auditory and visual enhancements that may be used with young children who are in the process of establishing a language pathway.

Factors such as age of loss, age of first language intervention, level of hearing loss, use of hearing technology, and amount of parental involvement, among others, should be considered when assessing language code preference. All instruction, no matter which pathway the child is using, should:

- be play-based for very young children,
- be meaning-based at all ages,
- be developmentally appropriate at all ages,
- take into consideration the cognitive and social development of the child,
- provide a bridge between the child's basic communication skills and the communication demands of the regular education curriculum,
- engage the child in pragmatically based, meaningful activities, and
- serve to help students access the regular education curriculum.

According to Vygotsky's *Zone of Proximal Development* (1978), adults working with a child should provide language input that is at a higher level than the child's present functioning challenging her to acquire greater levels of language understanding. This cannot happen when parents, teachers, and instructional

TABLE 5.3 *Activities to Enhance Auditory and Visual Development*

Auditory Enhancements	Visual Enhancements
Social reinforcement for responses to audition	Social reinforcement for responses to visual stimuli (e.g., smiles, touch)
Focus on speech rather than nonspeech sounds, as speech sounds require less auditory intensity to elicit a response than nonspeech sounds.	Enhance nonverbal communication through facial expression to convey feelings.
Vary auditory stimuli to maintain interest and attention.	Gain and direct attention (reduce divided attention) by using touch, movement, and placement of your body to break child's line of gaze.
Stress intonational patterns.	Use pointing to direct attention while still permitting language input.
Reinforce all attempts to imitate sounds as well as attempts at conversational turn-taking, even if the turn-taking attempt is gestural.	Make language visually salient.
Use short utterances.	Use short utterances.
Make sure that the meaning of your utterances is salient.	Link language and meaning. Use bracketing. Sign label or new information, point or describe, then sign label again.
	Modify signs by placing them closer to the object, repeating them, or enlarging and prolonging them.

Sources: Estabrooks, 1994; Mayne, Yoshinaga-Itano, Sedey, & Carey, 2000; Mohay, 2000.

aides have minimal communication proficiency. No child should be placed in an impoverished communication and information environment.

There are three major pathways by which the child with a hearing loss learns a first language:

- the auditory pathway for spoken English,
- the visual pathway for English, and
- the visual pathway for acquisition of ASL and English as a second language.

The degree to which a child uses each pathway depends entirely on his or her unique abilities. Some children who are deaf and hard of hearing are candidates for learning spoken English. Children who learn auditory approaches best are often described as hard of hearing, may have postlingual hearing loss, have received cochlear implants, or have high levels of usable hearing. Teachers generally use techniques of "motherese," which include modeling and self-correction practices (see Modeling and Self-Correction Practices later in this chapter). Teachers of young deaf and hard of hearing children learning language through an auditory pathway need to know:

- use and maintenance of auditory equipment such as auditory trainers, personal aids and cochlear implants,
- acoustic management of the classroom environment, and
- scope and sequence of auditory, speech, and language skills.

Teachers may also use visual means to support oral language instruction such as the use of patterning, color codes, language experience stories and charts, and computer programs.

Some children will combine both the auditory and visual pathways to learn English using English-based sign systems or Cued Speech. Children who learn best through a dual pathway are those who: (1) have some residual hearing or are postlingually deafened; (2) mediate language primarily through the auditory pathway, enhanced by the visual pathway; and (3) learn well sequentially. They are able to fill in the incomplete language code by hearing and seeing elements of the language presented simultaneously. Sometimes a child will receive her first exposure to any kind of signed language when she enters formal schooling. This child often enters school with little language because the parents may have been learning to sign themselves. When one is learning to sign, he tends to think about the signs rather than about the intention of the communication. This often ends in utterances that lack affect (Wolkomir, 1992). The older the child is when she begins to learn signs or cues for English, the more challenging learning a first language will be. When instructing the child who is learning English through a visual pathway, teachers should:

- understand auditory enhancements,
- understand visual enhancements,
- be fluent and proficient in the signed or cued system that the child is using,
- provide a complete message by enhancing the spoken message with signs or cues,
- enhance the affective component of communication that is often lacking in these systems, and
- use fingerspelling.

Finally, some children will learn a first language at school that follows a visual pathway leading to ASL. Many students learn ASL while receiving instruction in English. Teachers may do this as a simultaneous language-learning task (L1 and L2 at the same time). Simultaneous instruction generally occurs in the preschool years with young children. Teachers may also teach ESL based on ASL as a successive language-learning task (L1 first, then L2). Children who learn best through a visual pathway tend to have little or no usable hearing.

While there are many bilingual frameworks for teaching hearing students who are operating in two languages, there are few language-acquisition models of teaching a deaf or hard of hearing child a second language; however, models that teach ASL/ESL are in the process of development (Nover & Andrews, 1998).

It takes from five to seven years to acquire academic proficiency in English if the child has a good base in his first language (Collier, 1987; Cummins, 1984). Similarly, it takes a hearing individual many years of intensive instruction to learn ASL to a sufficient level of proficiency. ASL is classed as a Category II language, putting it on par with Indonesion, Malasian, and Swahili in terms of difficulty to learn (Kemp, 1998) (French, German, Spanish, and Italian are considered Category I languages). Why, then, would we expect deaf children to learn the language fast and easily, without direct instruction and without proficient language models? We recommend that all students who are learning ASL receive specific, sequential instruction throughout their years of schooling just as hearing students are required to learn about English. This is happening in Norway, where all deaf students receive 2,033 hours of instruction in Norwegian Sign Language (Handberg, 2000). Teachers in bilingual-bicultural programs (Evans, Zimmer, & Murray, 1994; Nover & Andrews, 1998) will need to:

- be proficient in ASL and in English,
- understand the importance of eye contact and linguistic uses of eye gaze,
- understand the process of first language acquisition,
- understand how to bridge from ASL to English and other strategies of teaching English as a second language,
- provide culturally sensitive instruction, including Deaf role models and studies of Deaf culture (i.e., history, storytelling, and community events),
- use culturally appropriate discourse (e.g., the *discourse diamond*, where the topic is identified first (the point), is expanded through examples and explanation, and concluded with a repetition of the topic),
- provide appropriate lighting and reduce glare as a Deaf student's eyes may become sensitive,
- provide appropriate assistive devices (e.g., TTYs, visual alerting systems, captioning, etc.),
- use appropriate attention bids such as tapping the child on the shoulder, flashing lights, waving, etc.,
- teach students to use interpreters, and
- sign at all times (e.g., no spoken side conversations while a deaf student is within visual range).

A problem that occurs often in regular education programs has to do with the signing level of the educational staff, whether the signs are ASL or English. Many regular education programs place a teacher's aide who has beginning knowledge of signs into the regular education classroom with a deaf or hard of hearing child. This is poor practice as it presents the illusion that the child is receiving instructional support and language intervention when probably he is not. The aide may not be providing a complete model of language and most likely is not using the intuitive parenting techniques that foster early language development. The child's communication skills may be too limited to benefit from the presence of the signer. At best, he is gaining some basic vocabulary, but this masks the need for intensive communication instruction.

Learning about Language: A Challenge to All Pathways

In the regular education curriculum, students receive instruction in "language arts." This involves reading, writing, and developing a metalinguistic understanding of language. For example, they are asked to identify parts of speech, to diagram sentences, or to explain how to fix a grammatical error. This subject is tested regularly throughout the school years and at graduation. From elementary through high school, hearing students learn the components of English at the metalinguistic level. They are able to do this because they have a rich and fully functioning language that they use for communication with others. The problem for students who are deaf and hard of hearing is that they may not have these underlying language skills. More often, children with hearing losses are learning language arts and a first language simultaneously. Metalinguistic analysis usually requires students to memorize rules. This may work for children who can hear, but it is counterproductive for children who can't. Analytic study of language begun before children have a level of language readiness may actually hinder the language-learning process.

At some point along the road to language-learning all students begin to learn about their language through the printed medium. Print becomes a powerful tool for helping deaf and hard of hearing students learn language as well as learn about language. Reading eventually becomes a powerful tool for assisting students to learn vocabulary incidentally through context (deVilliers & Pomerantz, 1992; Jenkins, Stein, & Wysocki, 1984). Hard of hearing students may be successful at learning to read and write phonetically, but most children with significant hearing losses will have difficulty encoding the spoken language and will, therefore, require other strategies.

Language and literacy development is intertwined. Learning to read and write is perhaps *the* most important language-dependent task children face. Most deaf adults become dependent upon the written word for access to everyday information (e.g., closed captioned news, emails, newspapers, journals, and magazines) and for informal interactions with hearing people. For a review of current language and literacy practices, see Paul (1998), French (1999), and McAnally, Rose, and Quigley (1994), and Schirmer (2000).

Learning Information through Language

One of the most important tasks that a teacher of students who are deaf and hard of hearing must perform is to provide a bridge between a student's present level of language understanding and performance and the language demands of the subjects being taught in the classroom. If the student who is deaf or hard of hearing is having difficulty grasping a subject, look beyond the content to the language needed for understanding. For example, Ashley may be studying the similarities and differences between the Allied invasion of Europe and the surrender of the Japanese after the bombing of Hiroshima and Nagasaki. Perhaps the teacher has used a timeline to show temporal relationships. In this situation the student will need to understand such language as *before* and *after* time phrases and clauses, time clauses representing simultaneous action (i.e., *while*), and specific time denotation of *until*. If the student does not understand these adverbial forms, then she will not understand the teacher's instruction or test questions.

Math. Specific semantic and syntactic skills are associated with math. For example, students must understand comparative language (Chamot & O'Malley, 1994) such as *as many pieces as, is taller than,* and *three times as much as.* Semantically they must understand inferred concepts (Kessler, Quinn, & Hayes, 1985) and must be able to use such connector language as *if . . . then, if and only if, because, for example,* and *either . . . or.* Time concepts are often presented as spatial metaphors (e.g., *over the weekend*). Word problems require students to understand important versus extraneous information, to understand sequences of events, and to understand inferred relationships inherent in the problems. Luetke-Stahlman (1999) described a ten-step model for examining math problems that is useful when working with students who have hearing losses. Culatta, Long, and Gargaro-Larson (1998) identified the following techniques, among others, to circumvent the language problems associated with math.

- Represent concepts with manipulatives.
- Solve problems in authentic contexts.
- Provide key words to help students discern the math process needed.
- Help students differentiate between necessary and extraneous information.
- Help students learn that there may be some missing information in a word problem.
- Relate new concepts/vocabulary to old or known.

- Rephrase the word problem by verbally mapping it with another language.
- Consider other forms of representation including counters, pictures, graphs, notations, and symbols.
- Help child build a vocabulary implicitly related to different processes (e.g., *share* and *distribute fairly* imply division.)

Vocabulary. Semantic development in students with hearing losses is challenging for many reasons. These include:

- *Amount.* The hearing child learns new vocabulary at a rate of four to six words a day. Students who are deaf and hard of hearing have a great deal of difficulty catching up and closing the vocabulary gap. This is especially true once the teacher's focus is on the general education curriculum.

- *Abstract nature.* It is easy to teach the meaning of words when we can show their referent, but most vocabulary past the first couple hundred words or so is abstract. The challenge is to visually highlight their abstract nature.

- *Multiple meanings.* Most words have multiple meanings. In fact, the smaller words are the ones with the greatest variety of meaning (e.g., *on*: on the wall, on a dime, continue on, talk on and on, on a bet, take on faith, a collar on its neck, a book on bugs, etc.). We tend to teach the most common meaning and leave the rest up to chance, although it is most likely that the secondary or tertiary meanings are equally as important (e.g., *base*: first, second, third, and home; bottom, crude, or nasty).

- *Idiomatic uses.* Many verbs and most prepositions are used idiomatically as often as they are used literally (e.g., *You are way off base. That's a strange get up. You were on target from the get go.*)

- *Derived forms.* Once we learn the base form (e.g., base) of a word, it is assumed that we can comprehend compound (*baseball*), noun adjunct (*base hit*), and derived forms (*basement, baseness*), but these must be taught to the child who is deaf or hard of hearing.

Vocabulary development is a challenge because students often do not pick up enough word meanings incidentally; on the other hand, you cannot teach every word and every innuendo there is to know. For this reason you must teach children a process for learning new words. The most effective process, and one that relates significantly to later development of reading (Paul, 1998) is a morphographic process.

- Students will benefit in the long run from any knowledge they gain about the relationship between root words (base words) and their morphographic derivatives (i.e., prefixes and suffixes), including Latin derivatives.

• Teach students how to use the dictionary as this is an essential tool for later vocabulary clarification.

• Highlight visually the primary concept represented, its opposites, its secondary meanings, and non-exemplars of the word.

• Determine an appropriate amount of words to cover each week and focus on developing a depth and breadth of knowledge about each word through use in text and experiences rather than on memorizing one meaning for a long list of words isolated from meaningful context. Coordinate efforts with other service providers as well as the student's parents.

• Help students develop their own personal dictionaries of words they frequently encounter that give them trouble. Some teachers for young deaf and hard of hearing children have them create their own dictionary or file box of words they need/want to know. This is very effective and helps create beginning dictionary skills.

• Choose one or two words a week to highlight as the "Word of the Week" or on a word wall and explore it in all its forms. Focus on using the word in all its meanings throughout the week. Table 5.4 provides two examples that you might use with a student like Kevin.

• Choose reading materials that contain the words, or read to the students, explaining the story to them while incorporating the new words into your discussion.

• Use the new words in daily classroom or on-line chat sessions.

• Do not give students a list of definitions to memorize or make them write sentences using the words without meaningful context. Use the words in meaningful ways throughout the week in activities such as those listed above.

Another procedure to increase vocabulary is to use context to aid acquisition of new vocabulary. Luetke-Stahlman (1993) suggested introducing novel vocabulary couched within contexts of known vocabulary or by contrasting it with known vocabulary. For example, "Benjamin, would you like to go to the zoo this afternoon? We can ride the train. The train is pulled by a big, black engine. The man driving the train is called an engineer. He drives the train at the zoo."

Language Learning Principles

No matter whether you are teaching language in and of itself, helping students bridge the language gap, or facilitating language development through learning about subject matter, meticulous and careful attention to their needs is essen-

TABLE 5.4 *Word of the Week Examples*

Word: hit	*Word: class*

Monday: dictionary meanings

| *Monday: dictionary meanings* |

1. To make forceful contact with your fist on someone or something else
2. One thing makes forceful contact with another
3. Something that is very popular
4. Successfully hitting a ball with a bat
5. The act of trying to kill someone

Monday: dictionary meanings

1. Group of students
2. Category
3. Sophistication
4. A period of time during which a teacher teaches
5. Social status

Tuesday: compound words/noun adjuncts

1. Hit and run
2. Hit parade
3. Hit man

Tuesday: compound words/noun adjuncts

1. Classmate
2. Class trip
3. Class act

Wednesday: verb idioms

1. "Hit on" someone
2. "Hit up" for money
3. "Hit it off"

Wednesday: verb idioms

1. "Class up" a place
2. "Outclass" someone

Thursday: figures of speech

1. Hit the books
2. Hit the road
3. Hit the roof
4. Hit your head against a brick wall

Thursday: figures of speech

1. A touch of class
2. In a class of your own
3. Head of the class
4. Class is out (he's not too bright)

Friday: derived forms and morpho-graphic variants

1. Hit (as a noun, a verb, and past tense)
2. Hitting (verb)
3. No-hitter (noun)
4. Switch-hitter

Friday: derived forms and morpho-graphic variants

1. Classy (adjective)
2. Classify (verb)
3. Declassé (adjective)
4. Classic (noun and noun adjunct)
5. The classifieds (noun)

tial. What the hearing child learns automatically will take some deaf and hard of hearing children years and years to acquire. Good instruction is essential for all children, no matter what their pathway. Good language instruction considers the following:

- *Comprehension and production are separate issues.* Some approaches work on these sequentially. Some approaches work on them simultaneously. All approaches recognize that the language-learner must have a firm knowledge of the meaning behind what is being communicated. What varies is the timing at which that is addressed.

- *The communication needs of the child provide the semantic and pragmatic base for instruction in grammar.* The child tells us in many ways why we should teach what we are teaching. If the child needs to know how to ask for help (pragmatic skill), we have the context (role-playing, asking for help) within which to teach comprehension. If he is trying to ask for an eraser, we now have information regarding the sentence pattern he needs.

- *Normal language development forms the scope and sequence of instruction in the grammatical aspects of language.* Some approaches adhere strictly to this sequence. Some approaches modify this sequence based on the child's incidental needs for form, function, and use (the what and when). Some approaches follow the scope and sequence of English, and some follow a scope and sequence modified by natural development of ASL.

- *Teachers need to help students generalize language skills to novel situations.* Some children are able to do this on their own. Some children need direct instruction on how to do this, and some children need to have teachers show them the generalizations.

- *To impart language in its richness and usefulness, there must be two-way communication.* Some approaches place a heavier emphasis on conversation than others, but all address it as an important element.

- *The child must experience the meaning of language in many ways.* These include but are not limited to demonstration, role-playing, showing pictures, and relating to another language.

- *Input must be comprehensible.* Although all philosophies agree that in principle input must be comprehensible, they differ in how they see this accomplished. The oral philosophy stresses maximization of residual hearing through hearing aids, cochlear implants, and the use of clear speechreading to provide comprehensible input. The total communication philosophy stresses accurate signed English in combination with speech, residual hearing, and the printed word to provide comprehensible input. The ASL bilingual philosophy stresses the need for a deaf child to have a fully accessible language through the visual pathway.

Language Instructional Approaches, Practices, and Techniques

There is much confusion regarding the terms *philosophy, approach, practice,* and *technique.* A philosophy is a belief system based on how one feels that children who are deaf and hard of hearing can and should learn language. Philosophies are highly controversial, mutually exclusive, and global. An approach is a set of practices and procedures that teachers follow to impart information. They tend to be associated with certain philosophies, but generally they are used across philosophies. Approaches are also controversial, tending to come in and out of favor. Approaches are made up of a series of practices associated not only with instruction but also with equipment maintenance, parental involvement, choice and use of materials, and other issues. Practices are specific procedures teachers follow to engage in actual lessons. Techniques are specific strategies that teachers use to address specific problems. In a previous chapter we discussed philosophies and approaches to the overall instruction of children who are deaf and hard of hearing. In this chapter we address language approaches, practices, and techniques.

Language Instructional Approaches

Three language instructional approaches are found routinely in schools and classes for students who are deaf and hard of hearing. They are the Language Experience Approach, the Whole Language or Balanced Literacy Approach, and the Project or Unit Approach.

Language Experience Approach.   The Language Experience Approach (LEA) has a long history based on early theories of natural language and emphasizes that language must be experienced, hands on, and relevant to the child's world. The teacher using the LEA plans activities in which language is practiced and used in meaningful ways (Johnson & Roberson, 1988). For example, a preschool teacher might prepare a lesson on butter. The class might take a field trip to a farm to get some cream, then churn it until it forms butter. During the activity the children are actively engaged in learning. There is much discussion and the teacher records each step as well as the class's comments. Back in the classroom she transfers these to a flip chart. For younger children the teacher usually draws pictures in addition to providing English text. Sometimes a class will dictate the story together following an experience while the teacher writes it on a flip chart or overhead projector. Often the teacher will reproduce the experience story as a booklet for the child to read independently. There are other techniques used in the LEA. (For more information about the Language Experience Approach see Schirmer, 2000).

Whole Language. The whole language approach differs from traditional teaching in many ways (see Table 5.5). Most whole language approaches are literature based; that is, the class learns to read and write based on material from a particular story, usually from a trade book rather than a basal reader. In the 1980s many public schools adopted the whole language philosophy, but by the 1990s whole language fell into disfavor as high-stakes testing became the driving force behind curriculum. Although abandoned by regular education, the whole language approach has merit in the language instruction of deaf and hard of hearing students (Schleper, 1997). Mason and Ewoldt (1996) stated that whole language and bilingual-bicultural education are very complementary. "Whole language provides learners with access to complete, natural language (through-the-air and in print) and offers them many and varied opportunities to experiment and choose their own strategies and their own learning goals" (p. 294). To become proficient language users, students need opportunities to use language in meaningful ways. Whole language has been adapted by some programs for deaf and hard of hearing students into *balanced literacy* approaches (Schirmer, 2000), which combine the strengths of whole language with skills-based instruction. (For more information see the May/June 1999 special literacy issue of *Perspectives* prepared by the staff at Gallaudet University's Pre-College National Missions Programs.)

The Project Approach to Teaching Language. The project approach to teaching language is similar to the whole language approach in many ways, but instead of being literature based it is topic based. The project approach strives to engage students in activities that have relevance to their lives and in which they are genuinely interested. Projects have been referred to as thematic units or topic-work. Regardless of the label, the project approach is an in-depth study of a particular topic. Use of the thematic or project approach varies from a couple of afternoons a week to the central focus of the instructional day. It varies by the age of the children and the school's policy. Typically projects in early childhood start by the students' learning about themselves and their immediate family. From there learning becomes more abstract and remote. By middle school students are learning about national and world events and by high school students are engaging in projects that revolve around critical issues relevant to their lives. The project approach takes into consideration the unevenness of students' development by planning for a wide range of activities at varying levels of complexity. Projects encourage students to work along side one another and to collaborate in their learning. There are three stages of project work: project planning, engaged learning, and concluding activity.

In project planning the teacher selects developmentally appropriate topics of interest to the students. Planning usually begins with a graphic organizer such as a topic web that identifies all the concepts that have potential for study. As the planning proceeds the teacher identifies the skills that will be developed

TABLE 5.5 *Whole Language vs. Traditional Teaching*

Traditional Teaching	Whole Language
Based on behaviorist theories	Based on constructivist theories
Class periods are broken down into discrete segments. Children usually rotate from subject to subject.	Class periods are organized into large chunks of time. Emphasis is on language immersion and integration of subjects, especially the language arts.
The curriculum is presented in a lock-step manner and is skills based.	The curriculum is presented from a whole-to-part perspective and is literature based.
Teachers teach basic skills often in isolation.	Skills are taught in mini-lessons as the need arises with application of the new skill immediately.
Teachers use drill and practice to reinforce concepts. Students who memorize easily do well in this instructional approach.	Teachers believe that instruction should be in authentic contexts and relevant to the students' lives.
What children learn is based on a prepared curriculum often connected with national achievement tests.	Teachers believe the "need to know" is the most powerful prerequisite to learning. When the need arises students tend to grasp the concept quickly.
Children tend to work alone.	Children work in groups on collaborative projects.

through the project study ensuring that state competencies are met. Next, the teacher makes plans for resources, materials, experts, and field trips that will be a part of the project. He also develops authentic assessment instruments (e.g., rubrics, checklists, interview forms, surveys) that will be used as the students proceed in their learning. When planning is completed, the teacher introduces the project and helps students select items to study.

During the active learning stage, students discuss, investigate, inquire, interview experts, and search for information. Students prepare classroom displays of their work and findings (e.g., students write articles, make posters, and construct models that reflect what they have learned). The length of the project will vary depending on the topic of study and the number of hours/weeks assigned to project work. For example, an elementary project that studies weather may last two weeks while a middle school project that examines global warming might take an entire semester. The project ends with a concluding activity during which students present their findings in a formal way in order to reflect and rehearse what they have learned. They celebrate their learning through a special, concluding activity. The ending activity can be a stage production or a poster session in an exhibit hall to which parents and other classes are invited. It can be a newsletter, a video, or a web page that explains the project and what was learned. A by-product of this activity is increased self-esteem and confidence.

Language Instructional Practices

There are three stages associated with most instructional practices: *exposure*, *comprehension*, and *production*. Before beginning instruction, the teacher may spend weeks, sometimes months, exposing students naturally in conversation to the language objective. Next, she focuses on helping the child understand or comprehend information presented through the language. This means that the teacher uses the language and the student does some activity to demonstrate comprehension. If the student does not comprehend or understand information presented through the language, internalization cannot occur. Only after the student has mastered comprehension do we expect production of the language. This process occurs over time.

Three major language instructional practices are listed then described below.

- Modeling and self-correction practices
- Practices using visual representation of English structure
- ASL/ESL practices

A web-based presentation of these practices is available by going to *http://www.gsu.edu/~wwwtod*. You will find it in the *Lessons* section. View it while you read the next section. You will see a clip of the different practices in action. The presentation is intended to demonstrate the practices associated with modeling and self-correction, visual representation of structure, and ASL/ESL practices. The focus on practices rather than on philosophies is intentional because many practices that we associate with a specific philosophy are not really philosophy specific. In fact many are applicable across philosophies. During the presentation you will see specific practices being used by teachers who support different philosophies.

Modeling and Self-Correction Practices. The foundation of modeling and self-correction practices is the relationship between mothers and their children who are learning language. Normal mother–child interaction is developmental. The mother naturally models needed information at the most opportune time. Mothers repeat what children say and provide an expanded, more adult-like model. Mothers tell children what to say. For example, at a birthday party they say, "Say, 'Thank you, Grandma.'" They model conversations during pretend play. Later, they hold the child responsible for his or her errors by directly correcting the child (e.g., "You said, runned. You're supposed to say, ran. What are you supposed to say?") (Ling, 1989; McAnally, Rose, & Quigley, 1994; Oliver, 1998; and *The Volta Review* [Special issue], 1992). Modeling and self-correction practices are based on patterns of motherese. Muma (1998) described this process as including the processes of expansion and replacement. Expansion allows the parent or teacher to take advantage of the active locus of learning which is present in the child's developmental repertoire. Replacement allows the parent and teacher to scaffold on to developmentally appropriate loci. The following teacher/child or parent/child interactions are key to modeling and self-correction practices.

- *Modeling.* Presenting an appropriate model of language for the child to repeat
- *Expansion.* Repeating the child's utterance, then expanding it to a more grammatically or semantically correct model
- *Expatiation.* The sequence of modeling, expanding, then returning to the nonexpanded form
- *Expounding.* Modeling, expanding grammatically, then expanding on the content of the sentence

The major features of modeling and self-correction include:

- Meaningful situations are used rather than drills or rote memorization.
- Functions of language are learned best through conversation. Later they are learned through writing and academic subjects.
- Principles are practiced in games, stories, and conversation.
- Teacher models, child imitates with reduction, teacher expands child's reduction. (In normal development, this allows the parent to reassess her hypothesis about what the child is saying so she can alter the expansion.)
- Teacher encourages a feedforward system and a feedback system associated by helping the child listen/attend to himself as he communicates (Say/sign that again and listen to/watch what you say.)
- Teacher helps the child to self-monitor through decreasing teacher cues with the goal being self-monitoring or self-correction.

The steps to modeling and self-correction are:

- Teacher provides direct correction ("Say/sign, TRAIN").
- Teacher presents an option for self-correction ("Is it TRAIN or SHORT?").
- Teacher presents the error ("You said/signed SHORT"). Child corrects.
- Teacher presents the type of error ("Your grammar/placement was wrong").

- Teacher presents the category of error ("Your verb/sign formation was wrong").
- Teacher gives meaningful clues to help child discern the error (e.g., trains run on tracks that are flat).
- Teacher calls attention to an error ("You signed something wrong in that sentence. Can you fix it?"). Or, teacher repeats answer with questioning facial expression. Child self-monitors and self-corrects.

Teacher's expectations of the child will vary depending on the objectives. Teacher addresses all aspects of communication: concept (idea or meaning), representation (speech/listen, sign/watch), and form (language: ASL/English).

Practices Based on Visual Representation of Structure.   Practices that use a visual representation of structure are based on the notion that the child will learn English when the teacher presents the rules via a metalinguistic symbol system (Paul & Quigley, 1994) such as the structured and combined approaches discussed in a previous chapter. Zorfass (1981) found that her subjects "exhibited varying metalinguistic abilities that generally increased with age and that were similar to the developmental pattern found in hearing populations" (p. 333). Most of the techniques and procedures associated with the visual representation of English require metalinguistic ability. Common practices associated with the visual representation of structure are:

- Use of signs, key symbols, icons, patterns, color codes, gestures, and other visual and metalinguistic representations of the structure of language.

- Use of familiar vocabulary to teach new grammar and familiar grammar to teach new vocabulary.

- Presentation of unfamiliar skills in the context of numerous examples.

- Evaluation of new skills in the context of numerous unfamiliar situations.

- Explicit teaching of rules and strategies.

- Explicit application of rules and strategies.

- Careful selection of examples. Start with examples that follow the rules, then teach exceptions to rules.

- Careful sequencing of examples.

The following is an example of the teaching sequence for a particular language pattern.

- Exposure to a variety of examples of the language pattern.
- Substitution of one element for another.

- Written, signed, and spoken production of the structure.
- Successive elimination of visual clues to encourage internalization of rules and principles.

Students begin to experiment with the language they have acquired by producing it with a visual pattern as a clue or guide. These are slowly reduced. Such experimentation often proceeds thus:

- Production with a visual pattern or clue in the visual field as a guide.
- Production with clues shown then removed.
- Production after teacher points to location where clue was located in space.
- Production without clue or prompt.

ASL/ESL Practices. ESL approaches to the instruction of English are not new to the field of deaf education. Goldberg and Bordman described the use of ESL practices with students at Gallaudet College in 1975. However, the resurgence of interest in recent years has brought new approaches, insights, and clarification to this process. Nelson (1998) described the components of a successful bilingual-bicultural program based on Rare Event Learning Theory. He felt that this theory appropriately explained the success of bilingualism with students with hearing losses. Rare Event Learning Theory "looks at social, attributional, emotional, and self-concept conditions as dynamically interacting with traditionally more 'cognitive' and 'linguistic' components of learning" (p. 80). This theory sees language instruction as dynamic, identifying "multiple, interacting conditions required for significant developmental steps forward in any language mode" (p. 79). These multiple conditions are presented by the acronym, LEARN. *L* stands for *launching conditions*, which surround the way we present a new language challenge to students. *E* stands for *enhancing conditions*, which are the strategies and catalysts used to garner attention, motivate the student, and make the lesson fun. *A* stands for *adjustment conditions*, which Nelson describes as the process of making continual adjustments in instruction to account for the emotional, attentional, socio-cultural, perceptual, motor, motivation, and self-esteem needs unique to each child. *R* stands for *readiness conditions*, or the unique skills of each child relative to the tools of speech, mode, fingerspelling, language, literacy, and learning strategies. *N* stands for *network conditions*, where information is stored in redundant, overlearned, consolidated, highly interconnected representations.

Nelson described the LEARN process as involving a "tricky mix" of conditions that must be satisfied and monitored closely from the perspective of each individual child since the necessary mix of conditions will vary from learner to learner and from attribute to attribute. One key tool of the LEARN process is that of *recasting*. "Recasts are new structural displays of the same information, as when the same basic ideas are expressed in one signed sentence by a child then recast into a structurally different signed sentence by a teacher" (Nelson, 1998, p. 81). Recasting is consistent with pragmatic theory, which tells us that there are numerous ways of expressing the same intent. In recasting, students and teachers take turns representing concepts by saying something in a different way, by demonstrating graphically, by writing it in yet a different manner, and by commenting on the recast, among other actions.

Teaching English through ASL is one component of an overall bilingual-bicultural approach. Philosophically this approach encourages the development of context, knowledge, and academic skills through ASL (Strong, 1988). Common approaches used in schools involve either simultaneous or successive language instruction as well as print-based English instruction.

Crutchfield (1972), Luetke-Stahlman (1998), Nover, Christensen, and Cheng (1998), Paul and Quigley (1994) and Strong (1988) among others described various elements of this practice. In addition, interviews with teachers using this technique and the authors' personal observations of ASL/ESL instruction helped to hone the description that follows. Common practices associated with ASL/ESL are:

- Teachers discuss all instructional issues in ASL.
- Teachers make it clear that students are studying two different languages.
- Teachers develop understanding or comprehension in ASL as the foundation for comprehension in English.
- Teachers use ASL to discuss features of English, and English is expressed primarily through print.
- Teachers use direct comparison of equivalent and nonequivalent structures.
- Teachers use space to convey grammatical structure.
- Teachers directly compare the languages from easiest comparisons to hardest comparisons.
- Teachers show the language-learner forms existing both in ASL and English (e.g., pluralization either through reduplications in ASL or the "-s" morpheme in English).
- Teachers show the language learner forms that do not exist either in ASL or English (e.g., *Much dogs* vs. *many dogs*).
- Teachers show the student the mismatches between ASL and English and instruct in compensating for this mismatch.

  - ASL has/English doesn't (classifiers)
  - English has/ASL doesn't (passive voice is shown by sign directionality)

- Student demonstrates in some manner (e.g., manipulative, role-playing, ASL) that he understands the meaning of the English printed word before trying to print it himself.

- Teachers use code-switching, a process of switching between languages, for clarification. "Code switching between ASL and English is extremely common in classrooms where the teacher is fluent in both languages" (Nover, Christensen, & Cheng, 1998, p. 68).

Language Instructional Techniques, Strategies, and Activities

Techniques or strategies refer to actual instruction or plans of action. By activities we mean the actual experience in which you are engaging the children. The experience may be a game, a trip, a role-play, or a paper-and-pencil task, but it is an actual task or activity in which you and the child participate. You can see it. You can demonstrate it. You can outline its steps. Techniques, strategies, and activities are devoid of content; that is, they may be used with many different objectives. Most teachers, no matter which philosophy they espouse, will use some or all of these activities at one point or another in their instruction. This next section describes several of the more common categories of techniques or strategies for language instruction. It is not intended to be a comprehensive curriculum but to present examples only. (For more information on language curriculums contact your state's school for the deaf).

Natural/Authentic Experiences to Support Language Intent.   If intent is the heart of communication, then students must be given important reasons for wanting to communicate. The most important content for instruction is real, authentic, and actual experience. All other learning depends on a solid base of world experiences. Unfortunately, many students with hearing losses lack this base. This is due in part to lack of exposure, but more importantly, to the lack of a communication system that the child may use to gain information from the significant adults in his life and to share ideas and ask questions. It is critical that teachers of the deaf provide their students with authentic and meaningful experiences to form the base for language learning.

Field Trips.   Field trips are an important way to share information with students. They occur within a time frame and can be used as a point of reference for the development of time concepts. They have the potential to provide topics for conversation for many days after the actual event.

Experiments.   Experiments are a useful way to demonstrate properties of the natural world to a child. As such, they assist in the child's understanding of math, science, and social studies concepts. Experiments are also fun, which is a very important component of good instruction. There are many language lessons that are learned through involvement with experiments such as the concept of why/because and cause-effect relationships.

Cooking.   Cooking is like taking a field trip without leaving the building. Concepts of number, sequence, texture, color, and other descriptive terminology are easily represented through cooking activities.

Demonstrations.   Demonstrations, or "how to" activities, are good opportunities to work on question forms, especially "how" questions involving sequence. They are also a good way to impart new skills. Demonstrations of creating, designing, building, and completing a project of some nature allow the teacher to discuss a wide range of vocabulary as well as to encourage sequencing and memory activities. While most demonstrations begin with the teacher, they should be predominately a child-manipulated activity.

Vicarious Experiences.   We cannot teach students everything they should have learned at home. Unfortunately, we must teach within the confines of the classroom. For this reason, we must create vicarious experiences for language learning by using our creativity and imagination. Here are several ways teachers accomplish this.

Toys and Other Manipulables.   The mainstay of the preschool, toys and other manipulable materials provide the opportunity to represent real-life events in miniature and through pretend. These are especially important when helping students learn to engage in conversations. Toys can also be used as props for plays and for development of scripts. Pretending to go to the doctor's office, police station, restaurant, post office, church, grocery store, or airport are excellent sources for initiating and practicing communication.

Role-playing.   Role-playing is another excellent tool that teachers can use to encourage the development of conversation. Role-playing can be done with great preparation and practice or it can be done spontaneously and off-the-cuff. Role-playing can be used with students of all ages, not just with young children. Glasser (1998) uses role-playing as a powerful tool for developing a comfort level in dealing with social and emotional issues. Easterbrooks and Miller (1986) developed a series of role-playing activities and objectives for students who are deaf and hard of hearing based on Glasser's Choice Theory and related to the development of language skills associated with students' transition from school to the world of work.

Storytelling.   Most programs for deaf and hard of hearing children use storytelling as a language technique. In bilingual programs ASL storytelling is the mainstay of a preschool language program. ASL storytelling provides a rich opportunity for deaf and hard of hearing children to participate in an enjoyable activity that fosters language skills. Early experience with reading often begins at a storytelling level, then proceeds along a continuum to storyreading (Schleper, 1997).

Visual Experiences to Enhance Language Learning. Many students need visual enhancements to help organize information in a way that it is understandable, codable, and retainable.

Maps, Diagrams, and Other Spatial Representations. Hyerle (1996) described the use of visual maps as a means of visual learning. Visual maps provide the visuospatial sketchpad necessary for working memory in children who do not have the phonological loop for working memory. One example of a visual map is the *affinity diagram.* Affinity diagrams tap both the left brain and right brain. They involve the creation, categorization, and synthesis of information. An example of a simple activity for early elementary students is to have them brainstorm all the names of animals they know. The teacher writes the names in large letters on large Post-it™ notes and sticks them randomly on a blank space. After the children have depleted all ideas, they work together to separate the animals and form categories or classifications. Depending on their existing knowledge of animals, the students might form simple categories such as (zoo and farm animals) and rearrange the Post-it notes to form these two groupings. Older students might form categories for mammals, amphibians, reptiles, carnivores, etc. Once the animals are in categories the students work in teams to write a statement that describes the grouping. Students may also write how the animals in the groupings are the same and how they are different. Older children will be able to write on the Post-it notes without the teacher's assistance.

Games to Support Language Learning. Games are an important way of interacting with deaf and hard of hearing students who are past the early language development years but are still developing a first or second language. Games are useful because they meet a major psychological need: the need for fun (Glasser, 1998). Games are also useful because they have the inherent quality of repetition. Most games have a set and predictable sequence of actions, eliminating any confusion the child may have regarding expectations. They are also enjoyable, so the child will want to play them again and again, thus reinforcing the language skill being worked on. For example, barrier games have been used to evaluate the student's ability to ask for clarification in conversation when they do not understand the message (Jeanes, Nienhuys, & Rickards, 2000). In a barrier game, students sit across from one another with a screen obscuring the materials that each student has. Each student has a corresponding set of materials such as Tinker Toys™, Legos™, arts and crafts materials, a tic-tac-toe board, etc. Students attempt to make an exact duplicate of each other's object without seeing the object. The leader gives instructions to his partner, and the partner must ask for clarification.

Paper-and-Pencil Tasks. The use of paper-and-pencil tasks to teach a first language violates all the principles of instruction previously discussed. However, from time to time the teacher needs to document progress or assign a grade.

Paper and pencil have little or no application when instructing students in pragmatic language, although they are used commonly when working on metapragmatic skills. Table 5.6 describes common paper-and-pencil tasks.

Technology, Media, and Materials to Support Language Learning. Having students use technology is effective practice in classrooms for deaf and hard of hearing students. Students need to be confident users of technology because their future will most likely be heavily dependent upon it. Every deaf education classroom should have a TTY or nearby access (and TTY trainers for young children). Interestingly, young deaf and hard of hearing students learn much language from TTY conversations. Captioning, once considered cutting-edge, is now commonplace. Every classroom should have access to captioning. In some cities, computer assisted real-time captioning (CART) is provided for students, especially those who do not know sign language and do not use an interpreter. In some cases the deaf student uses both an interpreter and CART. Every classroom should have ample access to word processing technology and to the Internet. Every teacher should know the benefits and applications of appropriate programs and CDs for language instruction. A variety of age- and language-appropriate programs should be available. Students who use assistive listening devices should have access to services that keep these devices functioning optimally at all times. New programs become available routinely that may have application to the language classroom. Teachers should keep abreast of these and should know how to evaluate their effectiveness. Technology allows us to make the language visual.

Considering the Needs of the Individual

Once the primary pathway for language learning is determined, the teacher plans how language instruction will proceed. She must take each student's individual needs into account. Some students will need language-intervention strategies and some will need language-enrichment strategies. Others will be precocious and learn language with little effort. Nothing works with all students all of the time. Some practices and procedures work best with one language skill while others work best with other language skills. Some children learn best with one technique while others learn best with another. Some students will learn best in small groups while others will learn best by individualized instruction. And, some students will have additional learning problems that complicate the language-learning process. Do not look for *the* one answer that will work with all your students. It is important to keep pragmatic intent in mind. For example, six-year-old Montel's primary intent might be to win the attention of his playmates while thirteen-year-old Jahan's primary intent might be to persuade others of his opinions. Also, we use different approaches depending on whether the child is addressing language skills at the normal developmental age or at a

TABLE 5.6 Paper-and-Pencil Tasks for Documenting Metalinguistic Understanding

Task	Description	Example
Synthesizing shorter sentences via sentence combining	Student combines two simple sentences into one new sentence that matches a target linguistic goal specified by the teacher. Can be used any time that students are combining simpler sentences into more complex sentences.	Teacher gives list of sentences such as *The potted plant crashed on the floor. The kitten knocked it over* followed by the instruction to combine the two sentences correctly using a "when" clause.
Judgment of grammaticality	Student is given sentences that contain either grammatically correct or incorrect examples of the linguistic skill from class.	Teacher says, "Put a plus by the sentences that use 'before' clauses correctly and a minus by the sentences that use them incorrectly." Give list of sentences such as *The man shaved before he went to work. Before be shaved, the man went to work.* Students indicate a + or – beside each sentence.
Sentence completion	Students are given a carrier phrase of a pattern and are asked to write correct ending to a sentence using newly acquired language skill.	Students are working on "because" clauses, teacher gives the carrier phrase *Summer is my favorite time of year _____*. She instructs students to use "because" correctly to complete the sentence.
Cloze procedure	Students are given partial sentences and fill in the correct linguistic item to make the sentence complete. There are many modifications to the basic cloze procedure.	Students are working on backward pronominalization. Teacher writes *Because _____ bad a toothache, Mary called ber dentist.* Students fill in correct pronoun.
Unscrambling sentences	Similar to sentence combining only in reverse	Given the sentence, *The boy who won the marathon was given a hero's parade,* students break sentence into its constituent parts: *The boy was given a hero's parade* and *The boy won the marathon.*

(continued)

189

TABLE 5.6 *Continued*

Task	Description	Example
Direct rule application	Students are told a specific rule and asked to generate a sentence containing the rule. Rule is shown explicitly on the board, a chart, or a sentence strip. After the student can apply the rule with the clue, the clue is removed, and the student writes a sentence spontaneously. In whole language classrooms rules such as these are taught during mini-lessons, as students need them. Students immediately use the newly acquired skill in their own creations (i.e., written stories). Avoid teaching rules in isolation, removed from meaningful application.	Teacher writes on the board "Change the -*y* to *i*, then add -*ly* to change an adjective to an adverb."Students receive a list of words such as *happy* or *mighty* to change to the adverb form.
Replacement of components	Used when working on morphological skills. Students are given sentences and asked to change one component to another. Initially teacher provides a correct model on the board, chart, or sentence strip, but eventually removes this and expects change from memory.	Students are working on past progressive. Teacher gives list of sentences containing present progressives, such as *The boy is running.* Students change from present to past progressive.
Paraphrasing	Student is given a sentence and asked to rewrite it in different language maintaining the same message. Sometimes the teacher tells students what she expects, sometimes not. Students are free to create any paraphrase.	Given a sentence such as *I like to swim*, teacher tells students "Use a gerund as in *I like swimming.*" Or, students create paraphrase such as *Swimming is something that I like to do very much.*

Sources: Muma, 1998; Wiig and Semel, 1977.

later age. We would use modeling and self-correction techniques with four-year-old Sissy, but would not with Colton. He would need a lot of visual structure because he has additional learning problems.

Keep different interests and backgrounds in mind. Although Mercedes and Jorge are both thirteen years old, Mercedes has had very different academic experiences, is highly oral, and has lots of friends whereas Jorge has poor communication skills, comes from an impoverished linguistic background, and has few friends. They are also of different genders. While Mercedes might be interested in studying about music, Jorge might be more interested in learning about basketball. Take into account individual students' learning styles when choosing instructional approaches and materials. For example, Kevin shows a very strong propensity toward holistic, visual learning strategies, and is still learning the basic building blocks of communication. Trisha, on the other hand, has a lot of residual hearing, strong auditory skills, and a propensity for oral and written English. ASL-to-ESL practices might be successful with Kevin but would not necessarily benefit Trisha, whose spoken communication skills are excellent. Take into account each individual student's communication style. Mercedes, for example, is a popular, bubbly young lady who loves to communicate, to interact with her peers, to be the center of attention, and to express herself at every opportunity. She would do very well with role-playing activities. Jorge, on the other hand, is somewhat shy and lacks self-confidence. He might find role-playing too challenging or embarrassing, and his need to stay out of the limelight would interfere with his ability to benefit from such activities. Take into account the presence of additional language processing problems. While Ashley and Martin are approximately the same age, there is evidence of neurological problems in Martin's history that would cause us to suspect that he has additional language processing problems. Even though his hearing is better than Ashley's, we can expect his progress to be slower. In addition, we can expect that he will need more structure, more opportunities for repetition and mastery, and considerably more assistance in generalizing the communication skills he has gained.

Most students who are deaf and hard of hearing learn language best when instructed early and in natural situations that serve a pragmatic function. However, some students, especially those with neurological impairments, require additional effort. You may want to explore the appropriateness of behavior modification, which as a rule works more effectively when nonlanguage behaviors are the objective. For example, Montel has problems with interrupting others' conversations. A behavior modification approach to reducing this behavior would be appropriate. Ashley has problems with talking to her friends too much and not paying attention to the teacher. She would benefit from behavior modification to reduce this behavior. Colton has problems with impulsivity that cause him to answer questions before thinking. The teacher might work with him to put his hand up before blurting out an answer. In limited situations, direct correction might be helpful. Jorge is bright enough to know the difference between right and wrong, and even though he has not internalized more than a basic vocabulary, he understands proper behavior. If his cousin were to teach him to say "Hey Baby" to the girls, direct correction along with an appropriate substitution would clarify for him that he should not use this conversation initiator with his female teachers.

Planning Language Instruction

At this point, we reiterate that there are many different ways to teach a single language skill. Students have different needs. Different philosophies promote different approaches, but the creative teacher is aware of all of them and is flexible enough to use whichever approach, practice, or technique meets the needs of an individual student. Table 5.7 outlines the steps in the language planning process to help you think about teaching a specific word or particular structure to young children.

Sample Examination of a Language Objective

The following example is provided to illustrate how a particular language structure could be taught to deaf and hard of hearing students after using the language planning process. In this case the target structure is the English word *have*. Some students will be learning English or ASL via through-the-air communication. Other students will be learning English primarily through print. This example serves only to provide an idea of how the language planning process unfolds and should be adapted based on students' needs.

IEP Objective Statement.   Begin by determining the appropriate objective based on assessment of the student's present levels of performance. This step may occur simultaneously with the next as your choice of objective will require not only an examination of the student but also an examination of the language objective itself. For example, Martin will use the English word *have* in simple sentences given a box of items.

Evaluate the Language Objective.   *Have* is a very complex word in the English language. By contrast, in ASL the concept of HAVE is considered a plain verb. A plain verb does not provide information about the subject or the object: the subject and the object are all signed separately. In English it is found in the following sentence pattern (subject + *have* + object). ASL uses the same structure. It is also found in the auxiliary system of the verb in English as a helping verb to represent perfect tense (ASL does not use this structure) and as a quasi-modal (hafta) to represent intent (also shared by ASL as in HAVE + TO). In addition, in English noun–verb relationships of tense and number require the user to understand the difference between the uses of have, has, and had. This does

TABLE 5.7 *Steps in the Language Planning Process*

1. Identify the IEP objective statement. Often the IEP language objective will be provided by the school's language curriculum guide or will be included in the state's mandated curriculum.
2. Evaluate the language objective. Compare how the structure functions in English and in ASL. Consider how to teach the targeted structure. Think about problems associated with the structure. Why might it be difficult?
3. Consider pragmatic uses for the language objective. Brainstorm ways in which the structure is used in the real world. Brainstorm activities you could do with the students to help them develop the underlying experiences necessary to understand and use this structure.
4. Identify the semantic contexts in which you will find the language skill. What semantic/discourse skills might you need to use this structure? (descriptions, direction, explanation, narration, persuasion, conversational interaction)
5. Identify ideas for exposure. Brainstorm activities that expose the students to a language skill before actually teaching it. Students vary in the amount and length of exposure they need. (conversations, historical charts)
6. Identify ideas for comprehension. Brainstorm activities that are based upon pragmatic intent and semantic context. If the student does not understand what you are trying to convey when you use a particular language skill, then anything you do afterward that depends on his knowledge or understanding will be unsuccessful.
7. Identify ideas for production (through-the-air or print). After you are sure that the student understands the language skill, then it is appropriate to ask him to produce the language on his own. Activities in this section assume that the child has mastered comprehension of the skill.
8. Identify modeling and self-correction techniques that might be used to teach the skill.
9. Identify how to visually support teaching the structure. How will you provide visual representation of the lesson other than through-the-air communication in order to heighten the visual salience of the rules associated with a language skill? (use of visual tools, maps, webs, charts, overhead, print-on cards)
10. Consider how to teach the target structure using ASL-to-ESL practices. How does this structure compare in ASL and English? What techniques and strategies will you use to teach English through ASL?

not occur in ASL. Further, use of these words in question form requires the user to understand the application of the auxiliary *do* (e.g., *Do you have . . . ?*). In ASL, *do* is not signed, but rather implied in the question IX (*you*) HAVE COKE OR PEPSI. Table 5.8 compares the use of *have* in ASL and English.

Pragmatic Intent of the Objective. Next, determine practical, pragmatic uses for this language skill. The better job you do of identifying authentic purposes

TABLE 5.8. *Comparison of English and ASL Use of* HAVE

Semantic Meaning	English Structure	ASL Structure
To show possession/concrete	I have a nickel.	_____t CENTS FIVE, IX *(me)* HAVE
	I have a Toyota.	____t TOYOTA, IX *(me)* HAVE
To show possession/abstract	I have an idea.	__t IDEA, IX *(me)* (implied HAVE)
To show guardianship	I have a son.	__t SON, IX *(me)* HAVE
	I have a dog and a cat.	____t CAT, DOG, IX *(me)* HAVE
Part–whole relationship	A table has legs.	___t TABLE, IX *(it)* L-E-G-S FOUR HAVE
State or condition	I have a headache.	_____t HEADACHE, IX *(me)* (implied HAVE)
Figurative use	She had a baby last week. Have a go at it. I've had it!	No comparative use of HAVE in ASL

for the language, the more activities you will be able to plan. Labeling, calling attention to an object, and expressing feelings (e.g., pride and delight) are some of the main purposes for using this language skill. Activities that will allow the student to share his pride in a possession are appropriate and motivating. Activities where students must share game pieces and can use their game pieces to make real contributions to the group activity are appropriate.

Semantic Contexts.   Next, determine the real-life contexts within which you would most likely experience the need to meet the pragmatic intent. For example, sharing something new, sharing something that is your favorite possession, calling attention to something unusual, cooking, playing games, and going on treasure hunts are all appropriate contexts within which to use this language. Determine the vocabulary associated with the activity you plan to do and pre-teach this if appropriate or incorporate it into your overall lesson.

Ideas for Exposure.   After bringing to conscious thought the different ways you might use this language, choose the ones you plan to use during the exposure phase. For example, bring something different for lunch each day. Tell the students what you have. Try unusual food items with which the students will be unfamiliar. Special treats will enhance their sense of delight. Ask what they have in their lunch boxes or bags. Bring a surprise box every day. Say, "I have something in the box. What do you think I have?" When a child makes a guess, share it with others. Say "William thinks I have a kitten in the box."

Ideas for Comprehension.　Most children will intuitively learn the meaning of *have* through conversation. If not, you will have to develop their understanding of its meaning and use by comparing the state or condition aspect of the verb with action verbs. Keeping the subject and object of the sentence the same, use pictures to demonstrate the differences between *have* and action verbs (e.g., *The girls have a doll. The girls washed the doll. The boys have a ball. The boys played with the ball.*). Use pictures of the sentence pairs. Help children sort pictures by category of *have* versus action. Next, choose a sentence pair. Say either of the sentences and have the child choose the appropriate corresponding picture. Repeat with all sentence pairs. Do this also in the context of fun activities such as the games mentioned here. For example, help the student describe his contribution to the cooking activity.

English: I have the sugar. It tastes good. I have the butter. It is yellow.

$$\overline{\quad t \quad} \qquad\qquad \overline{\quad (nod) \quad} \quad \overline{\quad t \quad}$$

ASL: SUGAR, IX *(me)* HAVE.　GOOD IX *(it)* TASTE.　BUTTER, IX *(me)* HAVE. YELLOW IX *(it)*.

Ideas for Production.　With this amount of exposure and direct work on comprehension, most students should be producing *have* in this context. If not, and if you are sure the child comprehends the meaning and use of *have*, then the child may need an opportunity to practice its use with guidance and encouragement. Give the child a box of interesting items. Have him pull one out and hide it behind his back, and ask for clues. ASL is provided in the following dialogue in small caps following the English sentence.

Is it green? Is it soft?	$\overline{\qquad\qquad q}$　$\overline{\quad q}$ IX *(loc)* GREEN.　IX *(loc)* SOFT.
Do you have a Pokemon card?	$\overline{\qquad\qquad\qquad t}$　$\overline{\quad q}$ P-O-K-E-M-O-N CARD, IX *(you)* HAVE.
I think you have an army man.	$\overline{\qquad\qquad t}$ ARMY MAN, IX *(me)* THINK IX *(you)* HAVE.

When the child finally shows you the item, say with enthusiasm,

A worm. You have a worm.	$\overline{\qquad\qquad t}$ WORM!, WORM, IX *(you)* HAVE.

Repeat the activity, this time allowing the child to guess while you hide the object behind your back. Encourage him to use the word *have* the way you did. Make sure that you have put meaningful and exciting items into the bag.

Ideas for Modeling and Self-Correction.   Recall that there are a variety of practices used to teach language. If you are using modeling and self-correction practices, you might use the following activity:

> Give a special, secret toy to each child in the group. Go to the first child and say,
>
>   <u>   t   </u>
> "You have a duck (DUCK, IX *(you)* HAVE)." Tell the class, "Keith has a
> duck <u>   t </u>
> (DUCK, K-E-I-T-H IX *(he)* HAVE)." Then ask, "What does Keith have?
>   <u>   wh-q </u>
> (K-E-I-T-H, IX *(he)* HAVE WHAT) " If students respond with "Duck," expand
>   <u>   t </u>
> and say, "Right. Keith has a duck (RIGHT. DUCK K-E-I-T-H IX *(he)* HAVE)."

Expect students to repeat your sentence, expanding and rehearsing as necessary. Go around the room asking each child to say what the first child has. Go to the second child and repeat the sequence, using that child's object. Take up the toys and give them back to different children.

>   <u>   t   wh-q </u>
> Ask "Who has the bunny? (BUNNY WHO HAVE)." The person in possession
>   <u>   (nod) </u>
> must say "I have the bunny (IX *(me)* HAVE BUNNY)." Use modeling and
> expansion techniques to elicit better approximations.

Ideas for Visual Representation of the Objective.   Another option is to use visual representation of the language. For example, place the pictures used in your comprehension activity on either side of a pocket chart, with *have* pictures on left and action verb pictures on right. Write the word *have* on several sentence strips and write the action verbs on other strips. Describe each picture emphasizing either *have* or the action verb, then place the verb under the picture. Next, take picture pairs and have the child place strips with the *have* or the action verb with the picture. Go through all sentences this way. Next, show one of the picture pairs to the child and have him choose between the *have* card or the action verb card, all the while providing a clear model of complete sentences. Next, give the child a choice of picture without the card cue. Finally, ask him to tell/sign to you the corresponding sentence. Alternately, place the pattern "<u>*(who)*</u> have/has____" on a sentence strip or write it on the board to indicate to the students that this is the pattern you want them to follow. Make the game more exciting by having students pass around an imaginary item. For example, pretend you are using an egg beater. Say, "I have an egg beater." Pass the imaginary item on to the next student who must invent another imaginary item. Ask him "What do you have?" When he shows his imaginary item (e.g., a pogo stick), ask other students to try to recognize it. Have them describe the item using the pattern.

Summary

Students who are deaf or hard or hearing are very diverse. They bring to the classroom a wide range of backgrounds and linguistic abilities. They learn language in different ways. Some students are monolingual, some students are bilingual, some students negotiate several languages at the same time, and others are languageless. All of them require different communication approaches. The teacher of language must first determine the most efficient pathway in which the child encodes language, then she must individualize each lesson to meet each child's needs.

We discussed in the first section of this chapter how important it is to provide language instruction via the pathway that affords the child the most rapid language growth. This decision made along with the family will determine future language instruction. We also discussed how important it is for the teacher to be proficient in the language of instruction. When a teacher is not language proficient then the students are at a severe disadvantage.

Decisions surrounding how to teach language skills to students who are deaf and hard of hearing must not be made cavalierly. Careful assessment of present levels of performance as well as monitoring of students' language development is critical to the language planning process. Language planning requires sensitivity to the differences and needs of each child along with skill in a wide array of procedures, techniques, strategies, and activities.

Questions for Critical Thinking

1. What approaches and practices would you use with each of the children in Chapter 3 and why?

2. For which of the children would it be appropriate to teach micropragmatic, macropragmatic, or metapragmatic skills?

3. Identify an English grammar structure. How would you respond to each of the components of the planning model if this structure were an objective for a preschooler, an elementary-age child, a middle schooler, or a high schooler? What student-related factors would you need to consider before beginning this task?

6

Answering and Asking Questions: Keys to Conversation

What to Expect in This Chapter _____

In this chapter you will read about the art of conversation and the complexities of the system of English questions. You will see that there is a mutual relationship between the two, with questioning skills fueling conversation and conversation providing the need to ask questions.

The purpose of this chapter is to describe the connection between question development and conversation development. Questioning skills are challenging for children with hearing losses to master. Conversation skills provide a similar challenge. Although most of the discussions in this chapter use English question forms as examples, understand that the issues of pragmatic intent, conversational development, repair strategies, classroom discourse, and incidental language learning described herein apply whether the language is ASL or English.

English question forms are difficult for children who are deaf and hard of hearing to master. Most of the information we have about this topic relates to the syntactic challenges of question formation in English. We begin this chapter with a discussion of the comprehension and use of question forms then proceed to a syntactic examination of the basic question forms of English and of ASL. The key element in helping children who are deaf and hard of hearing learn to use and answer questions is this: *Make sure they have an authentic question in mind.* This statement seems simplistic, yet its realization requires us to expand our notions of what language and instruction encompass. The intent to communicate, to gather information, and to understand and be understood are the foundation for all efforts toward conversation. The force that keeps con-

198

versations going, that allows us to interact with others, and that repairs misunderstanding is the ability to ask questions. In this chapter we build the case that question development must occur pragmatically, intentionally, and purposefully within the context of conversation.

The Relationship between Questioning and Conversation

Consider the two everyday scenes below. One takes place in a classroom of children who are deaf and hard of hearing. One takes place between a hearing child and hearing mother. They provide background for a discussion of what constitutes good instruction in the development of questioning skills through conversation.

Questioning Scene 1: Hearing Parent–Hearing Child Interaction

A mother and her son have just finished lunch. "Outside!" says little William. "Do you want to go outside?" asks Mom. "Well," says she, "You'll need your shoes." William stares at his stockinged feet. "Go get your shoes, honey," encourages Mom. "No shoes," replies William. "Where are your shoes? Are they in the bedroom? Are they in the bathroom? Where'd they go?" queries Mom. "Where go?" intones William. "Shoes. Shoes? Where go, shoes?" calls William entreatingly as he begins his search. "Shoes ober dere," says William as he toddles over to retrieve his sneakers.

Questioning Scene 2: The Typical Classroom of Children Who Are Deaf and Hard of Hearing

The teacher is sitting on one side of a kidney-shaped table with five eager preschoolers on the other side. She brings out a Fischer-Price™ Farm Set and places animals in various locations, describing what she is doing through simultaneous communication (e.g., "Tractor. The farmer is on the tractor. Fence. The rooster is on the fence."). Next, she begins to question the students regarding the locations of the various farm members. "Misty," she says, "Where is the rooster?" "Fence," replies Misty. "On the fence. The rooster is on the fence," says the teacher, providing an expansion. "Where is the rooster?" "On fence," is Misty's final reply. The teacher says, "Now you be the teacher. Ask Antonio about the animals. Use a 'where' question."

Both of these scenes involve the development of questioning skills. Their differences, however, highlight the relationship between question development and conversation development. Obviously there is no interaction between questioning and conversation in Scene 2. Questioning skills normally develop within conversations. No natural conversation is occurring in Scene 2. According to Bruner (1971), "One of the most crucial ways in which a culture provides aid to intellectual growth is through a dialogue between the more experienced and the less experienced" (p. 107). Young hearing children learn how to ask and answer questions because: (1) they overhear adult models asking and answering questions in conversations with one another; and (2) their primary caregivers engage them in routine conversations that blend information and questioning. Also, conversational questioning provides both the question and a possibility of an answer. The teacher in Scene 2 is not providing sufficient information for the child to be able to develop the use of questions. In Scene 1, the mother provided not only the question form to the child but also a possible set of answers. She didn't know it, but she was using *scaffolding*, a process where the child is given assistance in reaching higher levels of language. This process goes above and beyond the basics of modeling and expansion, providing the model for both the question and the answer but leaving it up to the child to think through the relationship rather than requiring imitation. The conversational process in Scene 1 is also flexible. In Scene 2, only inflexible, rote learning is occurring. Lastly, the child best develops the use of questions on an authentic, realistic, need-to-know basis rather than through contrived, teacher-driven activities. Because the child in Scene 1 is the initiator of the question/answer sequence (William's comment, "Outside!"), pragmatic intent is naturally built into the process. He wants to go outside (desire). His mother informs him that he needs his shoes (condition). He can't find his shoes (need to meet a condition), so the stage is set for him to practice questions and answers to meet this need.

We use questions when we need to know something. One can feign this need, as in Scene 2, but true need is elegantly powerful. It is elegant because of its simplicity and realness. It is powerful because it is based within pragmatic intent. In other words, we formulate a question when we have a true and real question, and questions arise most naturally during conversation. Not only do questions arise in conversation, but also they are the driving force behind conversation. If we automatically understood everything that another person said, we would be telepathic and there would be no need for conversation. Conversations are inherently dependent upon questioning. It is in the process of sharing information, experiencing complete or partial misunderstandings, and repairing conversational breakdowns that we learn to ask and answer questions. Unfortunately, the amount of time that anyone spends engaging children who are deaf and hard of hearing in real, mindful, intentional conversations is grossly insufficient to promote conversation and question development. Rogers, Perrin, and Waller (1987) stated that without extended classroom conversations, "language becomes primarily a device used to 'guess' the right answer rather than a tool the child uses to construct his or her own knowledge" (p. 17).

Limited conversational experiences lead to limited conversational and questioning skills, which lead to limited conversations. Such reduced conversing in turn leads to limited opportunities to learn questioning skills. It is a vicious cycle that takes children who are deaf and hard of hearing nowhere. The teacher must reverse this cycle by increasing real, open-ended opportunities for conversation. This will promote a pragmatic need for questions as tools that will increase the conversational experiences that in turn will improve conversational skills (see Figure 6.1). Regular curricular content can serve "as the substance of educational conversations, helping us meet curricular or administrative goals while promoting both language learning and learning through language" (Kretschmer & Kretschmer, 1997, p. 5). We propose that teachers minimize the amount of time spent on manipulating sentences through drills and worksheets and instead maximize dialogue-oriented, meaningful conversation aimed at problem solving.

Purposes of Conversation

Conversation in the classroom primarily serves two goals: a social goal and a classroom discourse goal (Bloom & Knott, 1985; Tattershall & Creaghead, 1985). The classroom discourse objectives of conversation are teacher directed and include behavior management, attention-getting, directing, informing, converging, and evaluating. In the classroom teachers control the conversation and as a result control the students. Look in any typical content-oriented classroom and you will see few free-flowing conversations. Weiss (1986) stated that certain behaviors in the classroom may be the result of students' attempts to get by with only partial communicative competence. In contrast, when students converse with one another for social purposes, conversations are purposeful, mutual, supportive, divergent, and spirited. Look in any cafeteria or on any playground and you will see lots of free-flowing conversations. When communicating among themselves, deaf children adhere to all the discourse rules associated with natural conversation (Prinz & Prinz, 1985). Why, then, is it that conversations with teachers and parents are so impoverished? Given the right reasons, children who are deaf and hard of hearing will converse. The academic, instructional discourse style was not intended to replace the natural, social style of human interaction that fosters the development of conversation.

Why Children Have Difficulty with Questions and Conversations

The main source of a child's inability to engage in conversation is the lack of opportunity. Most young children who are deaf and hard of hearing have parents who are in the process of learning how to communicate with their children, either through highly structured auditory and oral practices, through an English system of signs or cues, or through ASL. Because they are not yet proficient, young children often miss out on everyday conversational experiences. At school, language teachers tend to think in terms of the individual pieces of language (i.e., specific phonemes, vocabulary development, the development of connected language), and they tend to work on communication development in a fragmented manner. This does not leave much time for conversation. However, children develop conversations when and only when someone converses with them. Teachers absolutely must make a point of spending a large part of their day in conversation with all students, not just young children. It is only through attempts at the give and take (called "turn-taking") of communication that communication can grow. Even the youngest child with limited conversational skills will benefit from being drawn into conversations.

The second reason conversational skills are limited is that most children who are deaf and hard of hearing lack general knowledge of the world around them. This is a double-edged problem. Children communicate best about what they know, yet the child who has a limited communication system has been deprived of basic world knowledge, and, therefore, of the source for acquisition of basic world knowledge. This has implications for the development of questions. If a child does not know the answer, how can he answer the question? For example, if you want to teach deaf children how to answer English questions, then you must teach them to understand adverbs. Aside from simple *who, what, what category* (e.g., what color), and *what . . . doing* questions (which we answer with nouns, verbs, and adjectives), we answer many questions with some form of an adverbial: when, where, why, how, how often, with what, in what manner, by whom. Students must know these adverbial forms before they can answer a question such as *How did the boy carry the bowl of soup? (Carelessly.)* If a child is not interested in this kind of information or does not have the prerequisite experiential base, then language instruction in this area will be meaningless.

According to Raphael and McKinney (1983), there are three sources of information available to answer questions. *Explicit* information is that which is directly stated. *Implied* information is another source and is difficult for many students to grasp. The final source of information comes from the *individual's knowledge base*. Children who are deaf and hard of hearing need to learn that these three sources are available to them.

The ability to converse allows us to gather information to share with others so we can improve our skills in communication and in turn learn more about the world. Figure 6.1 demonstrates this relationship. Conversation is essential in the acquisition of world knowledge and accounts for a significant portion of the information children learn incidentally. Warren and Kaiser (1986) make a distinction between *incidental learning* and *incidental teaching*. Incidental learning occurs in multiple situations and with multiple partners. Incidental teaching is "the interactions between an adult and a child that arise naturally in an unstructured situation, such as free play, and that are used systematically by the adult to transmit new information or give the child practice in developing a communication skill" (p. 291). They further stated that the "contiguity between the child's attention to an event and its linguistic representation" (p. 293) captures natural, intuitive learning principles. Without conversation, incidental learning does not occur. Without incidental learning, the child's fund of world

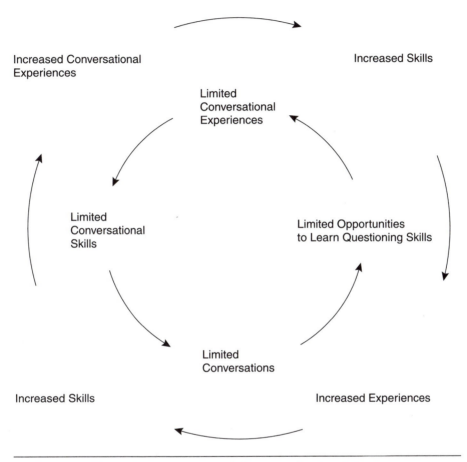

FIGURE 6.1 *The Cycle of Conversational Poverty in Deaf and Hard of Hearing Children*

knowledge remains limited. Conversational ability and incidental learning are highly intertwined, and questions fuel the process.

Reversing the Cycle of Conversational Poverty

Increasing a student's experiences with natural conversations happens in two ways. First, we must assist the child in observing conversations between others. This is not easily done; thus, literature is a powerful tool for deaf and hard of hearing children—the literature written for young children contains conversations. While the child might be shut out of overhearing a conversation between adults, the skillful parent or teacher can use storytelling as a means of demonstrating conversations. Second, we must engage the child in real conversations that are open-ended in multiple settings. One setting, *peer triads*, involves an older student who is a mature communicator interacting with two younger students who are developing communicators. Children look up to students who are just a year or two older than they are. Perhaps they feel that the challenge to communicate is easier with an individual whose skills are just a stage or two higher. Whatever the reason, younger children need lots of opportunities to converse with older children. Two younger children in a triad is an ideal mix; more than two may induce sub-conversations. Two children work well because they vie for the attention of the older student. This encourages the desire to communicate. Another setting, *parent–child dyads*, involves conversations between parents and their children. Most children have their needs met by their parents, and, as we discussed, getting one's basic needs met is a powerful motivation to communicate. Tye-Murray (1998) provided an excellent guide to help parents in developing conversational skills with their children who are deaf and hard of hearing. A third setting, *teacher–child dyads*, involves conversations between the teacher and one or two children whose conversational and questioning skills are on the same level. This allows students to practice their developing skills with one another in the presence of an individual skilled in spotting and encouraging language at the active locus of learning (Muma, 1998). It also allows the teacher to model accessible conversations to one child while engaging in conversation with the other. The final setting, *teacher–class conversations*, involves teacher-facilitated conversations among the members of the class. In classroom conversations the teacher can:

1. *Teach new conversational and questioning skills.* This occurs through instruction and practice with specific question forms. This kind of instruction should take place with real purposes in mind. The desire to ask a question must be a prime feature of instruction.
2. *Increase conversational experiences in assisted conversations.* Activities such as scripts, scaffolding, scenarios, and role-plays allow students to practice new skills.
3. *Practice developing skills directly and indirectly.* This involves focusing on a skill from one of the previous activities and helping the students practice it in meaningful experiences.

The teacher must make sure that he provides students with opportunities for conversations in a variety of settings because different sets of social language are expected in different settings. For example, the kind of language used at a Girl Scout meeting differs from the kind of language used at home. Contexts for communication include but are not limited to home, classroom, playground, social groups, the community, and the media. Students also need to know that the rules of conversation vary from formal to informal conversations depending on the setting. For example, in classroom discourse, teachers control turn-taking whereas in general conversations, both speakers negotiate turns (Bullard & Schirmer, 1991).

Conversation is a logical place for communication skills to begin. "Because it is only in conversation that all aspects of language come together in authentic settings, conversation should be the essential basis for developing language in hearing impaired students" (p. 21). A conversational approach to language development is appropriate whether the language you are teaching is spoken or signed, English or ASL.

The Johnson Conversational Model

What is a conversation? Johnson (1988, 2000) described the components of a conversation as a tool for evaluating and intervening in a student's conversational development (see Figure 6.2). This model defines the necessary elements of a conversation. Key to this model are the concepts of occurrences, segments, tasks, behaviors, and channels. According to Johnson, during the course of a day, an individual engages in numerous conversations, or *conversational occurrences*. Each occurrence, or *conversational segment*, follows a similar pattern of exchanges including a beginning, a middle, and an end. Specific *conversational tasks* occur within each segment of the conversation. The ten tasks are identified in Figure 6.2.

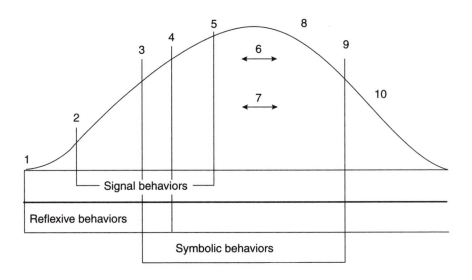

FIGURE 6.2 *The Johnson Conversational Model*

Reflexive behaviors: 1–4; Signal behaviors: 2–5; Symbolic behaviors: 3–9

Task 1 (Beginning): Noninteractional events.   These are the actions or events a person is engaging in prior to the conversation. They may influence the next conversational task (e.g., a fire starts, causing an individual to call for help) or they may have nothing to do with the next conversational task (e.g., a person is daydreaming and is interrupted by a new conversational partner).

Task 2 (Beginning): Gaining the individual's attention.   Conversations don't occur *at* someone but with someone. For this reason, a conversation cannot begin until both partners mutually agree to share a conversation. If you have ever tried to start a conversation with someone who is unaware of your effort, then you understand the importance of this task. Conversational partners engage in any number of ways to open a conversation such as recognizing the other's presence, using a simple greeting, using a nonverbal signal (e.g., "ahem") to garner attention, tapping the person on the shoulder, or any number of other attention-gaining behaviors.

Task 3 (Beginning): Onset of the conversation.   A conversation begins when the individual whose attention was sought indicates recognition that conversation is sought. This may be done by facial expression, body language, or a variety of verbal indicators (e.g., "Oh, hi!") to let the person seeking the conversation know that mutual attention has been negotiated. When analyzing a conversation, it is important to note the onset of the conversation.

Task 4 (Middle): Exchange pleasantries.   Most conversations begin with pleasantries. These can be very simple or very elaborate. A simple, "Yes?" or an elaborately acted out greeting, such as ritualized greetings that include touching and dancing moves, serve the same function. The nature of the pleasantry is determined by the relationship between the communicators, the pragmatic purpose of the conversation, the setting, and even the gender or social affiliation of the communicators.

Task 5 (Middle): Establish the topic.   There was once a conversation held between two sisters who were in a nursing home. Both were elderly and had noticeable hearing losses due to presbycusis. The first sister established a topic, but the second sister misunderstood and responded to a different topic. The first sister misunderstood her and continued with the same topic. Neither sister paid sufficient attention to the other to realize that the topics differed. As a result, their "conversation" continued until the second sister's remark about the first's topic irritated the first sister, who made a rude comment to the second sister. The second sister queried "What's wrong with her?" and both sisters went their separate ways. Although each sister relayed information, the sisters did not share a mutually agreed upon topic, and a true conversation did not occur. The topic one establishes is based on one's prior world knowledge, one's relationship with the communication partner, the context of the situation, the demands of the environment, and many other factors.

Task 6 (Middle): Exchange information.   A second problem with the sisters' conversation above is that information was not actually exchanged. Information exchanged may be minimal (e.g., a nod) or elaborate (e.g., a treatise), but there must be transmission of information from one individual to another for a conversation to have occurred. The information exchanged depends on the same pragmatic constraints already mentioned and is also dependent on the perspective of the initiator of each conversational turn.

Task 7 (Middle): Recognize and repair conversational breakdown.   Had the sisters above realized that each did not understand the other, they would have taken the opportunity to repair their conversation. When conversations break down, the communicators may or may not attempt to fix the problem. We fix problems that either we notice (the sisters did not) or are important to us or to the conversation we are having. Students who are deaf and hard of hearing need to be encouraged to watch for the signals of communication breakdown and to choose those breakdowns that are important to them and to the conversation at hand (see Strategies for Repairing Conversations later in this chapter).

Task 8 (Middle): Negotiate ending to the conversation.   As with the other components of a conversation, we engage in certain conventional practices to negotiate the end of a conversation. A variety of communication behaviors are available at this point in the conversations, and endings can be negotiated well or negotiated poorly. The way we extricate ourselves from a conversation depends on the setting, the relationship of the partners, the context, the content, and the purpose of the conversation. The process of agreeing to end a conversation may result in an abrupt ending, an extended ending, or with newly agreed-upon topics of conversation that put off an ending until later.

Task 9 (End): End the conversation.   Once both conversational partners agree to end a conversation, an ending takes place. Endings can be simple or elaborate, polite or rude. They are determined using the conditions described in Task 8.

Task 10 (End): Leave the conversation.   Once a verbal exchange has been made that closes the conversation, the conversational partners must break their mutual attention. This may be done simply (e.g., turning away) or elaborately (e.g., slamming the door behind you). Should either conversational partner choose to reconvene the conversation, simple repair strategies are not sufficient. Rather the initiator must begin the process of establishing attention again.

According to Johnson, these conversational tasks are accomplished via the use of three types of *conversational behaviors:* reflexive behaviors, signal behaviors, and symbolic behaviors. Reflexive behaviors are those that naturally occur all the time. They include such actions as blinking, being startled, or sneezing. These behaviors represent the external manifestation of internal states. They are not intended to convey communication. Prior to initiating the conversational sequence, most individuals are engaging in reflexive behaviors. In fact, reflexive behaviors occur all the time and are out of our conscious control. The difficulty comes when someone interprets a reflexive behavior as a signal behavior. Signal behaviors are those that occur toward the beginning of a conversation. Mistakenly interpreting a reflexive behavior for a signal behavior occurs most frequently between individuals who are unfamiliar with one another and between individuals from different cultures (e.g., Deaf versus hearing cultures). They are purposeful behaviors that are designed to convey communicative intent (e.g., a wave of the hand, a shrug of the shoulder, a head nod). They require a supportive physical context to be correctly interpreted. The intended meaning of the behavior cannot be correctly interpreted outside a narrow range of settings. Signal behaviors occur all the way throughout the conversational process and include behaviors to garner attention, behaviors to acknowledge what the speaker is saying without actually taking a turn, behaviors to indicate communication breakdown (e.g., a puzzled look), and behaviors to indicate affective response to the message (e.g., boredom, surprise). Symbolic behaviors are those purposeful behaviors of conversations which convey the message intended through required choices of vocabulary and grammar. These can be presented concretely (e.g., obvious choice of vocabulary) or abstractly (e.g., metaphorically, euphemistically). All three behaviors occur simultaneously, but one predominates depending upon the conversational task in which the communicators are engaged.

Communicators have several options for *conversational channels* that they may use to convey their message: the visual channel (e.g., gesture, sign, facial expression), the motorical channel (e.g., body language, showing, pointing, taking), or the verbal channel (e.g., speech). Johnson stated that the essential purpose of the conversational model is to provide an observational template through which a teacher can observe and document a student's conversation use of language. The focus of the teacher's observation is to determine

1. where within the conversational task the student is experiencing the frustration,
2. why that frustration is occurring, and
3. what others in the environment do to address such frustration.

The basic goal of observational work is to increase the students' communication competence, that is, their ability to convey effectively and to comprehend communicative intent. This may be done by increasing the number and range of topics, tasks, contexts (physical and interpersonal), pathways (face-to-face, spoken, signed, e-mailed, conveyed through text-based technology), communication repair strategies, and languages (English and ASL) that an individual can use both to understand and to be understood (Johnson, 2000).

Promoting Conversation and Questioning Skills

Table 6.1 lists the important points to remember when encouraging conversation development and questioning skills. First, consider the conversational environment. Background noise, poor room acoustics, visual noise and distractions, and poor lighting may seem like minor issues, but they contribute to the difficulty that children have in engaging in conversation. Children with poor questioning skills are stressed and strained enough when trying to learn new skills. Be sure that you are working in an environment that does not add to the problem. Second, consider your message to the student. Tye-Murray (1994) suggests the following:

1. Avoid verbosity and excess words. Be clear yet concise.
2. Avoid telegraphic speech (or signs). Provide a complete message.
3. Repeat important keywords and phrases. Make information available more than once.
4. Use precise vocabulary. Avoid using generic terminology. Words such as *this, them, that,* and *it* are important but develop more naturally when the child is comfortable conversing.
5. Pause between your utterances. Give the child time to think. Most children receive an incomplete message and must engage in mental closure, which requires extra processing time.
6. Avoid run-on sentences. Remember that the young child who is just learning to participate in conversations may be confused easily. Do not exceed the student's length of memory.

TABLE 6.1 *Factors to Consider in Promoting Conversation and Questioning Skills*

- Consider the conversational environment.
- Consider your message to the student.
- Maintain flexibility in questioning students.
- Understand the sequence of development of questions and the factors influencing these.
- Know well your student's present level of skill.

Third, maintain flexibility in how you question students during conversations. The purpose of questioning students is to promote conversation and to provide a source of material about which children will want to question you. Although it is fun to play the old game of "Twenty Questions," a rigid set of questions will not promote their use in natural situations. To maintain flexibility, incorporate the following into conversations:

1. Talk about topics that the students bring up. Do not impose a topic. Students ask questions when they have a question in mind, and they converse about things they know. Students are more likely to have information about their own topics, and you can keep conversations going longer than if you choose a topic about which the student has limited information.

2. Listen carefully to what the students are saying, and take advantage of opportunities to provide additional information. The more information you provide, the more likely it is that a child will ask a question. If possible, leave out partial information so that the students will want to ask a question.

3. Avoid comments that are likely to truncate a conversation (Rogers, Perrin, & Waller, 1987). For example, comments like "Interesting" and "Oh, really?" are conversation killers and do not invite the child to continue.

4. Avoid questions where there is an obvious or distinct answer. The more open-ended the question, the greater the chance that you will get a response. By open-ended we mean something other than "What is your favorite color?" because even though you are not expecting a particular answer, the question is likely to result in a one-word answer. Questions whose answers are nouns, verbs, or adjectives are more likely to be answered in one word.

5. Avoid asking question after question after question. This leads to a teacher–student mindset rather than a communicator–communicator mindset. Be sure to alternate information with questions. Wood and Wood (1984) found that as the number of questions a teacher asked increased, the amount of conversation children who were deaf and hard of hearing displayed decreased. "A great many questions produced a great many answers, but little else, whereas fewer questions and more comments and phatics (oh really, how lovely, mm-hmm) were met by children giving more spontaneous contributions, elaborated answers, and asking questions themselves" (Wood & Wood, 1984, p. 46). A good rule of thumb is to provide no less than two pieces of new information for every question you ask. For example, if you start a conversation by saying "How was Boy Scout camp this summer?" you will probably get the answer "Fine." Our tendency next would be to say, "What did you do?" which might lead to "swim," causing us to have to ask "What else?" Instead, provide information after each question. For example, after the initial ex-

change, contribute your own experience such as "I went to Girl Scout camp when I was your age. We did lots of fun things." The child may simply answer "oh," but he may ask what you did. By sharing information you give him the opportunity to be inquisitive. Remember the rule of thumb: give no less than two pieces of information anytime you ask a question.

6. Allow the student sufficient time to think about your comment and to formulate his response. If the student does not answer you right away, he may be taking extra time to process what you said. He may be thinking about the experience he wants to describe and weighing which answer to give, or he may not realize that you are expecting a response. Instead, use questioning behaviors such as raising your eyebrows, tilting your head, or raising your shoulders to indicate that you are patiently awaiting a response.

Fourth, understand the sequence of development of questions and the factors influencing these. Spend time learning about the developmental sequence of question forms that children pass through. By asking questions at the appropriate locus of learning, you increase the likelihood that the child will learn a new skill. Different purposes of communication foster different question forms. Understanding this relationship will help you think carefully about the question you pose and try to elicit. Finally, know well your student's present level of skill. Conversational skills develop along a continuum, as does the ability to ask and answer questions. Focus on the child's active locus of learning (Muma, 1998) to get the most mileage out of your conversational time.

Tools for the Enhancement of Conversation and Questioning

The relation between conversation and question development is paradoxical. On the one hand questions are learned through conversation and aid in keeping conversations on track by assisting in repairs and by requesting information. On the other hand too many questions can kill a conversation between a teacher of the deaf and the student with whom he is conversing (Wood & Wood, 1984). The challenge is to provide sufficient information, structure, and support without being too controlling.

Three tools for enhancing conversation and the ability to ask questions are scaffolding, scripts, and role-playing conversational scenarios. They all have as an objective the presentation of good models of conversation, but each is slightly different from the other.

Scaffolding. Scaffolding is an interactive process of guiding communication interchanges that would not have been possible without support. Scaffolding is often thought of as a tool for reading instruction (Merritt, Culatta, & Trostle,

1998). In reading, scaffolding involves teaching a structure (e.g., story grammar or maps) to enhance the student's ability to make sense of what he has read. Scaffolds are prior knowledge of a story structure that the student applies to a new story. The concept of scaffolding also applies to conversation because it, too, involves guided communication interchanges—the teacher provides conversational material necessary to ask and answer questions. Scaffolding for communication and questioning differs from scaffolding for reading in that the student does not necessarily know the structure of information prior to engaging in the conversation. Structure would be difficult to impose because conversations are free-flowing, and one can never predict where an actual conversation will lead.

There are two ways to use scaffolding. First, demonstrate the structure of other conversations (e.g., conversations from stories) to provide a scaffold upon which the child may base a newer version, or a recasting of the conversation and questions. Recasting is an important tool in language development and was discussed in Chapter 5. Second, scaffolding can present new bits of information upon which the student can build his conversation and questions. The following exchange, which demonstrates this practice, is with Ashley, who is struggling with asking "why" questions.

Scenario:

Teacher is talking to Ashley about a classmate who has been out for a very long time. The teacher models questions about the student's absence and provides information from personal experience to give Ashley the opportunity to ask questions. The following dialogue would actually transpire via a combination of speech, English signs, and ASL, given Ashley's history. We make no attempt to gloss this conversation since our point is to demonstrate scaffolding.

T: *Was Shontay in your mainstream class today?*

A: *No. Shontay still out.*

Teacher: *I wonder . . . Why is she out?* (Modeling question formation.) *Do you know?*

Ashley: *No.*

Teacher: *A long time ago a student of mine was out for a month. Many people asked me "Why is he out?"* (Modeling question formation.) *Guess why he was out.*

Ashley: *I don't know.*

Teacher: *He broke both of his legs.*

> **Ashley:** *Did he have car wreck?*
>
> **Teacher:** *Yes. I was out for six weeks once.* (Providing leading information.)
>
> **Ashley:** (Following model from her previous question.) *Did you have a car wreck?*
>
> **Teacher:** *No.* (Uses a pause to encourage Ashley to continue.)
>
> **Ashley:** *Sick?*
>
> **Teacher:** *No*
>
> **Ashley:** *Lazy?*
>
> **Teacher:** *No.* (Avoiding temptation to answer the question before it is asked.)
>
> **Ashley:** (Following teacher's model from earlier part of conversation.) *Why were you out?*
>
> **Teacher:** *I had a baby.*

In order to engage in this interchange, the teacher followed three steps:

1. Paid careful attention to the student to find out the question form that she needed to know (active locus of learning). Chose to provide a scaffold for this particular structure because of an immediate, pragmatic need: requesting information.
2. Relayed a personal experience or provided information as a vehicle for modeling the question forms the student needed.
3. Provided several examples of the model in context. The teacher does not directly instruct the student in the formation of the sentence.

This form of scaffolding conversations takes knowledge of the student's present level of performance, willingness to listen to the student, and quick thinking to find appropriate information as a vehicle to convey the question form. Conversational scaffolding requires a sincere effort to master, but the payoffs in conversational development are worth it.

Scaffolding is also applicable to the development of written language. Imagine now that the teacher is talking with Kevin, who is struggling with "how" questions. You might see the following interchange regarding Kevin's writing assignment:

Scenario:

The teacher is conducting a lesson on written language, in particular, describing a procedure. Prior to writing, she wants to refresh Kevin's memory regarding "how to" questions. Notice how she models both the question and answer.

Teacher: (Modifying her signed English to the level of comprehension she thinks he will understand.) *I see you are working on your writing assignment. What are you are thinking about?*

Kevin: (Signing and voicing.) *Me write dog vet.*

Teacher: *Oh, was your dog sick or hurt?*

Kevin: *Yes, leg break.*

Teacher: *Oh dear. That is sad. What happened?*

Kevin: (Describes events.)

Teacher: *What do you want to say in your story?*

Kevin: (Explains the best way he can that he wants to say how to care for a dog in a cast. However, the teacher knows that he does not use the embedded question form using "how to.")

Teacher: *Did I ever tell you that my father was a veterinarian?*

Kevin: *No.*

Teacher: (Providing model at active locus of learning.) *Yes. My daddy taught me how to clip an animal's toenails.* (Lists the steps in " first, next, then" format for Kevin.) *He taught me how to give a dog a bath.* (Lists steps in "first, next, then" format.) *He taught me how to give a dog a pill.* (Lists steps in "first, next, then" format).

Kevin: *My vet show me clean cast.*

Teacher: *Oh. He taught you how to clean the cast? Tell me the steps.*

Kevin: (Tells steps using "first, next, then" format.)

Teacher: *I can't wait to read your story. I'd like to know how to clean a cast.* (Calls other student into conversation.) *David, come here. Kevin, tell David what you are writing about.*

Kevin: *My dog, leg break. I write how to clean cast.* (David tells Kevin about the broken arm he had several years ago.)

This exact conversation could transpire in ASL. Pretend now that Kevin is an ASL user rather than an English sign user. We might gloss the conversation like this:

_____q   _____wh

Teacher: IX (*you*) WORK WRITE+++ TELL ME IX POSS (*your*) TOPIC WHAT.

Kevin: IX (*me*) WRITE STORY TAKE DOG V-E-T.

_____q _wh_

Teacher: IX (*your*) DOG SICK OR HURT. WHICH.

Kevin: DOG, IX (*his*) LEG BREAK.

_____wh-q

Teacher: SAD.   WHAT HAPPEN, WHAT.

Kevin: (Richly describes whole event in ASL.)

_____wh

Teacher: IX (*you*) INCLUDE+IN IX (*your*) STORY WHAT.

Kevin: (Explains in ASL that he wants to describe how to care for a cast.)

Teacher: (Seeing this as an opportunity to model "how to" so he can use

_____t

it in written form, explains that ENGLISH, USE HOW+T-O THEN 1, 2, 3. Proceeds to give an example through conversation, code-switching between English and ASL when necessary.)

_____q

IX (*me*) TELL IX (*you*) BEFORE, IX POSS (*my*) FATHER V-E-T.

Kevin: NO.

_____t

Teacher: TRUE. IX POSS (*my*) FATHER, TEACH IX (*me*). (Code switches to English and signs "How to." Code switches back to ASL indexing to thumb, first finger, and second finger before listing each activity.)

___t

Kevin: IX POSS (*my*) VET, SAME. TEACH IX (*me*). (Code switches to English signs "How to clean cast."

_____q

Teacher: V-E-T TEACH IX (*you*). (Code switches "How to clean a cast?")

_____t

(Switches back to ASL.) IX POSS (*your*) STORY, IX (*me*) WANT READ.

Dialogue Journals.   A second technique to assist conversational development is the use of *dialogue journals*. Dialogue journals are a vehicle for writing down conversations: two people write back and forth about a topic of mutual interest. Dialogue journals have been used successfully in helping deaf students to understand printed English. Scaffolding is not only appropriate for through-the-air conversation but also is applicable to print. As with through-the-air conversation, the teacher provides a model and sets up the situation for the student to write questions to her. The same principles apply: model correct language, give more information than questions, and do not directly correct the student's attempt to communicate. Dialogue journals promote an integrated language/literacy practice that helps students to learn English through print.

Scripts.   A *script* is a talking routine that parents impart to their hearing children in very specific ways. Parents direct scripts by telling the child very specifically, "Say . . . ." Bashier, Conte, and Heerde (1998) indicated that "students must be able to understand and participate in school scripts and in instructional discourse routines to be successful learners" (p. 7). Hearing children pick up scripts incidentally by modeling themselves after successful or admired peers. Students who are deaf and hard of hearing will benefit from instruction in specific scripts (Whitesell & Klein, 1997). Scripts include the use of three components: typical roles, typical props, and scripted language (Whitesell & Klein, 1997). Scripts for younger children include those surrounding actions at home, in the preschool classroom, and in the community. Scripts for elementary-age children include those surrounding actions in the regular classroom, at PE, in the cafeteria, in the hallway, at after-school events, and in community activities such as church or clubs. Scripts for older students include those surrounding actions leading to greater independence, handling peer pressure, keeping and getting out of tense situations, dating, and communicating with parents. Later, scripts for seeking and maintaining employment are useful. Table 6.2 is a checklist for monitoring progress of a script developed for visits to the doctor.

Scenarios.   Yet another technique for developing conversations is the use of scenarios. *Scenarios* are a type of conversational scaffold. They are like scripts in that we provide the student with the format for the conversation. They differ in that they are more open-ended. Scenarios involve role-playing. The roles are discussed in advance, and students who need suggestions for what to say are given help. The student is given a context and the vocabulary, and concepts involved are discussed and described. Scenarios are role-played again and again. This allows students to engage in recasting the language. Stone (1988) described a variety of scenarios through which children who are deaf and hard of hearing can practice their conversational and, therefore, questioning skills. Teachers may need to start off by suggesting appropriate language, but the actual information and questions involved should flow from scenarios the students choose. Remember to allow students to recast the language in multiple ways.

Johnson (2000) summarized the preconditions for effective intervention. "Effective language intervention is that which (1) creates an authentic need for the child to communicate within the context of a conversation exchange; and (2) focuses upon those elements of the child's communication behaviors that cause *him*, not his teacher, the greatest frustration" (personal communication). The source of intervention must come from a need the child has made evident. All test data pale in importance relative to this source.

TABLE 6.2 *A Script Progress Checklist*

Student's Name: _____ Doctor Script

	Did	Not Yet
1. Follows instructions/directions: For example:		
Have a seat, the doctor will be with you as soon as possible.	___	___
Please come over here. I need to see how much you weigh.	___	___
2. Gives directions if germane to particular role	___	___
3. Asks for clarification if needed	___	___
4. Provided clarification when requested	___	___
5. Narrates/tells series of events that led to accident, illness	___	___
6. Explains cause and effect relationships		
e.g., eating too much junk food led to stomach ache	___	___
7. Describes illness, medicine, etc.	___	___
8. Compares and contrasts		
(e.g., Different roles, different medicines, procedures, etc.)	___	___
9. Engages in well-structured conversations		
(e.g., Opens, closes, takes turns, stays on topic, etc.)	___	___
10. Answers the questions appropriately	___	___
11. Directs others via language	___	___
12. Persuades others via language	___	___
13. Participates in shared reading in waiting room, writing of		
forms, checks, prescriptions, etc.	___	___
14. Retells written/signed narratives that have been shared	___	___
15. Demonstrates ownership in script by voluntarily bringing		
and/or sharing related texts, experiences, props, etc.	___	___

Source: Whitesell, K., & Klein, H. (1995). "Facilitating Language and Learning Via Scripts" (*The Volta Review*, November 1995, Volume 97, Number 5). Reprinted with permission from the Alexander Graham Bell Association for the Deaf and Hard of Hearing.

Strategies for Repairing Conversational Breakdowns

Schirmer and Woolsey (1997) studied the relationship among the different types of questions (literal, analytic, synthesizing, and evaluative). They found that the students in their study who were able to answer higher-order questions about reading material did not need to answer simpler, literal questions because literal information was embedded in the higher-order questions. The implication for conversational questioning is that we should challenge children with questions that require them to analyze, synthesize, and evaluate. This, of course, will promote higher-order thinking, but it will also allow the teacher to model conversational repair strategies if the student's meaning is unclear and there is communication breakdown.

    Tye-Murray (1994) defined a communication breakdown as an interruption that occurs when the child or adult says something that the other does not understand. She defines a repair strategy as "a course of action taken by one of the conversational partners after a message has been misunderstood or not recognized at all" (p. 87). Use repair strategies when a conversation breaks down (Griffith, Johnson, & Dastoli, 1985). Caissie and Gibson (1997) identified eight strategies deaf adults use to clarify conversation when the partner indicates a misunderstanding: full repetition, partial repetition, paraphrase, elaboration, elaboration with repetition, confirmation, confirmation with elaboration, and confirmation with paraphrase.

When the child does not understand what you are asking, use a reduction sequence that makes the information increasingly evident. Begin with the simplest reduction, reducing complexity further if needed. Once you determine the level where the child can independently answer questions, then reverse the process and work toward the next higher level question strategy. Table 6.3 presents the appropriate sequence of question reduction.

When you do not understand what a child is saying, then you must also apply repair strategies. Use the following strategies to help the child to repair his own conversational breakdowns.

- Ask child to repeat the message.
- Encourage child to provide more information to help you discern his meaning. Elaborations may allow you to form mental closure on the intended message.
- Restate what you think the child said. This will provide him with information about what part of the message you misunderstood so he can choose repairs.
- Ask the child to rephrase or recast his statement.

Older students may benefit from direct, metalingluistic instruction in conversational repair. Discuss the components and role-play strategies. Analyze classroom breakdowns and identify the aspect of communication lost. Help the student decide what strategy he could have applied. Role-play a successful interchange based on a revision of the broken interchange.

Question Forms in English

English questions are quite complex. They emerge through a sequence that is similar from child to child, although as you will see in the following discussion of the developmental sequence, this is dependent upon the pragmatic function that the language structure serves.

A Morphosyntactic Look at Questions

Researchers who studied question forms from a morphosyntactic perspective found the following sequence of development (NcNeill, 1970; Klima & Bellugi, 1966; Menyuk, 1969; deVilliers & deVilliers, 1978):

TABLE 6.3 Reduction Sequence for Questioning

Strategy	Description	Example
Repeat the question	If student was distracted or missed part of the question, repeating helps him form mental closure.	Simply repeat the question as originally stated.
Rephrase the question	If repeating is insufficient, rephrase or recast question maintaining semantic content and pragmatic intent. Proceed from known to unknown by adding information leading to the answer.	Change "Which space shuttle launch caused the death of the first civilian in space?" to "Which space shuttle that blew up caused the first civilian to die in space?"
Simplify the question	If rephrasing is not sufficient, simplify the question. Break it into two sentences. Put more difficult questions into their *what* equivalent. Put more information up front. When your modifications become too wordy, move to the next level.	Change "When is your Dad picking you up?" to "What time is your Dad coming?" Change "Why do the tides rise and fall?" to "What object makes the tides rise and fall?" Change "Where did Talia hide the golden feather when she entered the castle?" to "First Talia entered the castle, then she hid the feather. Where did she hide the feather?"
Put question into *yes/no* form	If simplifying the question is insufficient, put some of the information in statement form up front and ask a *yes/no* question.	Change "Where did you leave your jacket?" to "You do not have your jacket. Is it on the playground?" Change "Why do the tides rise and fall?" to "Does the moon's gravity make the tides rise and fall?"

(continued)

219

TABLE 6.3 *Continued*

Strategy	Description	Example
Give choices	If the child cannot answer question in *yes/no* form, provide options. Use the natural gesture of an upturned open palm for one choice and the other upturned palm for the other choice, indicating that he should pick one or the other.	Change "What happened to your jacket?" to "You do not have your jacket. Is it on the playground or is it in your cubby?" Change "When does daylight savings time start?" to "Does daylight savings time start in the fall or in the spring?"
Write question into a multiple choice format	If asking/signing the question fails, try writing the question. If necessary, provide a word bank.	Change "Which of the space shuttle launches caused the death of the first civilian in space?" to "The launching of the _____ space shuttle caused the death of the first civilian in space." Choose from: Luna, Challenger, Eagle.
Model the answer	If the child still does not answer, provide a model to imitate. This is only done as a last resort. Tell the child the form of the answer or model the form in the first part and have child fill in the second part.	Change "Where did Talia hide the golden feather when she entered the castle?" to "Use 'under' to finish this sentence. "Talia went into the castle and hid the golden feather _____." Change "When do we set our clocks forward?" to "We set our clocks backward in the fall and forward in the _____."

1. Yes/no questions are simplest because they can be answered with a yes or a no. Initally they are in the form of a statement with rising intonation *(Daddy go?)* followed by the un-inverted subject-auxiliary *(I can go now?)*. The true yes/no form emerges last. Sixty percent of the questions used by two- and three-year-olds are yes/no in form (Tyack & Ingram, 1977).

2. The protoypical "wh" question, "Whuzat?" develops about the same time as do yes/no questions, although some researchers have found it to emerge earlier (James & Seebach, 1982). The pointing gesture both precedes and accompanies this form.

3. Yes/no questions beginning with the copula *be* emerge next *(Is that mine?)* and yes/no questions beginning with the auxiliary *be* emerge last *(Is Daddy coming with us?)*.

4. True "wh" questions appear next. Their order is related to pragmatic intent.

5. Tag questions follow next. They require an understanding of negation and contraction. A tag question is more often used as an affirmation of the base statement rather than an actual question (Child: "I was a good boy today, wasn't I?"). Here, the child is looking for the adult to reaffirm his belief rather than provide new information. Eventually the child will use this form both for new information and affirmation.

6. Subject-auxiliary inversions form the next category. They require the child to comprehend modals, "do-support," and the auxiliary aspect *have*. Initially the child will make a statement and use rising inflection, as in *I can go?* By inverting the modal *can* of the auxiliary system with the subject, the question form becomes *Can I go?*. When a simple subject and base verb are used, we add do-support to hold the tense, as in "Do you like ice cream?" When the word *have* is in the sentence (e.g., *You have a ball.*), we add do-support to hold the tense, as in *Did he catch the fish?*

7. Embedded questions are the most complex forms. They require knowledge of relative clauses and subordination (e.g., *He asked if we would go to the beach.*).

A Pragmatic Look at Questions

The emergence of question use is tied to pragmatic functions. James and Seebach (1982) studied the questions of twenty-four hearing preschool children, ages two to five years, during utterances that had the pragmatic functions of information-seeking, conversation, and directives. Information-seeking questions are those that request new information not in the child's repertoire. Conversational questions are those the child uses to initiate or maintain verbal interactions. This includes stereotypical openers (e.g., "You know what?") and "test questions" (p. 4), which were produced when the child already possessed the information (e.g., "What's that for?" pointing to a known object). Although they are not sincere requests for information, they serve to keep conversations going. Children used directive function questions to request action or permission from the listener. They found distinct patterns of emergence of questions as a function of age and pragmatic category. Table 6.4 provides a rank order of question forms from most commonly used to least commonly used based on pragmatic function. The top three forms used for seeking information were when, what, why. The top three forms for initiating and maintaining conversation were who, how, what. The top three question forms used for the directive function were yes/no, why, where. Most curricula for children who are deaf and hard of hearing do not take this into account. Bullard and Schirmer (1991) found that beginning a questioning sequence with Who is often out of context and abstract. For example, when looking at pictures, *who* questions may not lead children to observe the information that is most salient. Countless teachers around the country tack up *who* and *what* charts, asking children to categorize pictures and to paste them on the appropriate chart. Invariably children will mix up *who* and *what*. Invariably the teacher will become frustrated, saying "Who" in a louder and louder voice, or signing WHO in larger and larger circles surrounding first the mouth, then the face, then the upper torso. Children use "who" to seek information during conversations. James and Seebach (1982) also found that the earliest questions children used were for asking and practicing new words (e.g., *Zat? Whuzat?*). Absolutely *the* most critical question for all children to learn, and to learn very early, is an equivalent of *What's that?* Whether it is *dat*, *dis*, or the ASL equivalent <u>wh</u> THAT, communication development depends on the child's curiosity about how the world is labelled. Adults must recognize requests and must provide the requested information.

TABLE 6.4   *Rank Order of Question Form Use from Most Commonly Used to Least Commonly Used as a Function of Pragmatic Category*

Information Seeking	Conversational	Directive	Combined Pragmatic Functions
when	who	yes/no	what
what	how	why	where
where	what	where	why
yes/no	why	how	yes/no
who	when	who	when
why	where	when	how
how	yes/no	(did not use *what*)	who

Source: James & Seebach, 1982.

The two-year-olds in James and Seebach's study primarily used *yes/no* questions and *what* questions. The three-year-olds added *where, why,* and *who* questions. The four-year-olds added *when* and *how* questions to seek information and for conversational purposes, and the five-year-olds asked all question types, but primarily for information-seeking purposes and directives. These researchers concluded that "the major pragmatic function for which children use different question types is information-seeking. Second, some questions are more likely to be used for the directive function and others for conversational purposes." Additionally they concluded that "children used new question types to serve the information-seeking and sometimes conversational function, but . . . only old question types to serve the directive function" (p. 7). In other words, only well-known questions are used for directive functions. Children apparently add new question forms for the purpose of seeking information and engaging in conversation. This provides clear direction for instruction. New question types are best learned through conversation and for seeking information. Conversation provides a fertile ground for helping the child seek new information. Children use old question forms to direct the other's actions.

The Special Case of *How* Questions

How questions are notoriously difficult to answer. For this reason we give them special attention. First, there are many sub-categories, each requiring a different type of answer. Unlike *who* and *what* questions, where the answer is always a noun, the answer to a *how* question might be a partitive, an adjective, a prepositional phrase, a sequence, or even no answer at all. When promoting the use of *how* questions, be sure the child has the necessary language skills and information needed to answer the question. Categories of "how" questions include:

1. Using *how* when the answer is a partitive. This usually occurs with mass nouns.

   How much (mass noun) do you have? (e.g., a bag of, a box of, several tons of)

2. (a) Using *how* when the answer is a number. This usually occurs with count nouns, and the answer is a number or a description.

   How many (count noun) do you have? (e.g., two, a bunch)

   (b) The second answer form using a number with the semantic category of the answer.

How tall is he?	5 feet tall
How old is he?	7 years old
How fast can your new boat go?	55 miles per hour
How much (money) does it cost?	15 dollars
How much (how many pounds) does she weigh?	145 lbs.

3. Using *how* when the answer is an adverbial.

The answer depends on the adverbial requested.

(a) Adverbial of frequency.

How often do you go to a movie?	Annually (adverb)
How many times a day do you brush your teeth?	Three times a day (NP)
How routinely do you change your oil?	Somewhat routinely (adv)

(b) Adverbial of manner. This form often requires do-support.

How did you get here?	By bus (conveyance)
How do you open this package?	With scissors (instrument)
How did you find out about the murder?	On TV (source)
How does he write his name?	Messily (manner)

4. Using *how* when you mean *why did*. The answer usually requires either a *because* clause or a complete sentence for explanation.

How come he gets to stay up late and I don't?	Because he is older than you.
How come your shoes got wet?	I guess I walked through a puddle.
How could this have happened?	You have a wild 3-year-old in your house.

5. Using *how* when the answer is a simple sentence.

How did you bruise your knee?	I fell down.
How did he get an A on his paper?	He studied.

6. Using *how* when the answer describes a multi-step process. The student must be able to answer questions in category #5 before he can answer multistep questions.

How do you tie a shoe?	First you . . . , next you . . . , last you . . . .
How do you make a peanut butter sandwich?	First you . . . , next you . . . , last you . . . .
How do I get to the train station from here?	First you . . . , next you . . . , last you . . . .

7. Using *how* when you are actually offering someone a choice of action. A *yes/no* type of answer is required.

How about ordering the shrimp?	Sure. That sounds good.
How about giving me a hug?	OK. Just one.
How about a soda?	No thanks.

8. Using *how* when checking reading comprehension. This is very difficult to understand because it questions *thoughts* rather than asking for information about objects, traits, or actions. It usually means *what happened* or *what evidence do you have that* and requires a *because* clause.

How do we know that Jason was responsible?	Because he tried to hide the evidence.
How can you tell what she was thinking?	You can tell by the look on her face

9. Using *how* as an embedded question (without a question mark) when no answer is expected. This is difficult because we are not asking a question. Instead, we are "listening in" on a person asking a question of himself or thinking a question to himself. The word *how* follows a verb, indicating that the person is engaged in a thought process.

He *wondered how* he *would* get home.
She *thought about how* things were between them.
The tornado left its victims *asking how* it could have happened to them.

10. Using *how* as a rhetorical question (with a question mark) when no answer is expected. We often use rhetorical questions when no one else is around and we are talking to ourselves. They also are used in literature when a character is faced with a dilemma.

Now, how am I going to get that stain out?
How could this have happened to me?
How will Martin get himself out of this mess? Read the next chapter to find out.

11. Using *how* in idiomatic expressions. Examples are as vast as human creativity. Generally they will fall into one of the preceding categories.

How's the weather up there? (spoken to a tall person)
How now, Brown Cow!

There are some special considerations to consider regarding the use of how question forms.

1. As with all question forms, teach the student the pragmatic uses behind the *how* question.

2. Start by giving the student a *closed set* of answers. (e.g., The answer will be "with a fork," "with a baseball bat," or "with a shoe." Ready? How did the woman kill the fly?)

3. After the child understands the above application, ask *open set* questions. In an open set question, the child does not know the answer.

4. When the child can answer this form of question, mix it with other "wh" questions. (e.g., Where did the boy live? How did he get home from school?)

5. Lastly, mix with other *how* forms where the child must show flexibility in choosing the correct grammatical form for the answer in addition to the correct semantic information. (e.g., How did the boy hurt his knee? How will he take care of it?)

6. Weave *how* questions into appropriate conversations.

English and ASL are very complex. Both languages require that the teacher study the linguistic target she is going to present in order to understand all the parameters involved in ensuring successful acquisition. Many components of language have multiple forms, meanings, and uses. This is true for question forms. When considering IEP objectives related to question forms, study each question form to discern the multiple ways it is used, ordering the forms from less difficult to more difficult. For example, we answer *when* questions in different ways. The answer can be a noun such as *yesterday* or a specific time on the clock. The answer can also be a simple prepositional phrase using a time/space metaphor such as *before lunch* or *through the holidays*. Further, we answer *when* questions with a dependent clause such as *when the snow starts to fall*. The more you understand the different ways a question is used, the better you will be able to provide appropriate interventions such as scaffolding during conversations.

Question Formation in ASL

This next section describes ASL question forms. In ASL environments, the development of questions has the same relationship to conversational development as in English classrooms. Pragmatic intent, incidental language, and the need to repair communication breakdowns remain the same. Only the language is different, and because two languages are involved, we see code-switching throughout instruction.

ASL Question Types

Non-manual markers play an important role in the formation of questions in American Sign Language. Valli and Lucas (1995) consider questions to be one of the five basic sentence patterns in ASL. Four categories of questions comprise the ASL question system: yes/no questions, "wh" questions, question mark wiggle, and rhetorical questions.

As in English, yes/no questions in ASL require a yes/no answer. Unlike in English, word order is not crucial. The important feature of yes/no questions in ASL is their nonmanual markers. These include the following:

- eyebrows raised
- eyes widened
- head and body tilted forward
- shoulders raised
- last sign held

For example, the question "Is that your dog?" is indicated by the gloss, _____q.
DOG YOUR.

Glosses are English words written in small capital letters with various markings to indicate the ASL equivalent. ASL does not have a writen form, so we gloss to show the English equivalent. The preceding glossed phrase means that an ASL yes/no question is represented (hence, the "q"). The capitalized words indicate that the signs used have equivalent words in ASL. What you do not see in a gloss are the nonmanual markers. An individual might sign DOG YOUR, but in addition to the signs he would use several or all of the nonmanual question markers listed above.

"Wh" questions form the next category of questions. As with English, the "wh" questions in ASL are *where, what, when, who, how,* and *why.* The nonmanual markers for "wh" questions are:

- eyebrows squinted
- head tilted
- body leans slightly forward
- shoulders may be raised
- slight side-to-side head shake
- palms oriented up, slightly clawed, slight side to side movement.

"Wh" questions are often located both at the beginning and the end of the question. To gloss the question, "Where is the dog?," we write _____wh
DOG WHERE

In English we use "wh" questions as embedded questions (e.g., *Who do you think will come to the meeting?* or *I wonder who will come to the meeting.*). In ASL the question is extracted from the embedded clause (Neidle et al., 2000). For example, we extract the implied question, *Who will come to the assembly?* from the larger sentence. First we engage in topicalization (Valli & Lucas, 1995) or the process of identifying the topic we are discussing, then we state the question as

$$\underline{\hspace{4cm}t} \qquad \underline{\hspace{2cm}wh} \qquad \underline{\hspace{4cm}wh}$$

in MEETING, IX (*you*)+THINK COME WHO or IX (*me*) CURIOUS COME WHO. In topicalization, the head goes down, eyebrows go up, the topic is signed closer to the body, and eye contact is made. After establishing the topic, there is a pause, then the extracted question is posed. Facial expression reflects the content of the questions (Lane, Hoffmeister, & Bahan, 1996).

The third kind of question in ASL is the question mark wiggle (QMwg). The pragmatic intent behind the QMwg is to express surprise at the information received or to verify the signers comment (Lucas & Valli, 1995). Nonmanual markers for QMwg are the same as for yes/no questions. For example, instead of saying "You mean I have to do this math problem again?," the ASL

$$\underline{\hspace{3cm}QMwg}$$

user might sign AGAIN MATH PROBLEM.

The fourth kind of ASL question is the rhetorical question. For example, instructors often use the rhetorical question to set situations up so that students will expect some information. For example, the instructor might say "And when would we use this procedure? We would use it in a preschool class." The question cues the listener to pay attention. A rhetorical question serves the same function in ASL but ASL conversations use it more frequently than English

$$\underline{\hspace{5cm}rhet}$$

conversations. For example, an ASL signer might sign CAT DIE WHY CAR RUN+OVER. The signs for *reason, when, who, why, what, where, who,* and *for-for* are all used in this manner. Nonmanual markers for rhetorical questions include raised eyebrows and a slight shake or tilt of the head to distinguish between true "wh" questions and rhetorical forms.

The purpose of this section was to identify the basic features of ASL questions, which are new to most beginning teachers of the deaf. We recognize that we have only scratched the surface and encourage teachers to continue educating themselves regarding ASL.

The Elephant in the Livingroom

Children learn to communicate from people who can communicate with them. Sadly, many teachers of the deaf have limited communication skills (discussed elsewhere in this text). To improve their conversations with children, teachers must improve their own skills first. Many teachers use a mix of communication ranging from sign-supported speech to speech-supported sign. Auditory-oral instruction is not simply the elimination of signs. It requires a set of skills and procedures from the teacher that make available the information the child lacks. An adequate signing environment is not one that simply follows speech production with the signs available in one's personal repertoire. It requires thoughtful attention to visual enhancements in the environment. Until all teachers who work with deaf and hard of hearing children meet standards of communicative competence themselves, whatever the pathway, they will continue to hold back the students they claim to teach.

Summary

The purpose of this chapter was to present an examination of the relationship between the ability to ask and answer questions and the ability to engage in conversations. Both skills are challenging to students with hearing losses. Further, they are mutually dependent upon one another for their continued development. This chapter examined the sources of the cycle of poor questioning skills and impoverished conversations and suggested ways to reverse this cycle. The chapter ended with an examination of the question forms of English and ASL.

Conversations must become an integral part of every teacher's interactions with students. Conversations form the basis for learning to communicate and for learning about the world. Without the ability to converse, students with hearing losses are at a great disadvantage. Conversational interactions must be based around the authentic need to communicate in real-life situations. Teachers of students who are deaf and hard of hearing must strive to improve their own communicative competence and must make conversational development a priority in all their interactions with these students.

Questions for Critical Thinking ———————————————

1. What is the relationship between conversation development and question development?

2. Why are some question forms more difficult to learn than others?

3. What is the relationship between a teacher's communicative competence and that of her students?

7

English and ASL Grammar

What to Expect in This Chapter

In this chapter you will read about the grammars of English and ASL. You will see the similarities and differences in the languages.

The purpose of this chapter is to describe the structures of English and ASL. In preceding sections we presented a discussion of *how* to teach communication skills. In this chapter we focus on *what* to teach. We include skill hierarchies to assist you in organizing your objectives. Languages are extremely complex. There is no quick way to master the content, so take your time. Recognize that you will be studying about this subject for a long time.

In this chapter you will find skill hierarchies. Presenting a hierarchy is a risky business for two reasons. First, for every suggested hierarchy, another exists that disputes the sequence of the first. This is because language is not simply a set of grammar or vocabulary skills but an integrated process with multiple components that act upon one another in various ways. Second, language develops in fits and starts. A child may be in one phase with one skill (e.g., verb tense) but in a different phase with another (e.g., negation). Any attempt to align all the components and systems of language into one overall sequence would violate this basic premise of child development. Be that as it may, teachers need a framework for decision making. You will use assessment information and your perceptions and knowledge of each individual child to choose appropriate objectives. The hierarchies presented do not represent hard and fast rules or inviolable sequences, but rather a point of departure to which the skilled teacher may refer. We present a hierarchy at the end of most sections (i.e., nominals hierarchy, verb phrase hierarchy, etc.). The hierarchies are written in terms of phases. The phases do not correspond with one another. That is, Phase 2 adverbials are not necessarily equivalent to Phase 2 verbs because students may be making rapid progress in one area but slow progress in another. If you are looking for an overarching hierarchy, contact the language coordinator of a school for the deaf.

In the 1970s and 1980s many schools developed comprehensive curricula that detailed sequences of morphology, phonology, and syntax, among other skills (Laughton, 1983). Referred to as "language scope and sequence charts," these were very popular. Many teachers had them posted on their classroom walls. Some schools still display these hierarchies. Others have changed to pragmatically based curricula, but language development is not an either/or issue; we don't teach either grammar or pragmatics. We teach it all, account for it all, and assist students in moving their communication skills forward in all areas.

This chapter takes a broad look at many of the components of English and American Sign Language (ASL). It is weighted more heavily toward English because we have a greater knowledge base about the scope and sequence of English. That is not to say that the scope and sequence of ASL is less important. However, we have only in the past decade seen the level of investigation into ASL issues that the topic warrants. We hope that future investigation will continue to provide increasingly sophisticated knowledge of ASL.

Orientation to English Language Structure

The English language is made up structurally of phrases (Brown & Miller, 1999). When we think of something that a person has said to us, we think in terms of a phrase. The phrase in English provides a meaningful unit of information that causes us to see a picture in our heads. For example, when someone

        NP   VP   Adv-P

says, "The little kindergartner/couldn't sit still/in his seat," our interpretation of that sentence unfolds through a series of pictorial changes in our heads. First we see a small child. Depending on our personal experiences (perception is relative to past experience), that picture in our heads might be of a little boy or a little girl. The picture in your author's head is of a little blonde-haired boy. If we change some of the features of the noun phrase, for example to *the brown-eyed kindergarten girl*, then the picture in our head changes as well. We do not interpret the sentence as *the* plus *little* plus *kindergartner*. We process this visually as one picture. Next, we modify that picture based on the gestalt, or whole feeling, of the verb phrase. We see that little child wiggling around because he "couldn't sit still." Again, where we think he is wiggling depends on our past experiences—perhaps we see the child wiggling at the dinner table or in the church pew. We modify the first chunk of words (i.e., the phrase), or the first picture in our head, by the second chunk of words, resulting in a second, modified picture. Finally, we get that last chunk of information, which tells us the location of where this is all taking place. The picture in your author's head is now of a blonde-haired little boy wiggling his bottom around on a rather uncomfortable classroom chair. In the real world of communication, all this information passes through our language systems so rapidly that we see the result rather than the transitional pictures. If we change a component of any of the phrase (to *the pretty little kindergartner*) or if we change an entire phrase (to *in the car*), our picture changes based on interpreting the whole phrase, not on interpreting the individual words.

Chomsky (1957) wrote extensively about the phrase structure rules of English. Many of the curriculum guides, test materials, and language instructional materials we have in classes for deaf children in North America today break language down into its constituent parts. One problem in application has been that we have taught the components of the phrases as discrete pieces of information rather than as visual chunks. The Apple Tree Program, for example, is based on the development of language through putting different structural components of language together. According to the Apple Tree Program, there are ten very common sentence patterns in English that are made up of these different chunks (or phrases or components). Everything else we do to language from a grammatical standpoint is an addition, deletion, substitution, or rearrangement of phrases and phrase components.

Remember that each English phrase provides a whole piece of information. A chunk can be as small as a phrase *(over the tree)* or as large as a clause (The boy *who has a new puppy* is my nephew). We do not process it as a single, discrete set of individual words but as a whole or gestalt. This is one of the reasons why using American Sign Language as a bridge to English is useful for many children who are deaf. ASL goes directly to the visual gestalt of the chunk, allowing the student to understand the meaning, and often the intent, of the message. It is when we get to the written form of English that individual elements become of overriding importance (*an* apple rather than *a* apple). We *understand* language when we see the whole phrase in our heads.

In English, there are five basic sentence types and their modifications (Anderson, Boren, Kilgore, Howard, & Krohn, 1980; Blackwell, Engen, Fischgrund, & Zarcadoolas, 1978). These are:

1. NP1 + VP i (intransitive) (Type 1)
   The kitten jumped.

2. NP1 + VP i + Adverbial (when, where, how, why) (Type 1 plus adverbial)
   The kitten jumped out the window.
   The kitten jumped because he was startled.

3. NP1 + VP t (transitive) + NP2 (Type 2)
   The kitten chased the bug.

   NP1 + VP t + NP2 + Adverbial (when, where, how, why) (Type 2 plus adverbial)
   The kitten chased the bug into the bushes.

4. NP1 + VP t + NP3 + NP2 (modification of #4) (Rearranged Type 2 with indirect object)
>   *The kitten caught his mother a bug.*

5. NP1 + VP be + Adjective (Type 3)
>   *The kitten is hungry.*

6. NP1 + VP be + NP1 (Type 4)
>   *The kitten is a boy.*

7. NP1 + VP be + Adverbial (Type 5)
>   *The kitten is under the bed.*

The phrases of English occur in sentences in a fairly prescribed, sequential manner. English is an auditory-sequential language. ASL, on the other hand, is a visual-simultaneous language.

Orientation to the Components of ASL

American Sign Language is a visuo-spatial language used by the Deaf community in North America (Brentari, 1998; Neidel, Kegl, MacLaughlin, Bahan, & Lee, 2000). It is "a complete natural language, quite independent from English" (Lane, Hoffmeister, & Bahan, 1996) with its own grammar. ASL varies among users because of the heterogeneity of the signing community (Neidel et al. 2000). Most ASL signers did not learn the language from their parents; instead, they learned it from other deaf children. In cases where deaf and hard of hearing children had no contact with deaf children, they usually learned to sign from their teachers who were hearing, non-native users. Only later as they began to interact with adult native signers did they develop near-native skill. Consequently, many adult signers use a hybrid form of ASL. There are also variations among cultural groups, and Deaf people code-switch depending on their communication partner. For example, African-American Deaf people sign differently when signing among themselves than when signing with others (Aramburo, 1989).

Glossing ASL

"Glossing means choosing an appropriate English word for signs in order to write them down" (Valli & Lucas, 1995, p. 20). Glossing from English to ASL is not merely translating one language into the other. Glossing is not ASL written down. Glossing provides English users with a way to represent how ASL is used. It takes training and exposure both to ASL and glossing to learn this skill. Following are basic glosses and what they represent (Neidel et al., 2000; Valli & Lucas, 1995).

- Signs are represented by uppercase letters (e.g., BOY).

- The pound sign (#) represents fingerspelled loan signs that are recognized as an individual vocabulary item (e.g., #DO).

- Hyphens (-) between uppercase letters indicate fingerspelled words (e.g., R-A-C-H-E-L).

- Lines above sign glosses have symbols to represent nonmanual markers such as "wh" questions (wh), topicalization (t), or head nod (hn). For example,

<u>   t </u>
MOUNTAIN, BIG.

- Two words combined into one signed movement are represented by a hyphen (e.g., not-yet, told-me).

- POSS is a gloss that refers to a possessive pronoun.

- IX refers to index (use of index finger to point to a location, represents a pronoun).

Fingerspelling

Fingerspelling is a process of spelling out English words where there is no sign equivalent in ASL. Proper nouns are often fingerspelled such as B-O-N-N-I-E. The fingerspelled alphabet corresponds to the English alphabet. "When fingerspelling, signers execute in rapid sequence handshapes that correspond to each letter in a word" (Padden & Ramsey, 2000, p. 173). Young children can recognize fingerspelled words early if they are important words such as names of family members and functional objects in their environment.

Loan Signs

When two cultures come into contact, it is natural for them to share their vocabulary, with each culture loaning vocabulary to the other. For example, the Spanish word *macho* is so commonly used that it is accepted as an English term. In ASL there are three kinds of loan signs. The first are those signs that begin as fingerspelled words but have become a signed word. An example is D-O, which is fingerspelled so rapidly that it is used as a sign. A second category of loan signs is the group borrowed from other signed languages (Valli & Lucas, 1995) such as the signs that represent country names. The third kind of loan sign is initialized signs, where the first letter of an English word is incorporated into the ASL sign (e.g., EXPERIMENT is made by signing SCIENCE with an "e" handshape).

Eight Types of Signs

There are eight types of signs in American Sign Language (Brentari, 1998).

- One-handed signs (e.g., UNDERSTAND)

- Two-handed signs (e.g., ENJOY)

- Fingerspelled borrowings (e.g., DO)

- Derived nouns or nominalized signs (often reduplicated as in SIT/CHAIR or trilled [see Gerund section, this chapter] as in DRIVE/DRIVING)

- Agreement affix (referring to someone or something at a location in space, as in indexing)

- Compound word signs (e.g., THINK + FREEZE = SHOCKED)

- Verbs that include aspect and tense—how objects and events relate in time (e.g., sign for GIVE presented once iteratively to mean "give to someone" or duratively to mean "give and give over a long period of time.")

- Classifier forms—an ASL handshape that is combined with location, orientation, movement, and non-manual markers to form a predicate (e.g., CAR 3-CL, movement from right to left).

Simultaneity Principle

In English, all the pieces of a sentence occur sequentially. In ASL, multiple pieces of a sentence can occur at the same time (Woll & Kyle, 1998). For example, a verb moved in a particular direction includes the preposition as in GO-TO. A verb signed more than once can mean a noun (e.g., GO BY TRAIN TRAIN). This important feature of ASL is initially difficult for English speakers to grasp because the sequential nature of English is so ingrained.

Five Basic Sentence Types

There are five basic sentence types in ASL (Valli & Lucas, 1995): question, negation, commands, topicalization, and conditionals. With the addition of facial grammar, fingerspelling, spatial markers, and other grammatical features, signers can express any content or sentiment expression by English speakers.

Questions.   Question formation is extremely problematic for many students with hearing losses. The questions systems of English and ASL provide great challenges. We feel that this topic is significant enough to warrant a chapter of its own (see Chapter 6).

Negation. In English the negative form modifies most of the parts of speech, but especially the predicate noun (e.g., *He is no friend of mine.*) or the predicate adjective (e.g., *He is not happy.*). When the negative modifies a verb, we add *do* in front of the verb (e.g., *I do not know.*) or a modal in front of the verb (e.g., *He can not remember her name.*). We say it is *prefronted.*

_____neg

In ASL, negation is applied across the sentence. For example, BOY HAPPY means that the boy is not happy; however, a headshake is used for the duration of the sentence. Non-manual markers of negation are: headshaking from side to side, frowning, squinting, etc. Other forms of negation include *none, nothing,* and *no.*

Commands. A command is also called an imperative and is glossed using an asterisk at either end of the word as in *stop*. Sometimes signers will point to the person, as in *stop* IX *(you)*. Non-manual markers of commands are: direct eye contact and frowning when appropriate.

Topicalization. Sometimes the object of a sentence is used as the topic. This allows signers to indicate the topic of a sentence prior to commenting on it. Topicalization is glossed using a "t" above the line. For example, *I like popcorn* is

_____t

glossed POPCORN, IX *(me)* LIKE. Non-manual markers of the topicalized word are raised eyebrows, a head tilt, and a short pause. The non-manual markers of the comment vary with the affect of the comment (i.e., negative, neutral, positive).

Conditionals. A conditional sentence in English is an *if . . . then* sentence. In ASL, #IF and SUPPOSE are used to set up a condition and means the same as the English *if . . . then.* For example, the sentence *If it snows tomorrow, school will*

_____cond

be cancelled would be glossed as TOMORROW SNOW, SCHOOL CANCEL. Some signers use the #IF or SUPPOSE sign up front. Some do not. Non-manual markers of the conditional are: raised eyebrows, a head tilt, and a short pause between the condition and the result.

An Examination of Nouns, Noun Phrases, and Nominalized Forms of English

A noun (Krifka, 1999; Payne, 1999) is a person (William), place (the lake), thing (a boat), idea (fun), state (happiness), or condition (relaxation). It can be concrete (oars) or abstract (contemplation). It can be something countable (life-jackets) or something we view in terms of a mass (water). Concrete nouns are relatively easy to teach because we can show pictures of them. Abstract nouns are less easy to teach. We cannot show pictures of faithfulness or happiness. The way we teach abstract nouns is by showing examples and non-examples of the concept. An abstract concept is within a *category* of experiences and feelings, which we can label with the word that identifies the category. The old TV game show, *$10,000 Pyramid*, is an example of the process of categorization of abstract concepts. The clue-giver gives examples of members of the category (e.g., cat, dog, hamster, canary) to the contestant, who must discern the *superordinate label* (pets) for the *subordinate members* of the category. For deaf children to win at the game of English vocabulary, teachers must provide sufficient examples of members (e.g., turtles, gerbils, parakeets) and nonmembers (bears, pythons), or subordinate categories, of a concept so that children may discern the superordinate label. This is easy to do with concrete nouns, and the creative teacher finds exciting ways to do this with abstract nouns, but things get a bit more challenging when we look at more advanced forms of the noun phrase.

A noun phrase is made up of components called the *determiner* and a *noun*. (Early syntactic theory held that the noun was the head of the noun phrase and used the abbreviation, NP, to represent this. Recent theorists declare that the determiner is the head of the noun phrase and use the abbreviation, DP [determiner phrase], to represent this segment of grammar [Payne, 1999; van Eijck, 1999]. Because this is not a text in linguistic theory, we chose to stick with the abbreviations most currently used in deaf education.) There are several categories of words that make up the determiner system. Very few of these, except perhaps for the adjectives, are observable. In fact, many determiners fall into a category called *functors* or function words. That is, they have a particular function in relating one word to another but do not have any real meaning themselves. It is more helpful to think of their semantic relations to the rest of the phrase than to think of them as syntactic features (van Eijck, 1999). The word, *of*, is an example of a functor. It has no meaning by itself but shows us the relationship between two other words, as in the noun phrase *several of the boys*. The function of the word *of* is to show a link between *several* and *boys*. Therefore, when we want to teach *of* we have to do it in the context of the noun phrase. So in order to teach functors, we have to teach them within phrases or chunks (i.e., thought units). This is the problem that arises when teachers try to use tools such as the Dolch Word List. The philosophy behind teaching words from word lists is that if the child knows certain words that are highly representative of utterances in English, then he should be able to understand and/or read English. This is too simplistic a treatment.

In addition to nouns and noun phrases, which can occur in multiple locations within an overall sentence (e.g., subject, direct object, indirect object, object of the preposition; see the basic sentence patterns described above), English uses what are called *nominalized* forms, words and phrases to which we have done something so that we can stick them in the noun or noun phrase position in a sentence (Muysken, 1999). For example, in the sentence, *The boy likes pizza*, we know that *the boy* and *pizza* are the noun phrases of the sentence. In English, we do many things to different parts of speech that turn them into nouns, or nominalized, forms. *Nominal* means name, or in other words, a noun. For example, we can take the verb *swim*, add the progressive tense "-ing," making the sentence, *The boy likes swimming*. In this context, *swimming* is a noun, specifically a gerund. We have nominalized the verb.

There are many, many examples of nominalized forms. In each case, the word, or more frequently, the whole phrase, actually becomes the noun in the sentence. Sometimes nominalized forms are necessary in order to complete the sentence. When this happens, they are referred to as *complements*. Some forms of complements complete a sentence by taking place of, or rather becoming, the noun phrase. For example, the *infinitive noun phrase complement, to swim*, can go in our sentence above as in *The boy likes to swim*. Here the preposition *to* plus a verb (the infinitive form of the verb) is made into a noun, or nominalized, and is stuck in a noun phrase position in a sentence, making it a complement and completing the sentence. Other complement forms act as dependent clauses.

One advanced nominalized form is the *noun clause* or *noun phrase complement*, which is located in the direct object position of a sentence. For example, in the sentence, *He saw the girl, the girl* is the direct object (NP2). We can substitute the noun phrase complement *she was crying* in the position of the direct object, adding *that* to make the sentence, *He saw that she was crying*.

Not all changes to noun phrases are complements. Some are just simple substitutions, such as *pronouns (she, them, itself, someone)*. Others are simple additions, such as *derived nouns*, where a prefix or suffix is added to a word to change the word into a noun (bake/baker, establish/establishment). Still others involve *word order transformations*, or changes, such as *indirect object/direct object preposing*, where the position (posing) of the indirect object is moved in front (pre) of the direct object. In this case, the sentence *Mother gave a movie ticket to her daughter* is changed by moving the indirect object in front of (preposing) the direct object, as in *Mother gave her daughter a movie ticket*.

Suggestions for Teaching Nouns and Nominals

There are two guiding principles for teaching nouns and nominals:

1. For nouns or noun phrases, give examples of what the subject is and what it is not. For young children, highlight this visually by placing pictures beside each word.

An Establishment	*Not an Establishment*
a building	a lake
a movie theater	a kiss
the post office	a letter

2. For more extended forms of nominalization, show multiple pictures of the gestalt, or whole impression, of the phrase. For example, to teach the noun clause (or relative clause) in the sentence *He sees that the girl is happy*, you might make a puppet of a boy look at a location on the page. Place eight or ten pictures of happy girls in several locations that would correspond to the puppet's line of sight.

Members of the Noun Phrase, Complement, and Nominalized System

The simple noun phrase is made up of a determiner and a noun. We find them in sentences as subjects, direct objects, indirect objects, and objects of the preposition. Some forms are made up of additions, some of substitutions, and some of rearrangements. Some are entire phrases and sentences unto themselves. Table 7.1 outlines the components of the noun phrase and nominal system.

Phases of Acquisition

As mentioned before, it is always risky to suggest a sequence of development because it is often disputed, and teaching from a strict hierarchy violates current best practices. However, it is still important for the teacher to understand what a child knows and what he needs to know. Without a road map, how will we know where we are going, and without a destination, how will we know if we have arrived? Table 7.2 is a hierarchy of the nominal system. Keep in mind the following rules of thumb when using the hierarchies in this chapter.

1. Each hierarchy is separate. Phase 4 verb issues do not necessarily correspond to Phase 4 negation issues. Language does not develop evenly in all children.

2. The phases are just that—phases. Phases flow into one another. Some children are ready to move on to a higher phase before mastering each skill in an earlier phase, but many are not. The teacher needs to use his or her discretion in deciding when to address a skill.

Noun Issues in ASL

American Sign Language represents nouns in distinctly different ways from English. The following is a discussion of the complexity of nouns in ASL.

Spatial Reference

In ASL the use of space is an essential linguistic feature. Often, the nouns of a sentence will be identified then placed at an abstract location in space. For example, you might sign BOY, then point to a place in front of you. After that, any

TABLE 7.1 *Components of the Noun Phrase and Nominal System*

Category	Types	Examples
Determiners	Pre-articles	some of, several of, a few of, none of, a lot of, one of, all of
	Partitives (describe a mass or group)	a pod of whales, a box of cereal
	Articles	a, some, the, null
	Adjectives	descriptive word of size, shape, texture, etc.
	Cardinals	one, two, several, no
	Ordinals	first, second, next, last
	Genitive (possessives)	his, their, our, your
	Demonstrative (pronouns)	this, that, these, those
Pronouns	Personal, as subject	she, he, it, we, you, they
	Personal, as object	him, her, them, you, us
	Direct object, also called accusative	
	Indirect object, also called dative	
	Object of the preposition	
	Possessive, also called genitive	his, her, hers, our, ours, your, yours, its, their
	Demonstrative	this, that, these, those
	Reflexive	himself, herself, itself, ourselves, themselves
	Indefinite	someone, anyone, somebody, anybody, anything, nothing
Derived nouns	Prefixes	anti-, bi-, de-, dis-, im-, un-, re-, pre-, ad-, ab-, tri-, omni-, dys-
	Suffixes	-able, -ed, -er, -en, -ing, -ly, -ness, -y, -s, -ment, -tion
	Latin roots	bio, geo, sect, dict, micro, script, phone, tele, struct, turb

Indirect object/direct object preposing	Indirect object moves in front of direct object	*Sara showed a book to Chelsea* becomes *Sara showed Chelsea a book.*
Passive voice	Involves both nouns and verbs. The two nouns in the sentence change position. Direct object (the recipient of the action) moves to the subject position. Four types: *Reversible passive* (semantically interchangeable) *Non-reversible passive* (not semantically interchangeable) *Truncated* (leaves off *by whom*) *Non-truncated* (uses *by*) *Derived adjectives* (*be* verb plus perfect tense verb)	*The judge kicked out the reporters* becomes *The reporters were kicked out by the judge.* *The record was broken by the swimmer* but not *The swimmer was broken by the record.* *The kidnapper was apprehended.* *The kidnapper was apprehended by a common citizen.* *He is exhausted.*
Gerunds	*"-ing"* is added to verbs and treated as if they are nouns	*Eating is not an Olympic sport.*
Infinitive complements	*to* plus verb (the infinitive) is treated as if it were a noun	*To run is his passion.* *To feel the wind on his face was the dog's greatest pleasure.*
For/to complements	*for* plus a specific noun and *to* plus a specific action becomes the noun. Can also replace the direct object noun	*For the cat to swim surprised us.* *He asked for her to help him.*
Possessive noun plus progressive verb	Possessive +"-ing" in the subject position in the direct object position with object of preposition with longer sentences	*Seth's driving scared his mother.* *She feared Seth's driving.* *She was worried about Seth's driving.* *Seth's driving the dilapidated Chevy made her nervous.*

(continued)

TABLE 7.1 *Continued*

Category	Types	Examples
Noun phrase complement (noun clause)	An entire sentence sits in the noun phrase position.	
	With process verbs: thought, felt, knew, understood, believed	He *thought that she was pretty.*
	Abstract verbs: wondered, asked, questioned	He *wondered where he should take her on their first date.*

Sources: Anderson, 1999; Blackwell, Engen, Fischgrund, & Zarcadoolas, 1978; Hargis, 1984; Heidinger, 1984; Paul, 1998; Roberts, 1999; van Eijck, 1999; Vincent, 1999.

TABLE 7.2 *Hierarchy of the Nominal System*

Noun Phrase and Nominal System Hierarchy	Examples
Phase 1 Early Determiners	
articles (a, an, the, some, more, null)	*the* boy
cardinal numbers (one, two)	*two* girls
Singular and plural count/noncount nouns	*trees/sand*
Personal pronouns about self and conversational partner (I, me, you, we)	I want
Possessive pronoun about self	*my* daddy
Phase 2 Demonstrative determiners (this, that, these, those)	*that* dog
Possessive nouns using the apostrophe	*John's* dog
Possessive pronoun (your, mine)	is *mine*
Third person personal pronouns (he, she, they)	*he* went
It referring to concrete objects	I want *it.*
Derived noun in agentive form: "-er" (farmer)	Driv*er*
Infinitive NP as direct object	I want *to play.*
Non-reversible passive	The truck *was broken.*
Phase 3 Early pre-articles (one of, some of, two of, none of)	*One of* the cats
Ordinals (first, next, last)	The *first* house
Possessive pronouns (their, theirs, her, hers, his, its, ours)	*her* doll
Object case personal pronouns (him, her, them, us)	I saw *him.*
Reflexive pronouns (myself, yourself)	I did it *myself.*
Multiple pronouns in one sentence	*He* saw *her.*
Demonstrative pronouns (this, that, these, those)	*This* is old.
Person's name in direct address	*Sara,* sit down.
It referring to weather and calendar	*It* is Monday

(continued)

243

TABLE 7.2 *Continued*

Noun Phrase and Nominal System Hierarchy		*Examples*
	Indirect object/direct object preposing	Give *Sandy* the *box*.
	For/to complement in direct object position	Ask *Dewey to help*.
Phase 4	Later pre-articles and partitives (both of, each of, every one of, any of, of, a few of, a lot of, a bag of, a piece of)	*a piece of* the pie
	Advanced articles (other, another)	*another* cookie
	Indefinite pronouns (someone, anything, nobody)	*Someone* is here.
	It referring to abstract concepts of time and season.	*It* is 3:00. *It* is winter.
	Noun clause complement with *that*	I saw *that you came.*
Phase 5	Complex pre-articles (either of, neither of, "-est" of, "-er" of	The *biggest* of the trees.
	Gerunds	*Swimming* is fun.
	Reflexive pronouns (herself, themselves, ourselves)	Do it *yourself.*
	Noun clause complement with *if*	He asked *if she had a cold.*
	Indirect discourse (asked _____ that, told _____ that)	He *told* Sally *that be did.*
	Reversible passive	*The dog was kissed by the boy.*
Phase 6	Noun clause complement with "wh-" form	He knew *where she lived.*
	Possessive + "-ing"	*William's singing* was sweet.
	For/to complement in subject position	*For you to try* is important.
	Noun phrase complement *that* in subject position	*That the baby needed changing* was obvious.

time you refer to the boy, you will point to that location in space. When discussing action between you and the noun, the direction of signing occurs between these two locations in space. When discussing the relationship between two nouns placed in space, the direction of the signing occurs between these two locations. The only limit to the number of locations you can set up is the memory capacity of the signer or receiver. Nouns are identified in many ways. These include *reduplication, classifiers, gerunds,* and *compounding.*

Reduplication is a process that allows us to make verbs into nouns (Brentari, 2000). For example, if you make the sign for SIT once, it means *sit* but if you repeat the sign it means *chair.* Noun classifiers are handshapes that represent classes of concepts. Classifiers can be used as nouns or as verbs. Nouns and verbs may be represented by the same distinct handshape, (Niedel et al., 2000), but the way you use the classifier determines if it is a noun or a verb. Kantor (1994) provided a description of common classifiers.

- General person—closed fist, index finger points upward representing the movement of the person or animal.

- By-legs—the V-handshape, fingers pointing downward representing the movement of the legs such as sitting, walking, standing, etc.

- Vehicle—thumb points upward, the index and middle fingers are spread and point in the direction of the movement (e.g., CAR PASSING BY).

- Plane—thumb, index, and pinkie finger extended, index finger points in the direction of movement.

- Stationary object, taller than wide (moveable)—closed fist, thumb extended at right angle to the palm of the hand (e.g., HOUSE).

- Stationary object, taller than wide (fixed)—arm extended upward from elbow to fingertips (e.g., TREE).

Lentz, Mikos, and Smith (1988) provide the following explanation of classifiers as used in the *Signing Naturally* curriculum.

- Descriptive classifier (DCL)—a sign used to describe an object or person (e.g., DCL CURLY HAIR).

- Locative classifier (LCL)—a sign representing an object in a specific place and sometimes indicating movement (e.g., LCL:B LEAF DRIFTING TO THE GROUND).

- Semantic classifier (SCL)—a sign representing a category of nouns such as vehicle or person (e.g., SLC:1 PERSON WALKING BRISKLY).

- Body classifier (BCL)—a sign in which the body "enacts" the verb of the sentence (e.g., BCL PUT ARMS AROUND FRIEND).

- Instrument classifier (ICL)—a sign in which part of the body, usually the hands, manipulates an object (e.g., ICL PLAYING JACKS).

- Body part classifier (BPCL)—a sign representing a specific part of the body doing the action (e.g., two handed, 2h BPCL:1 CROSSING LEGS).

- Plural classifier (PCL)—a sign indicating specific number or nonspecific number (e.g., PCL:4 LONG LINE OF PEOPLE).

A gerund is another form of noun. In English gerunds are made by using a verb plus "-ing" as a noun (e.g., *cooking is fun*). In ASL (Brentari, 1998) a verb stem is also used and is marked by trilling movement (TM). Trilling refers to small, rapidly repeated uncountable movements incorporated into the verb to change it to the noun. Whereas most English verbs can become gerunds, the number of ASL verbs is restricted (e.g., *Drawing* is acceptable as a noun in both languages. The word *loving* is not used as a noun in ASL).

Compounding in ASL refers to the process of combining two signs to make one concept (Brentari, 1998). Verbs and nouns may combine (e.g., SLEEP + DRESS = NIGHTGOWN). Adjectives and verbs may also combine (e.g., SILLY + FINISH = CUT IT OUT). Verbs and verbs may combine (e.g., THINK + FREEZE = SHOCKED; THINK + TOUCH = OBSESS). Adjectives and nouns may combine (YELLOW + HAIR = BLONDE), and nouns and verbs may combine (e.g., NAME + SHINE = GOOD REPUTATION). Other categories may combine as well to make compounds.

Pronouns

In English a pronoun represents a person, place, or thing that has already been identified. ASL pronouns do not make a distinction between subject and object pronouns (e.g., in English she/her). This distinction is shown by the sequence of the signs. For example: in IX *(me)* LOVE IX *(you)*, both IX *(me)* and IX *(you)* use the same handshape and orientation, but the difference is in the location with *(me)* pointing toward the chest and *(you)* pointing away from the signer.

ASL pronouns show number difference. When referring to one person the signer points one index finger away from his or her body. Referring to more than one person, the signer might use the same pointing index finger in a sweeping action. Number can also be shown by incorporating lexical numerals using a number handshape (e.g., TWO OF THEM) the movement is a quick back and forth sweeping action or (THREE OF US) in a circular movement.

According to Niedel et al. (2000) ASL pronouns show possession. Possessive pronouns, glossed as POSS, use the open palm orientation pointing towards a location in space. As with IX, POSS can be made plural by a sweeping movement. Reflexive pronouns and emphatic pronouns use a closed fist, thumb oriented upward pointing toward the location in space associated with the referent.

An Examination of Verbs, Verb Phrases, and the Auxiliary System of English

A *verb* is a word that expresses action *(throw)*, existence *(is)*, or occurrence *(appear)*. Verbs have semantic, syntactic, and morphologic characteristics. The morphological elements of verbs determine their *tenses*, or time frames. The semantic elements of verbs determine their meanings and how they are used. The syntactic elements of verbs determine how they fit together in sentences, how sentences are reordered, or how one sentence is embedded into another (Crookston, 1999). Specifically, we are concerned with the following information about verbs:

1. Verb forms—transitive, intransitive, or linking

2. Verb meaning and use—action, process, or stative

3. Verb auxiliaries—tense, modals, and aspect

4. Issues of noun-verb agreement

5. Phrasal verbs made of a verb plus a preposition (e.g., *stuck up* means snobby) that differ in meaning from that of the preposition or verb alone (e.g., *give up* means to surrender).

6. Embedding of verbs from two simple sentences to form one complex sentence (e.g., *He saw the girl. She was laughing* becomes *He saw the girl laughing*).

Suggestions for Teaching Verbs, Verb Phrases, and the Auxiliary System

The verb system of English is extremely complex. It goes way beyond simple morphological issues of "-ed," "-ing," and "-s" on the ends of words. For example, the tense structure represented in the sentence *He was playing* involves the interrelationship between an active time frame occurring within the context of the static time frame. Some tenses of English represent more than one time frame, and some time frames can be represented by more than one tense. Tense is only one of the features of verbs that make them so difficult.

When teaching verb tenses, teach them from the perspective of what is represented by the whole, or gestalt, of the phrase. The picture in our heads of when the action is happening is of overriding concern. Labeling the structure may or may not help some students; it depends on the students. For example, consider again the sentence, *He was playing*. We might analyze the syntactic use of *playing* and say that it is a past progressive intransitive verb. We might analyze it semantically and say that it is an action verb. Both pieces of information are helpful to the teacher. However, in terms of pedagogy, we are most interested in the active and static time frames represented and the interrelationship of the two. In this sentence, the static time frame is the past. Somehow in explaining this to the child, we must represent the past to him. The active time frame is progressive, or an action in the process of happening. To represent this, set up an activity where the child visits another room and sees others engaged in activities. Upon returning, that time frame is now static and in the past. However, we can talk about the active part, which is what the individuals were engaged in doing. We can show the child both the past time frame (in the other room) and the progressive aspect (playing). We show the child what the entire phrase represents. As a second example, suppose we are trying to teach the child what the sentence, *The racer chewed up the pavement* means. *Chew* is abstract in this context and *up* does not refer to a direction or location. The two words together mean something entirely different. In order to teach this, explain what the whole phrase means (i.e., driving rapidly).

Think of the word ending "-ing." In three sentences or less, explain to someone what "-ing"ness is. Couldn't do it, could you? That's because, as with all aspects of language, one piece doesn't make sense without the other. Consider the word *chewing* in the following sentences:

> *The dog is chewing the bone.*
> *Are you chewing the fat this weekend, or are you studying?*
> *The chewing dog got in trouble.*
> *Chewing is Sparky's favorite pastime.*

Chewing does not make sense unless it is in the context of a sentence. In the first sentence it is present progressive; in the second it represents future action. In the third sentence it is an adjective, and in the last sentence it is a gerund (noun). The same word can represent multiple syntactic categories and have multiple semantic connotations. No wonder English is so confusing to the new language user. When teaching verbs, keep the following principles in mind:

1. Always analyze the entire verb phrase to determine the underlying semantic connotation and pragmatic context. Use this to help students develop pictures in their heads of what the verb phrase represents. This is especially important with phrasal verbs.

2. For verbs other than simple past, simple present, and simple future (which actually appear in conversation and print relatively infrequently compared to the other verb forms), be sure to represent both the static and active components of the phrase, or the multiple perspectives represented by the verb. This applies both to advanced tenses and complex (or double) verb combinations.

Members of the Verb System

As with every aspect of the English language, the verb system is extremely complex. Table 7.3 provides a summary of the *major components of the verb phrase.*

TABLE 7.3 *Hierarchy of the Verb System*

	Verb Phrase and Auxiliary System Hierarchy	*Examples*
Phase 1	Basic transitive and intransitive verbs	The dog *chewed* the bone. The dog *barked*.
	Concrete uses of *have*	William *has* a new puppy.
	Predicate use of *be* verbs followed by an adjective, noun, or prepositional phrase of location	He *is* happy. He *is* a doctor. He *is* under the chair.
	The modal *can* to represent skill.	I *can* dress myself!
Phase 2	Simple past and future tenses	The puppy *chewed* my socks. Sara *will* play with me.
	Past and present progressive	Daddy *was laughing*. The puppy *is barking*.
	Understanding yes/no questions with *do* auxiliary	*Do* you like your puppy?
	May granting permission (meaning *yes*)	You *may* go with Grandpa.
Phase 3	Abstract *have*	Do you *have* a minute? I *have* a question.
	Sense verbs	The coffee *tasted* funny.
	Present progressive meaning *future*	Franklin *is going* to Grandma's soon.
	Using *do/did* as emphasis	I *do* have a loose tooth.
	Using *do/did* as a substitute for the verb	I *did* my homework on the bus.
	Idiomatic verbs	He *turned in* for the night.
	May referring to possibility	We *may* have rain tonight.
	Non-reversible passive	The toy *was broken* by the boys.

(continued)

TABLE 7.3 *Continued*

Verb Phrase and Auxiliary System Hierarchy	*Examples*
Phase 4	Special verbs (seem, cost, appear, weigh) Double verb sentences *There-* transformation Multiple uses of all complex modals and quasimodals (*would* as an activity in the past, as a yes/no question form, as a "wh-" question form, for emphasis)	Deanna *seemed* tired. The cat *sat watching* the bird. *There* were three birds. On rare evenings, she *would* sing us a song. *Would* you go with me? What *would* you like to eat? I *would love* to go.
	Reversible passive	The boy *was tickled by* his mom.
Phase 5	Perfect tense.	He *has taken* the train. Samantha *had eaten*.
Phase 6	Complex perfect tense forms with modals and double aspect	I *have been coming* here for 11 years. She *should have been driving* the car, not I.

The verb phrase is made up of verbs and of the auxiliary system. The auxiliary system is made up of tense and modals. Teach tense and modal semantically. Table 7.4 gives a description of the semantic relationship represented by the different verb configurations. Each verb configuration can represent many different time frames. Table 7.5 provides examples of *verb particles*. Some verbs take particles in the form of a preposition to make two-word verb combinations (Jaworska, 1999). These verbs are made up of a verb plus a preposition. The preposition is a part of the verb, not a part of the adverbial. Some of these verbs are highly idiomatic while other verbs with particles are not idiomatic at all. When teaching verb idioms to deaf children, it is helpful to put them on a continuum of most idiomatic to least idiomatic. You might also use the terms *concrete/abstract*, *normal/strange*, or any other indicator that will make sense to the child at that particular age. Both verb idioms and non-idiomatic verbs with particles in the form of prepositions have a similar syntactic characteristic in that the preposition (particle) can move away from the verb to the other side of the direct object. Verb idioms can occur with intransitive verbs *(He blew up at the suggestion)* and with transitive verbs *(He put out the fire)*. When a verb and its particle occur with a transitive verb, the particle can move after the direct object *(He put the fire out)*. When the direct object is a noun, particle movement is optional. When the direct object is a pronoun, particle movement is obligatory *(They pulled it off)*.

In addition to those components that modify verb tense, we make *passive voice* changes to the verb. Active and passive voice constructions are thematic paraphrases of one another (Roberts, 1999). Passive voice occurs only with transitive verbs because in all passive voice sentences, someone/something has done something to someone or something else (Heidinger, 1984). In the sentence *John loves Mary*, John is doing something to Mary. *Mary* is the recipient of the action of the verb. When *Mary* is moved to the position of the first noun phrase in a sentence, the sentence becomes passive in that the subject is passively involved with the action, not actually doing it himself or herself *(Mary is loved by John)*. We often use passive voice when we are vague about the subject of the sentence (e.g., *Something startled him* becomes *He was startled*). It is often used for brevity in newspaper headlines (e.g., *An avalanche trapped seven people* becomes *Seven Trapped in Avalanche*). The word *got* is often used informally as the passive, such as in the sentence *She got caught*.

Another transformation that occurs to the verb phrase is the *there-transformation*, often referred to as either the *expletive there* or the *existential there*. This transformation changes a sentence by adding the word *there* at the front of the sentence and moving the verb in front of the subject (e.g., *A bird is in the birdbath* becomes *There is a bird in the birdbath*). *There* has no actual meaning by itself. It does not refer to a location. It is used for drawing attention to something or for emphasis.

Serial, or double, verb sentences represent a highly overlooked component of the English language. Serial verbs "allow two or more verbs (other than

TABLE 7.4 *Members of the Verb System*

Category	Description	Examples
***Type Be* (Vbe)**	Also called linking verbs	is, am, was, were
Intransitive (Vi)	Used where the action is complete	She played.
Transitive (Vt)	Requires a recipient of the action of the verb	She fed the doll.
Have (Vh)	Requires a direct object defining what was had	She had a lollipop.
	Can be abstract	She had a baby.
Sense (Vs)	Verbs that act like linking verbs and for which Vbe can substitute; represent characteristics inherent in the five senses	The coffee tasted (was) bitter.
B (Vb)	Includes such verbs as *become, seem, appear, weigh*; acts like a linking verb	He seemed (was) tired. The baby weighed (was) 7 lbs.
Tense and aspect		
Simple past "-ed"	Completed action	jumped
Simple present	*Habitual*	jump
Simple future	with modal *will*	will jump
Past perfect	*had* + "-en"	had chosen
Present perfect	*have* + "-en"	have chosen
Future perfect	modal *will* + *have* + "-en"	will have chosen
Past progressive	*was* + "-ing"	was sleeping
Present progressive	*is* + "-ing"	is sleeping
Future progressive	*will* + *is* + "-ing"	will be sleeping
Past perfect progressive	*had* + "-en" + *be* + "-ing"	had been eating
Present perfect progressive	*have* + "-en" + *be* + "-ing"	have been eating
Future perfect progressive	*will* + *have* + "-en" + *be* + "-ing"	will have been eating

Modals

Modals are components of the auxiliary system. Teach semantically.

Modals		
Can	Capability	William can do 10 pushups.
	Assertion	I *can do* that!
	Permission (colloquial—see *may*—considered incorrect)	You *can have* dessert now.
Could	Capability	Chelsea *could walk* at 12 months.
	Possibility	We *could go* to Six Flags this weekend.
Shall	Future time (formal)	I *shall see* you tomorrow.
Should	Possibility	Daddy *should be* home anytime now.
	Expectation	You *should brush* your teeth after eating.
	Obligation	We *should write* a thank you note.
	Opinion	I *should think* you would be happy.
Will	Future time (informal)	Chelsea *will ride* the bus home with you.
	Promise	I *will take* you to the store after school.
	Capability	The jet ski *will carry* two passengers.
Would	Strong desire (formal)	*Would* that she *were* here.
	Strong desire (informal)	Sandy *would love* to go to the beach.
	Willingness (conditional)	I *would help out* if they asked.
May	Permission (formal)	You *may have* dessert now.
Might	Possibility	Sara *might help* me after school.
Must	Necessity	The cat *must go* out after she eats.
	Strong possibility (often implying concern)	She *must have bad* the baby by now.
	Emphasizing repeated activity	I *must have told* you that a thousand times!
	Assertion	You *must tell* me.

(continued)

TABLE 7.4 *Continued*

Category	Description	Examples
Quasimodals		
Have to (hafta)	Necessity	I *have to* (*hafta*) *go* to the bathroom. Applicants *have to earn* a 900 on the GRE.
Ought to (otta)	Requirement	Brian *ought to be* here by now.
Going to (gonna)	Expectation	He's *going to wash* the car this weekend.
	Future time (informal)	I'm *going to make* you some cookies.
	Promise	
Want to (wanna)	Wish or desire (object)	I *want to get* a new Barbie doll.
	Wish or desire (action)	Daddy *wants to remodel* the room.
Special Modals		
Had better	Pertinent action	We *had better go.*
	Mild warning	You'd *better stop.*
Would rather	Preference	Dewey *would rather remodel* the room.
Passive voice	Non-truncated	The bone was chewed by the dog.
	Truncated	The bone was chewed.
There-transformation	Existential	There's a fly in my soup.
Serial verbs	This structure takes on many different forms, but in all of them, the first sentence is dependent upon the second sentence either to complete it or to give it clarity.	S1: She saw _____?_____. S2: The boy was playing. Serial Form: She saw the boy playing. S1: He finished _____?_____. S2: He was doing his homework. Serial Form: He finished doing his homework.

Sources: Hargis, 1984; Heidinger, 1984; Palmer, 1999a, 1999b; Parker & Riley, 1994; Sebba, 1999; Smiley & Goldstein, 1998.

TABLE 7.5 *Uses of the Various Verb Tenses*

Tense	Uses	Examples
Simple past	Actions, states, feelings completed in the past; actions may: be continuous, habitual, or occur only once.	He lived in Georgia all his life. Some dinosaurs ate meat. He fished in the lake.
Simple present	Personal or sense verbs for states or feelings existing in the present time Actions that will occur in the future Activities that are relatively permanent (facts) Habitual or continuous actions	I am here. I play shortstop this coming Saturday. Turtles crawl. We breathe oxygen. I wash the dishes every night.
Simple future	Activities and events that will occur or exist in the future Requests Asking permission Asking for affirmation To draw attention, not as a question form	We will have a party this weekend. Will you buy that for me? Will you let me go with them? Will you agree to that? Will you look at that!
Past perfect	Action that began in the past and was completed in the past. Includes the use of clauses	He had run for office in the previous election. She'd tried the front door before she broke the window.
Present perfect	Action that began in the past and continued or was repeated up to the present time Action that was recently (just) completed in the past Actions that began in the past but the exact time is not known or not stated	I have lived here for two months. I have finished my homework. I have seen that movie.
Future perfect	Activities that begin or occur before another activity or point in the future	She will have gone by the time we get there.

(continued)

TABLE 7.5 *Continued*

Tense	Uses	Examples
Past progressive	Continuing action in the past that was interrupted by another action	I was washing the dishes when the phone rang.
	Ongoing action in the past occurring around a specific time	I was sleeping when the robbery occurred.
	Ongoing action that began in the past and which may or may not be continuing at the present time	When I called her she was cleaning her house.
Present progressive	Activities that will take place sometime in the future	I'm going to Hawaii for my vacation.
	Activities in progress at the moment the speaker is speaking	Your slip is showing.
		You must be kidding me.
Future progressive	Activities begun in the past and continuing into the present	He is spending the night at our house.
	Activities begun in the past that may continue in the future	We will be looking for a new house during our vacation.
	Activities that will be in progress in the future	
Past perfect progressive	Action in progress in the past interrupted by another action	They had been watching TV when the storm hit.
Present perfect progressive	Ongoing action that began in the past and continued or was repeated up to the present	I have been living here for four years.
	Ongoing action that began in the past, but the exact time is not known or not stated	She has been working here for quite a while.
Future perfect progressive	Activity that will exist or occur before another activity or part of time in the future	I will have been sleeping for only two hours by then.

256

auxiliaries) within a single noncomplex sentence or clause, with no overt signs of coordination" (Sebba, 1999, p. 334). Serial verbs occur when we embed one sentence within another. In the first sentence, a part of the information is unknown. Parts of the second sentence are needed to make the first sentence complete.

Hierarchy of the Verb Phrase System

Table 7.6 presents a hierarchy of the verb system. To reiterate, the purpose of a hierarchy is to provide guideposts for decision making about what to teach and when to teach it. Keep the aforementioned rules of thumb in mind when using the hierarchies in this chapter.

Verbs in ASL

It is essential to grasp the concept of simultaneity when trying to understand ASL verbs. In ASL, multiple components exist simultaneously.

Movement, Space, and Directionality

Verbs in ASL carry little meaning unless they are interpreted relative to movement, space, and directionality. Most action verbs in ASL contain some inherent movement, which represents the action of the verb (e.g., RUN, THROW, MOVE). The movement of the verb also occurs in the space between the subject and the object of the movement (e.g., IX (*you*), THROW-TO, BOY). When there is no object of the verb (e.g., BABY CRY), then use of the verb is iterative, that is, the verb states the action. In English *be* verbs link object and description as in *He is tired*. In ASL *be* verbs are deleted and directionality links to the object to the description. The sample sentence is glossed, IX (*he*) TIRED.

Classifiers Used as Verbs

Spatial verbs do not inflect for person, number, or aspect, but do accept locative affixes. This group of verbs has been determined to form a predicate classifier system. According to Valli and Lucas (1995), classifiers used with verbs are handshapes that are combined with location, orientation, movement, and nonmanual signals to form a predicate. A classifier predicate consists of a movement root and a classifier handshape together (i.e., the affix). Every classifier predicate has a location, usually represented in three-dimensional space and, if an object moves, location tells the initial and the final position. Woll and Kyle (1998, p. 865) described five subsets of spatial verbs:

TABLE 7.6 Verb Particles from Idiomatic to Non-Idiomatic

Highly Idiomatic	Somewhat/Vaguely Idiomatic	Not Idiomatic
Turn off (to disgust)	*Turn off* (break an electrical circuit)	*Turn off* (turn direction of a vehicle)
Green eggs turn me off.	Don't forget to turn off the lights.	Turn off Bay Drive.
Pull off (be successful)	*Pull off* (drive off)	*Pull off* (remove)
He pulled off the heist.	The car pulled off the road.	Pull off your wet socks.
Pick up (pay)	*Pick up* (clean)	*Pick up* (remove from floor)
He picked up the tab.	Please pick up your room.	Pick up that rock.
Dry up (disappear)	*Dry up* (become less moist)	*Dry up* (wipe)
"Ah, go dry up!" she yelled.	The paint will dry up.	I need to dry up the spill.

1. Predicates with locative affixes (MOVE, PUT)
2. Predicates with locative, instrument classifier, and manner affixes (CARRY-BY-HAND)
3. Predicates with locative, manner, and noun classifier affixes (VEHICLE-MOVE, PERSON-MOVE)
4. Predicates with locative classifiers on the body (HIT-IN-THE-EYE)
5. Predicates with locative affixes and body-part noun classifiers (CLENCH-FIST)

Intransitive Verbs

Intransitive verbs in English do not project their action onto an object (e.g., *The boy walked*), rather the subject is the experiencer of the action. In ASL, the experience of intransitivity is represented by the nonmanual markers of head tilt, eye gaze, or both (Neidle et al., 2000). For example,

<u>head tilt i</u>
LUCAS, SHOWER

indicates that Lucas took a shower, not that he showered something. In the sentence,

<u>eye gaze i</u>
CARMEN, SLEEP

we know that Carmen experienced the process of sleeping. Sometimes both head tilt and eye gaze are used simultaneously.

Transitive Verbs

English transitive verbs have objects and follow a subject + verb + object pattern. ASL uses this same sentence pattern; however, different combinations of word order are possible. When this occurs the sentences are marked in a particular way, with the subject of the sentence being marked simultaneously with a head nod (hn) (Valli & Lucas, 1995). For example, the English sentence *The*

<u>hn</u>
boy loves the dog could be signed in ASL as BOY LOVE DOG (subject + verb + object

<u>hn</u>
order) or BOY LOVE DOG BOY (with the subject repeated at the end) or LOVE

<u>hn</u>
DOG BOY (with the subject signed at the end). Often when signing the subject + verb + object sentence pattern, ASL users will topicalize the sentence. In this instance, the object is placed at the beginning of the sentence. The sentence

<u>t</u>
would then be DOG, BOY LOVE.

Tense and Aspect

Tense refers to the time frame (i.e., past, present, future) within which action occurs. In ASL, basic tense is displayed by forming signs in relation to an imaginary time line running through the body. "The area near the torso has a general meaning of 'present,' the area farther away has a meaning of 'future,' and the area over the shoulder has a general meaning of 'past' " (Valli & Lucas, 1995, p. 114). In addition, ASL uses more specific descriptions to mark the time of events than does English. For example, words like NOW, RECENTLY, TOMORROW, NOT YET, WILL, and FINISH are included in sentences to orient the recipient of the communication to the time frame being discussed. Another simple way basic tense is incorporated into sentences is the use of compounded signs for orientation. For example, TWO-WEEKS-AGO is made by using the sign for TWO starting with the movement for WEEK and flowing into the location for past action. Nonmanual markers provide additional information.

As with English, ASL can express simple past, simple present, and simple future. Simple past is described by the use of orienting words, the use of the sign FINISH, or by sign directionality (toward the shoulder). Simple present generally refers to actions that occur habitually (e.g., *I get up at 6 A.M.*), and to inherent traits of the subject or to things that usually happen (e.g., *Mosquito bites itch*). They are marked by orienting signs (e.g., EVERYDAY) or by a slower, deliberate, and repeated production of the sign. Simple future is represented by the sign WILL.

In addition to orienting the sign-reader to the time frame of a sentence, signers provide information about the time stability of actions. This is commonly referred to as *aspect* (Lehmann, 1999). According to Lehmann (1999), "time-stability of a situation is not its absolute duration in time but its volatility, its liability to change" (p. 43). English aspect occurs sequentially in the auxiliary system (e.g., *have gone; is going; might have been going*). ASL aspect occurs simultaneously.

Telicity refers to the time boundaries of an action (Lehmann, 1999). An action may be atelic, with no time boundaries (e.g., *The inner core of the earth contains magma*), or it might have a specific beginning and ending. Defined in English as progressive or perfect, ASL marks telicity by motion of the sign. Although simple ASL tense is relatively straightforward, ASL grammatical aspect is highly complex. Aspect in ASL describes "both the temporal unfolding of an event and the distributional properties of the objects and persons involved in the event" (Brentari, 1999, p. 19). The movements of signs, the use of various markers, the use of directionality, and spatial orientation are intricately interwoven. They describe whether an event is habitual, continuous, intermittent, durative, prolonged (protractive), of known or unknown starting time (inceptive), and of known or unknown time of completion (completive). These components of ASL perform the same functions as the perfect and progressive aspects in English, but a discussion of them is beyond the scope of this book.

An Examination of English Adjectives, Adjective Phrases, and Advanced Adjectival Forms

Basic, survival-level communication requires that we state a topic (e.g., *boy*) and make a comment about it (e.g., *boy run*). A simple verb is a sufficient comment to get across basic information. However, the lovely thing about communication is that it can be very rich, descriptive, and picturesque in nature. We get this richness by our ability to describe not only things, but also how things act. The words we use to describe nouns fall under the heading of *adjective and adjectival forms*. As with nouns and verbs, there are basic adjectives, advanced adjectives, and very ornate complexes of components that function like adjectives.

An adjective, according to Webster (New World Dictionary, 1966), is defined as:

1. any of a class of words used to limit or qualify a noun or other substantive, or
2. any phrase or clause similarly used, or
3. having the nature or function of an adjective, and
4. dependent or subordinate.

Adjectival refers to something:

1. having the nature or function of an adjective, or
2. added to an adjective base, as an adjectival suffix.

Given these definitions, our perspective on the topic of adjectives broadens considerably. The domain to which we refer by the word *adjective* actually covers a lot of territory. An adjective can be a simple word *(fuzzy)*. It can be something other than a *real* adjective; that is, it can have the nature of an adjective, such as a *noun adjunct (toy box)*. It can be something that is added to a different part of speech, which turns it into *derived adjective (wooden shoes, balding gentleman)*. It can be a phrase or clause used like an adjective, known as a *phrasal adjective (hot and cold running water)* or an *adjectival clause* such as a relative clause *(doll that had the rockabye eyes)*. *Parenthetical speech* is actually adjectival because it has a qualifying or explanatory nature *(My brother, John [John, as you know had been recently selected as candidate for class president] has recently embarked upon another quest)*. There are even some wild forms which look like adverbs (because they have "-ly") but act like adjectives *(lively horse, goodly sum)*. How *dare* they! Isn't the situation already confusing enough?

In addition adjectives have a very rich semantic domain, not to mention a very active social life. By that we mean that adjectives are highly susceptible to whatever the slang of the time wants them to be. An interesting and popular person can be referred to as *bad;* a person, an item or action can be *camp, groovy, tony, cool, outta sight,* or *awesome,* depending on the decade into which the speaker was born.

Suggestions for Teaching Adjectives, Adjective Phrases, and Advanced Adjectival Forms

When teaching early adjectives, choose those that are most important to the child. When teaching comparative and superlative adjectives, be sure to compare at least five to show that "-er" and "-est" are relative to the size of the neutral position (e.g., *a dog is bigger than a mouse but it is not bigger than an elephant*). Also, teach comparatives in a positive direction (e.g., *tall, taller, tallest*) before those in a negative direction (e.g., *short, shorter, shortest*). Use lots of pictures to show the meaning of the adjective. As a general rule of thumb, the more pictures and the more examples you give, the better. When teaching derived adjectives (e.g., *the swollen river*), incorporate these into conversations. For children who sign, fingerspell the word or write it down. When (and not before) children are comfortable with books and with basic issues surrounding print, you may begin to expose them to the variety of word endings associated with adjectives. When teaching more advanced descriptive language such as idiomatic expressions, similes, etc., directly instruct the student in the actual meaning of the phrase. Do not draw silly pictures of the concrete meaning (e.g., picture showing a smiling clam to represent *Mom was as happy as a clam at high tide*). Children who are deaf and hard of hearing are visually oriented. They may be more likely to retain a visually engaging silly picture than the actual meaning. Go directly to the meaning (e.g., say "Clams prefer to be in water. It means that Mom is happy because she is doing what she prefers. She is doing her favorite thing.").

Members of the Adjective System

Adjectives.   The first and most obvious member of the adjective system is the adjective itself. The adjective system is quite extensive. Semantically speaking, we use adjectives to describe a vast array of traits of objects such as size, shape, age, texture, and color, among other things. These are referred to as the *semantic case* of an adjective. Table 7.7 lists the most commonly used semantic cases of adjectives and provides an extensive outline of the multiple ways in which we describe nouns (i.e., people, places, things, ideas, and concepts).

Derived Adjectives.   Derived adjectives are those adjectives that begin as one form but end up as another after the attachment of a suffix. The most commonly known derived forms are the comparative *(bigger)* and the superlative *(biggest).* There are many derived forms of words (e.g. *derived nouns*), but we address derived adjectives in this section. Table 7.8 outlines common morphemes from which adjectives are derived.

TABLE 7.7 *Semantic Cases of English Adjectives*

Case	Description	Examples
Cardinal number	Actual or general number	*seven* birds, the *lone* Ranger, a *single* rose, *three* pigs
Ordinal number	Numerical system indicating relative position	*first* base, the *next* house, the *fourth* inning
Evaluational	Evaluative term	a *beautiful* sunset, a *nice* girl, an *okay* time, a *blatant* error
General quantifier	General amount or number	*many* trees, *any* car, *some* boys, *few* doctors,
Consecutive quantifier	Specific or forthcoming nouns	*each* puppy, the *next* item, *another* peach
Size or amount	Size or amount	the *big* lollipop, the *fat* worm, a *minuscule* amount
Color	Color	the *green* car, *cerulean* blue china
Hue	Shade of color	the *light* green car, a *dark* blue dress
Location	A direction in reference to the body or an object or location	his *right* hand, on the *left* side of the house, *front* yard, in the *back* of the closet
Physical length	Physical length or distance	the *long* boat, *short* haircut, a *far* journey
Temporal length	Length of time	a *short* trip, an *interminable* lecture, a *lengthy* discussion
Condition	Physical condition	the *clean* room, *fried* chicken, a *broken* mirror
	Mental condition	a *broken* psyche, an *ugly* attitude
Physical status	Physical state of an individual	a *deaf* child, a *dead* chicken, a *lame* horse
Emotional status	Mental or emotional state	a *happy* boy, a *disappointed* reader
Chronological age	Actual age of people, objects, events	a *forty-eight-year*-old woman
General age	General or relative age of people, objects, events	a *young* organization, *ancient* glaciers, an *old* man
Distance	Length or height of individuals, objects, events	a *high* wall, a *deep* river, a *long* nap
Variation	Equivalence or nonequivalence	the *same* book, *special* school, *various* situations, a *different* approach
General type: partitives	General type of individual, object, event	a *type* of personality, a *kind* of cheese, *sort* of a party
Specific type	Specific type	a *Ford* car, a *Maytag* repairman
General amount: partitives	General amount	a *can* of worms, a *bucket* of fried chicken, a *ton* of fun
Demonstrative determiners	Deictic relationship of individuals, objects, or events relative to one another	*this* book, *that* idea, *these* children, *those* ballgames

(continued)

TABLE 7.7 Continued

Case	Description	Examples
Physical metaphor	A physical adjective used to describe an emotion, event, or experience	*scratchy* voice, an *ugly* comment, a *hot* temper, a *blue* mood, a *square* meal, a *lame* idea
Wealth	Specific or general amount of money a person possesses	a *rich* man, a *wealthy* advocate, a *poor* nation
Cost or value	Specific or general amount of costs or value	a *$2.00* block of fudge, a *plug* nickel
Weight	Specific or general amount of weight	a *light* suitcase, a *77-lb.* boy
Climatic conditions	Weather conditions of events	a *rainy* wedding, a *dry* desert
Shape	Physical perimeter of an object	a *round* table, a *square* peg
Function	Function for which objects, individuals, or events are used	*educational* videotapes, *religious* symbols, *racing* equipment
Comparison or degree	Comparison of one object, event, individual to another	the *mild* salsa, the *gifted* child, the *early* flight
Powers	Physical or mental powers someone or something possesses	the *magic* lamp, the *clairvoyant* woman, a *guardian* angel
Auditory	Noise level or pitch produced	a *high* screech, the *low* rumble, the *soft* piano, a *loud* crowd
Presence/absence	Presence, absence, or completion of an object or event	the *end* result, an *empty* chair, a *done* turkey, the *late* Mr. Jones
Emotional intensity	Degree of emotional reaction	with *deep* sympathy, a *shallow* person, the *intense* artist
Tactile trait	Proprioceptive and tactile characteristics	a *scratchy* face, *slimy* soap, *soft* skin
Truth or falsity	Actuality of an object, individual, or experience	*virtual* reality, *fake* fur, a *true* friend
Identifier	Identifier which singles out one entity from a generic grouping	that *particular* test, *such* a person
Body parts	Parts of the body	*facial* hair, *ocular* pursuit, *nasal* congestion
Social condition	Sociological status	an *enslaved* culture, an *upperclass* club, a *third-world* nation
Fixture	Permanence or transience	*temporary* lodging, *permanent* fillings, *fleeting* memory
Nationality or section	National, regional, or state origin of an individual, item, or experience	*Yankee* ingenuity, *Canadian* coin, *Southern* hospitality, *Eastern* bloc

Rate	Rate of motion an object, individual, or event displays	fast tempo, lively beat, slow motion
Part-to-whole	Psychological or physical completeness or status of an object, individual, or event	the main point, the basic plan, an adjunct facility, an associate professor
Type	Specific type of individual, object, or event	mechanical bull, medical evidence
Flavor	Flavor	orange soda, vanilla pudding, lemon pound cake
Group purpose	Reason for a group to be one entity	a solidarity march, a charity ball, a political rally
Time relationship	Time relationship of one event to another	a future president, a past slight, a recent affair
Sex	Sexual/biological identity	boyish figure, feminine traits, male cat
Social/physical appearance	Social status of physical appearance	a formal invitation, a coming-out party
Time commitment	Amount of time available to events by individuals or objects	A free man for the weekend, the unencumbered funds, unfettered ideas
Physical needs	Physical state requiring satisfaction	The sleepy baby, the hungry puppy, the thirsty horse
Movement	General mobility	Moveable adverb, stationary bicycle
Statistical concept	Statistical characteristic	The average man, the slow learner, significant effect
Temperature	Temperature	A hot afternoon, a cool breeze, the temperate zone
Marital status	Marital status	The engaged girl, the divorced man, the single mom
Degree of difficulty	Ease or difficulty with which events are performed	A hard game, easy instructions, simple directions
Smell	Odors emanating from someone or something	Fragrant gardenias, musty room
Taste	Taste	A dill pickle, sour taste, sweet watermelon
Complexity	Relative complexity of an event or task	A simple question, a difficult answer, a complex problem
Salary	Amount of money earned	A high-paid model, a top-salaried executive, a low-paying job
Religious affiliation	Religious affiliation	An Episcopal priest, a Buddhist monk, the Baptist hymnal, a Jewish bakery
Seasonal	Associated with a season	Summer haircut, winter coat, the fall fashions
Public status	Availability to all or a few	A private plane, a public auction
Fuel	Kind of fuel objects and individuals require to maintain functions	A man-eating shark, the coal furnace, a diesel truck, a vegetarian secretary

Sources: Goldsworthy, 1982; Heidinger, 1984; Smiley & Goldstein, 1998.

TABLE 7.8 *Derived Adjectives*

Morpheme	Meaning or Source	Examples
-er	Comparative	A bigg*er* box
-est	Superlative	The bigg*est* box
-ed	Passive voice derivation	The box*ed* roses
-ed	Derived from *with*	A spott*ed* pony, dimpl*ed* cheeks
-en	Passive voice derivation	Stol*en* moments
-ened	Passive voice derivation	Her straight*ened* hair
-y	Derived from verb	Stick*y* buns, greas*y* hands
Multiple	Multiple	Sick*eningly* sweet
-ier	Comparative where adjective ends in -y	The luck*ier* twin
-iest	Superlative where adjective ends in -y	The lonel*iest* man
-ly	From noun, meaning *noun-like* (or not if un-added)	Heaven*ly* aroma, priest*ly* garbs, un-characteristi*cally* quiet
-ly	Old usage	Come*ly* wench, good*ly* sum, sloven*ly* habits
X + like	Seeming like a specific noun	Waif-*like*, wraith-*like*
X + person	Where X is a verb plus a morpheme defining function	The *washer* woman, the *delivery* man
-able	Added to verb	Wash*able* shoes, market*able* concept
-ing	Added to verb	Look*ing* glass, row*ing* venue
-tion	Added to verb	*Action* news

Noun Adjuncts.   Noun adjuncts are a special kind of adjectives. They are actually freestanding nouns with meanings unto themselves but which act as if they are adjectives. Just about any noun can pretend to be an adjective in one way or another. Following are a few of the possibilities.

love boat	road rage	lab coat	light bulb
rose water	traffic jam	plastic toy	fire wall
water meter	ghost town	shoe box	tin roof
glasses case	game show	bottle top	tax man
hat rack	bus tour	paper cut	power bill
toy box	hospital benefit	chocolate milk	window dressing

Adjectival Phrases.   Adjectives are like potato chips; it's hard to eat just one. Similarly it is hard to use just one adjective. Most of us describe things in an exuberant fashion using multiple adjectives. We talk about the fabulous, wonderful, highly entertaining, and amusing individual whom we recently met, or we complain about our terrible, miserly, crabby old neighbor. This requires the use of conjunctions and commas in writing. There is also an expected order of adjectives. We discuss this next, in relation to ASL.

Adjectival Clauses/Relative Clauses.   Recall that an adjectival form adds more information to or modifies some existing noun. This being the case, we could consider certain relative clauses to be adjectival. When the relative clause modifies a noun, this would be true (e.g., *Bob, who is an attorney, lives in Atlanta*). However, when the relative clause completes a sentence, or when it refers to *where, when,* and *how* concepts, it would be better understood as an adverb (see below). Relative clauses describe nouns by attaching a descriptive sentence to a noun using *who, which,* or *that* (e.g., *Malcolm, who bought a sailboat, is quite wealthy; The tree, which had been struck by lightning, was an historical landmark;* and *The policy that many opposed passed by a narrow margin*). Relative clauses can modify any noun, whether it is the subject, direct object, indirect object, or object of the preposition. Any noun in a sentence can modify a noun in another sentence. For example, in the sentence (S1) *Joe was a fisherman* we can modify the subject with a second sentence (S2), *She loved Joe.* Because *Joe* in S2 is a direct object, we use the object pronoun *whom* to create a relative clause within the first sentence: *Joe, whom she loved, was a fisherman.* When teaching the relative clause, explain that relative clauses add more information about the noun. Stress that *who* is not, in this case, a question. Stress that its purpose is to point to the noun being described (e.g., *Joe ← he/himself/who*).

Figurative Language.   The category of figurative language has many components, one of which we addressed in the verb section of this book: idiomatic verbs. Idiomatic verbs are an example of figurative language because a verb and a preposition together can imply a whole new non-literal meaning (e.g., *shoot off your mouth*). However, we chose to discuss idiomatic verbs in the verb section because of their unique construction.

Figurative forms in general are those forms of language that result in a non-literal meaning. *Idiomatic expressions* (e.g., *chip off the old block*), *similes* (e.g., *she looks like an angel*), *metaphors* (e.g., *my brain is a sieve*), *fables and morals* (e.g., The Fox and the Grapes), *personification* (e.g., *Mr. Toothbrush wants you to tickle him*) are just a few of many other forms that make up the figurative or non-literal system. Those forms for which we can provide a direct definition (e.g., *pulling my leg* means *teasing me*) are the easiest to teach. The longer the form (e.g., metaphors are shorter than allegories) and the more language involved, the harder it is to give a definition, and the harder it is to teach. One might even argue that some forms of *hyperbole* may be adjectival in nature *(She was as old as the hills)*, although an equal argument could be made in favor of calling this an adverb. While technically an adverb (because it answers the question *How old?*), we can reconfigure the sentence to *She was old* where *old* is an adjective. *Parenthetical speech* might also be considered as an adjective because it meets the criterion of adding new information (e.g., *Dewey went home after work [as you know, he recently started his new job] only to find that the boat had sunk*.)

Hierarchy of the Adjective System

Table 7.9 presents a hierarchy of the adjectival system. Once again we remind the reader that the purpose of the hierarchies presented here is to provide general guidelines for viewing the complexity of each topic area. Some children will progress more rapidly than others. At times children will have growth spurts in one area while seeming to make little progress in another. Remember also that the phases of one chart do not necessarily correspond to the phases of another chart.

Adjective Issues in ASL

In English, we expand our descriptions of nouns and nominals with adjectives and adjectival forms. Description in ASL occurs in a similar manner; although, sequence is not always an issue and much description occurs in simultaneity.

ASL Adjectives

ASL adjectives can occur before the noun (e.g., TALL BUILDING) for the purpose of specifying which noun you are referring to, or after the noun (e.g., GIRL, BEAUTIFUL) to describe the noun. When multiple adjectives are used to describe a noun they occur in the following order:

$$\overline{\qquad t}$$

topic, trait (UGLY), size (BIG), number (TWO): DOG, UGLY, BIG, TWO. This is the opposite of the adjective order of English: *Two big, ugly dogs.*

Numerical Incorporation

A second form of description occurs by the process of numerical incorporation (Valli & Lucas, 1995). In the English sentence, *I had my nails done three weeks ago* the cardinal number *three* precedes the word *weeks*, and is therefore an adjective. In ASL, numbers are not always necessarily used sequentially. Thus, the sign for THREE would be incorporated into the sign for WEEK. Numerical incorporation occurs with cardinal numbers and words and with ordinal numbers and words (e.g., EVERY OTHER WEEK, ALL NIGHT).

Relative Clauses

In English, relative clauses also describe nouns and nominal forms. These are confusing because (with the exception of the word *that*) relative clauses begin

TABLE 7.9 *Hierarchy of the Adjective System*

	Adjective System Hierarchy	Example
Phase 1	Simple predicate adjectives (in SP III)	Seth *is happy.*
	Simple nominative adjectives (before nouns)	The *happy* boy
	Early descriptive content (color, number, size, shape, temperature, and texture)	Blue, happy, soft, warm, hot, big, round, old, wet, green
	Series of two, then three adjectives	Big and red, old and dirty
Phase 2	Simple derived adjectives	gold/*golden*, mess/*messy*
	Comparative and superlative	big/*bigger*/*biggest*
	Noun adjuncts	*toy* boat
	Adjectives derived from passive voice with "–ed"	the *washed* puppy, *boiled* chicken
	Common idioms	
Phase 3	Adjectives derived from gerunds	The *meowing* cat
	Adjectives derived from passive voice with "–en" or null participle	*frozen* pizza, *cut* beans, *grown* children, *sworn* statement, *beaten* eggs,
	Hyphenated adjectives	*accident-prone* man
		well-spoken youngster
	Adjectives that look like an adverb	lively debate, comely wench
	Figurative adjectives	*blue* Monday, *sharp* wit, *soft* heart
	Restrictive relative clause where the subject of S2 modifies a noun in S1 and the relative pronoun is *that, who,* or *which*	The girl *who is laughing* is my sister. The dog *that won the race* is mine. The boy in the green wagon, *which has a red stripe*, is my son
	Adjectives with multiple morphemes	An enticingly spoken message
	Less common idioms	
	Frozen metaphors	

(continued)

TABLE 7.9 *Continued*

	Adjective System Hierarchy	Example
Phase 4	Restrictive relative clauses where the object of S2 modifies a noun in S1 and the relative pronoun is *that*, *whom*, or *which*	My boss liked the man *whom I hired.*
	Simile	He was *like a breath of fresh air.*
	Hyperbole	She was *madder than a wet hen.*
	Novel metaphor	
Phase 5	Non-restrictive clauses modifying nouns	Adolescents, *who can be frustrating,* are often in turmoil.
	Allegories	

with question forms *(which, who, when, where)*. In describing this to students who are deaf, we must make it clear that the question word is not asking a question but is relating one sentence to a noun in another sentence. This is accomplished by topicalizing the main noun, then using a pronoun form (e.g., *he, it, itself, himself,* etc.) as a substitute for the relative pronoun (e.g., *who, which, that,*

$$\underline{\quad t \quad}$$

when), then attaching the description. The glossed form BOY, HIMSELF LEG BREAK, IX *(he)*, POSS *(my)* FRIEND would equate with *The boy who has the broken leg is my friend.*

An Examination of English Adverbs, Adverb Phrases, and Advanced Adverb Forms

According to Webster's New World Dictionary (1966), an adverb is defined as:

1. any class of words used to modify a verb, adjective, or other adverb by expressing time, place, manner, degree, cause, etc., or

2. any phrase or clause similarly used.

Adverbs are extremely important to us in answering questions. In fact, most of the time when we are asking for information, we receive it in the form of an adverbial. We ask basic *who/what* and *what is X doing*-type questions about the nouns and verbs of sentences. If we want to ask a question about an adjective, we usually use the word *how* along with the semantic case of the adjective, as in *how old is* or *how tall is the*. Just about everything else we ask requires the child to answer with an adverb. This important area of English language learning was discussed in Chapter 6.

Suggestions for Teaching Adverbs, Adverb Phrases, and Advanced Adverb Forms

Always teach adverbs within the context of verbs because an adverb is meaningless without context, and teach categories of adverbs—teaching adverbs individually would be far too time consuming. Teaching categories of adverbs based on their semantic meaning allows the focus to be on meaning and use (the important stuff), and the nuts and bolts soon follow. Once children have *meaning* and *application* under their belts, they will be more likely to recognize new specific examples of members of that category. For example, when teaching the concept "Ways to Get Places" (i.e., adverbs of conveyance) we are actually teaching not only adverb categories (e.g., mechanical means, animal means) but associated nouns (e.g., *car, dog sled*), prepositions (e.g., *in, by*), and question forms (e.g., *how did X go*). But the primary reason to care about adverbs is that they answer the really big questions in life such as:

Mommy, why can't I go outside? *Because it is raining.*	adverbial of reason
Daddy, where do I come from? *From Philadelphia.*	adverbial of place
Grandpa, you weren't really in the war, were you? Actually, I was shot down over the ocean.	adverb of factuality, adverbial of place
I can't do this homework! That's because you're doing it too quickly.	adverbials of reason, manner, and an intensifier adverb

We can describe *things* in life with adjectives, and we can tell what we have done with verbs, but when we really, really want to explain just about anything, then we need adverbial forms. Adverbs hold the verbal building blocks for the larger questions of life. Without them, we would have a very concrete existence.

Members of the Adverbial System

Adverbs present us with two kinds of complexity: syntax and semantics (van der Auwera, 1999). Syntactically, members of the adverbial system come in the form of adverbs, prepositional phrases, and sometimes, special nouns. Semantically, adverbials describe many different actions of the verb such as manner (how), place (where), time (when), duration (how long), frequency (how often) and reason or purpose (why). Table 7.10 provides a list of the semantic cases of English adverbs.

Single Words.   Adverbs can take the form of single words, phrases, or entire clauses. Most simple adverbs are formed by adding "-ly" to an adjective (e.g., *He brushed his hair quickly*). However, there are some special "-ing"-word adverbs that do not use "-ly". These include but are not limited to: *often, everyday, very, never, ever, always, already, once, just, even* and *only*. The list goes on. Sometimes words such as *here, there, home, yesterday, tomorrow* and the like are adverbials (e.g., *The meeting is here*) because they perform the same function as an adverb, answering the same semantic questions (e.g., *where*) as other adverbials.

Prepositional Phrases.   In addition to single words and words that end in "-ly," *prepositional phrases* are found in the adverbial position in sentences, and they answer the same question forms as do other adverbs. For example, a prepositional phrase can make up an adverbial of manner (e.g., *He wrote his reply in a brusque manner*), an adverbial of place (e.g., *She lived in the desert*), an adverbial of conveyance (e.g., *They went on the bus*), or many of the other semantic cases. Words such as *before, during,* and *until* (e.g., *until tomorrow*) function in the same manner as the more commonly known prepositions (e.g., *in, on, under, over, around, through*). One word, *ago,* functions as a preposition but occurs in the postposition (e.g., *They leave in three weeks* versus *They left three weeks ago*) (Jaworska, 1999).

TABLE 7.10 *Semantic Cases of English Adverbs*

Case	Description	Example
Location—goal	Place of termination	William hid *under the bed.*
Location—stative	Location of one's being	Keith is *in the car.*
Location—source	Place where an action or event begins	Sara drove all the way *from town.* Steve pulled a rabbit *out of his hat.*
Location—action/process	Place where an action or event occurs	Sharon pondered her future *on the beach.*
Reason/function/purpose	Reason or purpose for an event occurring	Susan left *due to the lateness of the hour.* Dad bought a motorcycle *for the heck of it.*
Intensifier	Indicator of the intensity of an event	Samantha was *very* crabby.
Manner	Manner in which an event occurs	Mom arranged the flowers *artfully.* Chloe opened the letter *hopefully.*
Accompaniment	Resemblance	The sleeping baby looked *like a little angel.*
Means—method	Method by which something was accomplished	She plays piano *by ear.* Her teacher taught language *with the Fitzgerald Key.*
Means—conveyance	Method of transportation	Chelsea went to school *on the bus.*
Means—tool/instrument	Device used to accomplish a task	Steve cut the grass *with a lawnmower.* Sondra cut her steak *with a knife.*
Cause/result	Means by which events occur	Victoria made it *by hand.*
Repetitious time	Generic time occurrence of events	William fell *again.*
Non-existence	Non-existence or appearance	Chloe has *no* front teeth. There is *no* joy in Mudville.
Denial	Prevention from occurrence	That is *not* funny !
Uncertainty	Denial of all or any part of a sentence	*Maybe* lightning hit the TV. *Perhaps* Norma will call.
Exception/exclusion	Lack of certainty about an event	All the children are present *except* Virginia. The whole gang came *but not* John.
Inclusion	Indication that an event or experience occurred or applies to all but one	Bonnie wants ice cream, *too.* We *also* rode the roller coaster.
	Extension of an event to another time, person, or event	

(continued)

TABLE 7.10 *Continued*

Case	Description	Example
Rejection	Rejection or prohibition of an action	*Don't go* !
Approximation	Indication of approximate time or experience	I'll be there *around* noon. That's *about* right.
Confirmation	Affirmative response to a yes/no question	Headshake, *yes, yeab, uh-bub.*
Explication	Socially approved term or phrase used to segue into the next comment	*Well,* I guess you can. *If you ask me,* he's one brick shy of a load.
Evaluation	Judgment about an event	You did *well.* Sara drives *carefully.*
Similarity	Description of resemblance (simile)	William's mind is *like greased lightning.* Your dress *looks like* spun butter. He is *as sweet as* sugar.
Time—beginning	Specific or generic description of the inception of something	We *just* arrived. The game starts *at ten.*
Time—static	Time frame within which events occur	Sandy's birthday is *in September.*
Time—sequencing	Temporal order of an event	Cheryl went home *after work.* Norma finished *before* 3:00.
Time—frequency	Time frequency with which an event occurs	We worked on this book *every day.*
Time—duration	Temporal duration of an event or occurrence	Brian was in college *for five years.*
Time—continuation	Generic indication of time lapses	*Then* she drove home.
Indefinite time	Generic time frame	Victoria will meet us *later.*
Time—action	Time frame within which an action occurs	They went to the races *on Tuesday.*
Pathway	Path used to get from one place to another	They escaped *by the air ducts.* We went *down* I-85.
Availability	Availability of something	Jean keeps chocolate *bandy.* Barbara is ready to go *at a moment's notice.*
Conversion/change	End product of an action	The rain turned the front yard *into* a giant mud puddle.
Return	The return of an object or event to its source	Dad drove *back* home.
Time—ending	Time ending sequence or generic description of cessation	Stop, *NOW!* We'll arrive *at six.*
Remainder	Indication of what remains after the cessation of an event	Brian had $7 *left over.*

Standard	Standard against which something is compared	Sara compared her paycheck *to his*. The hotel was *like a palace*.
Complexity	Indication of the degree of complexity	The driver *simply* fell asleep.
Factuality	Indication of the truth	The Cougars *actually* won for a change. *To tell the truth*, I was bored.
Reciprocity	Indication of two points between which something occurs	Leasa drives *back and forth* everyday. The train runs *between* D.C. and NY.
Adversary	The opponent in an event	We played *against* their team.
Preference	Indication of preference	I would *rather* go to Disney World.

Sources: Goldsworthy, 1982; Heidinger, 1984; Smiley & Goldstein, 1998.

Adverbial Clauses in Subordination.   We can subordinate one sentence under another by the use of clauses. The subordinate clause is often called the dependent clause. It is introduced with a subordinator *(when, as if, until)*. There are many components to the subordination system.

Adverbial Clauses—Time, Location, Manner, Concession

Time subordinators:	*when, whenever, after, before, as, until, while, since*
Location subordinators:	*where, wherever*
Manner subordinators:	*as if, as though*
Concession:	*although, though, even though*

Causal Clauses—Cause, Effect, or Consequence Clauses

Cause subordinators:	*because, since, as, so that, in order that, because of, due to, on account of*
Effect subordinators:	*so, so that*

Conditional Clauses

Conditional subordinators:	*if, so long as, provided that, unless*

Relative Adverbs.   When a question word such as *where* or *when* introduces a sentence that describes action or relates information to the action, it forms a relative clause. For example, in the sentence *He drove where there was no pavement,* the relative adverb *where* introduces the sentence that tells us more about the action of the verb *drive.* The sentence *She died when the last leaves fell from the trees* tells us more about the verb *die.*

Hierarchy of the Adverb System

Table 7.11 presents a hierarchy of the adverbial system. As with previous hierarchies, we caution the reader to remember that language skills develop unevenly. Progress in one hierarchy does not equate to progress in another hierarchy.

Adverb Issues in ASL

In English, an adverb is a separate word that describes an adjective or a verb. In ASL the features of the sign that carries the description are often incorporated directly into the sign. Facial expression is an important component of adverb and adverbial forms. There are several grammatical forms of adverbials in ASL.

TABLE 7.11 *Hierarchy of the Adverbial System*

	Adverbial System Hierarchy	Example
Phase 1	Single word adverbials of place (*here, there, home*)	Get *down.*
	Prepositional phrase adverbials of place	Sit *in your chair.*
	Simple negation	No.
Phase 2	Simple adverbs of time (*yesterday, tomorrow, now*)	Put that *down, now!*
	Intensifiers	It's *so* big, *too* hot, *very* old
	Negation	*None, nothing, never*
	Negation incorporation (ASL)	*Don't want, don't like*
Phase 3	Adverbials of manner and frequency (*everyday, once, twice, sometimes*)	She laughs *daily.*
	Adverbs using -ly	They ran *swiftly.*
	Later adverbials of time (*before, after, already, always, finally, never*)	He left *before lunch.*
	Adverbials of accompaniment	He played *with the puppy.*
	Because clauses	They cried *because the movie was sad.*
Phase 4	Early idiomatic expressions	*In a rut*
	Adverbials of purpose or use	*With a knife*
	Qualifiers (*almost, about, rarely, hardly, barely, just, even, only, such*)	It's *about* ready.
	Common dependent clauses (*before, after, during, while, since, until*)	*After the game was over,* they went for pizza.
Phase 5	Sentence adverbs as modals (*probably, possibly, maybe, most likely*)	He will *probably* be late.
	Sentence adverbs providing evaluative component to the sentence (*fortunately, luckily, happily, strangely, hopefully, strangely enough, oddly enough*)	*Fortunately,* his luck held out.
	Relative adverbs	He lives *where the fault lines intersect.*
	Later idiomatic expressions	Get *out of my face!*

One-Word Adverbs and Adverbial Morphemes

When a single sign is used to describe an action (e.g., RAN+QUICKLY), corresponding intensity and stress are added to the movement of the verb. The nonmanual marker, mouthing, is an essential component as the lips purse, the tongue trills up and down, or the cheeks puff. Lentz, Mikos, and Smith (1988) identify the following adverbial nonmanual markers.

- _____ cs   close by in time or location. *cs* stands for cheek to shoulder
- far away   marker for "off in the distance"
- _____ stress   (marker for intensity)
- _____ mm   (normal or with regularity)
- _____ oo   (abnormally small or thin)
- _____ cha   (abnormally large or tall)

When used to describe an adjective (e.g., *very tall*), there is a deliberate, but more exaggerated movement and differently paced movement of the adjective.

Prepositional Phrases

English prepositional phrases are used to define the manner, location, frequency, intensity, and duration of a verb, among other descriptions (e.g, *Mother is in a hurry*). In ASL this is indicated by the reflexive pronoun as in MOTHER,
_____ r
HERSELF, HURRY. The corresponding nonmanual markers listed in the preceding section apply. Adverbials of time, such as *She went on Monday*, are indicated by setting the time frame first, then describing the action. Adverbials of place as in *He lives in Colorado* are indicated by the rhetorical question, as
_____ rhet
in (IX *(he)* LIVE WHERE, COLORADO).

Adverbial Clauses

The final adverbial form is the adverbial clause (e.g., *He left town after he was arrested*). While in English the sequence of actions is represented by the adverb used, in ASL the action is presented sequentially. Examples are:

Before	Let's pack a lunch before we leave for the beach.
	BEFORE GO + TO BEACH, TWO-OF-US LUNCH, P-A-C-K.
After	We ate dinner after the performance.
	FINISH PERFORMANCE, TWO-OF-US EAT DINNER.
While	While I waited in line, I read a newspaper.

_____ wh
IX *(me)* LINE WAIT, IX *(me)* #DO, NEWSPAPER READ.

During	I had a coke during my break.
	TIME BREAK, IX *(me)* DRINK COKE.
Since	I have been working since midnight.[1]
	MIDNIGHT SINCE, IX *(me)* WORK.
Because	Because I hurt my knee I can't run.
	BECAUSE POSS *(my)* KNEE HURT, IX *(me)* RUN, CAN'T.
Until	The school does not open until 7:00 A.M.

SCHOOL, IX *(it)* OPEN, TIME 7 MORNING, BUT NOT BEFORE TIME 7.

| When | When we were at the store, a robber came in. |
| | ROBBER, IX *(he)* ENTER STORE SAME + TIME TWO-OF-US IX *(loc)*. |

HAPPEN is an important adverbial in ASL. It is used to mark segments of activity. For example, we might indicate that an action was initiated with the sign HAPPEN, followed by a discussion of what transpired. It is also used to mean *it happened that . . .* , *once upon a time*, and *there was a. . . .* HAPPEN can also take the place of other subordinators as in:

A car hit me while I was crossing the street.

HAPPEN IX *(me)* SCL: 1 "crossing street," CAR SCL: Vehicle "hit me."

An Examination of the Negation System of English

We include a discussion of negation in this chapter because it uniquely cuts across nouns, verbs, adjectives, and adverbs. For example, in the sentence *Terry has no shoes, shoes* is a noun whose meaning is changed by the word *no*, so the negator functions like an adjective because it modifies the meaning of the noun. But in the sentence *Sandy never gains any weight*, the word *gains* is a verb whose meaning is changed by the word *never*, so the negator functions like an adverb. Negators are also found in the grammatical class of interjections as in *Oh, no!*

Suggestions for Teaching Negation

In teaching negation, be sure you have a firm understanding of the concepts you are teaching, and do not use them simultaneously. For example, *no* can be the answer to a *yes* question or it can mean *none* (e.g., *no luck*). Recognize that English negation can confuse students because the negator can be found in many different locations in a sentence. Recognize also that this aspect of language needs direct attention. Often negation is overlooked in instruction because it seems so simple, yet an examination of the topic reveals its complexity. We say

---

[1]The sign for SINCE more specifically means UP TO NOW in ASL.

"no" in many ways. For example, when a child asks the teacher, "May I go to the bathroom?" the teacher might answer, "I'd really rather that you complete your math page first," but she is actually saying, "No!"

Types of Negation and the Negation Hierarchy

Children tend to acquire negation skills in a similar sequence to one another. Following is the order in which the normally developing child acquires negation (deVilliers & deVilliers, 1978; Owens, 1996; Nelson, 1998).

1. The child shakes head or uses other recognizable gestures.

2. *No* or *not* precedes or follows a holophrastic phrase (*no cookie*).

3. The child develops sentences that include subject and object (*I eat*).

4. The negative element follows the subject of a sentence (*Doggie no eat*).

5. The negative element is added to the auxiliary or modal (*I can't do it? Don't*). *Can't* and *don't* are special words because they are learned for practical use before the child uses *can* and *do* as auxiliaries.

6. The negative element is used in combination with indefinite pronouns. Use is later refined to follow acceptable grammatical patterns. *I not doing nothing* is a double negative and requires higher-order cognitive development for the child to understand. Proper use of double negatives develops much later following a period of inaccurate usage.

7. Negation is used in tag questions (*He broke that, didn't he?*).

8. Negation is used with subject-auxiliary inversion questions (*Doesn't that hurt?*)

9. Negation represents a nonexistent time period (*Never go there*).

10. Negation is used in connected language (*neither . . . nor*).

11. Speakers say one thing but mean "No, don't" or "Stop" (e.g., when mother says to child "I think the kitty wants to stay on the floor" instead of "No. Put kitty down").

Negation Issues in ASL

Negation has a very important pragmatic function, which is "to correct states of affairs assumed by the speaker to be either shared knowledge or to represent the commonest ones to be expected in the context" (Ramat, 1999, p. 241). Negation keeps conversations on track. Negation is rarely used in starting a conversation but is frequently used in repairing them.

Negation in ASL represents the same semantic meanings as does negation in English: a response to a *yes/no* question, denial, and nonexistence. The difference between ASL and English negation is that ASL uses clearly different signs for each meaning. For example, *no* in English can be the answer to a *yes/no* question or it can mean *none* (e.g., *He has no money*). In ASL the signs for these two concepts are different, clearly marking the concept. Another difference is that *don't* and *not* are sometimes signed the same in ASL because ASL does not require an equivalent of *do*-support to hold tense as does English. Another difference is that ASL negation relies heavily on the nonmanual markers of headshake, frowning, squinting, body movement, and gesturing (e.g., LIKE becomes DON'T LIKE by a shake of the head). Also in ASL compounding of negation may occur, with incorporation of negation into the word it is negating. For example, the sign NOT and WANT may be signed; thus, the thumb pulls out from under the chin while the fingers pull toward the chin to represent DON'T WANT. All concepts of negation can be represented in some manner through ASL.

Summary

The purpose of this chapter was to present descriptions of the grammars of English and ASL. Nouns, verbs, adjectives, adverbs, and negation from simple to advanced forms were described. We provided hierarchies for the reader to use when trying to determine what to teach next. Wherever possible, we drew comparisons between English and ASL.

Grammar in any language is a challenge. Grammarians and linguists have studied English for centuries. In contrast, ASL grammarians and linguists have studied ASL for only a few decades. More research is needed to elucidate the grammatical forms of ASL to the same degree that English forms are. Sufficient information is already available to keep the novice to the field busy in his studies for years. We strongly advise and encourage you to continue studying both English and ASL. The more you understand them, the better you will be able to make decisions regarding the instruction of children who are deaf and hard of hearing.

Question for Critical Thinking ―――――――――――――――――

1. What are the semantic and syntactic complexities of the word *since* in ASL and English?

References

Ahlgren, I. (1994). Sign language as the first language. In I. Ahlgren and K. Hyltenstam (Eds.), *Bilingualism in deaf education* (pp. 55–60). Hamburg: Signum Press.

Akamatsu, C. T. (1998). Thinking with and without language: What is necessary and sufficient for school-based learning? In A. Weisel (Ed.), *Issues unresolved: New perspectives on language and deaf education*. Washington, DC: Gallaudet University Press.

Albertson, J. (1996). While the pendulum swings: Activities for a hard of hearing support group. *Perspectives in Education and Deafness, 14*(5), 4–5, 24.

American Speech-Language-Hearing Association (1998). *Directory of speech-language pathology assessment instruments*. Rockville, MD: Author.

Anderson, E. (1992). *Speaking with style: The sociolinguistic skills of children*. London: Routledge.

Anderson, J.M. (1999). Case. In K. Brown and J. Miller (Eds.), *Concise encyclopedia of grammatical categories* (pp. 58–65). New York: Elsevier.

Anderson, M., Boren, N., Kilgore, J., Howard, W., and Krohn, E. (1980). *Appletree*. Austin, TX: PRO-ED, Inc.

Andrews, J. (2000). To be or not to be monlingual or bilingual. *Odyssey, 1*(3), 56–57.

Anthony, D. (1971). *Seeing essential English manual*. Anaheim, CA: Educational Services Division.

Antia, S.D., & Dittillo, D.A. (1998). A comparison of the peer social behavior of children who are deaf/hard of hearing. *Journal of Children's Communication Development, 19*(2), 1–10.

Aoki, C., & Siekeutiz, P. (1998). Plasticity and Brain development. *Scientific American, 259*, 56–64.

Aramburo, A. (1989). Sociolinguistic aspects of the black deaf community. In C. Lucas (Ed.), *The sociolinguistics of the deaf community* (pp. 103–119). San Diego, CA: Academic Press.

Arehart, K.H., Yoshinaga-Itano, C., Thomson, V., Gabbard, S.A., & Stredler-Brown, A. (1998). State of the states: The status of universal newborn hering identification and intervention systems in 16 states. *American Journal of Audiology, 7*, 101–114.

Austin, J. (1962). *How to do things with words*. London: Oxford University Press.

Bachevalier, J., Malkova, L., & Beauregard, M. (1996). Multiple memory systems: A neuropsychological and developmental perspective. In G.R. Lyon and N.A. Krasnegor (Eds.), *Attention, memory, and executive function* (pp. 185–198). Baltimore, MD: Paul H. Brookes.

Baddeley, A.D. (1986). *Working memory*. New York: Oxford University Press.

Baker, C. (1978). How does sim-com fit into the bilingual approach to education? In F. Caccamise and D. Hicks (Eds.), *Proceedings of the 2nd national symposium on sign research and teaching* (pp. 3–12). Silver Spring, MD: National Association of the Deaf.

Baker, S. (1996). The Native American deaf experience: Cultural, linguistic, and educational perspectives. Unpublished doctoral dissertation. Oklahoma State University: Stillwater.

Barry, K.E. (1899). *The five-slate system. A system of objective language teaching.* Philadelphia: Sherman and Co.

Bashier, A.S., Conte, B.M., & Heerde, S.M. (1998). Language and school success: Collaborative challenges and choices. In D.D. Merritt and B. Culatta (Eds.), *Language intervention in the classroom.* San Diego, CA: Singular Publishing Group.

Bates, E., Camaioni, L., & Volterra, V. (1975). The acquisition of performatives prior to speech. *Merrill-Palmer Quarterly, 26,* 407–423.

Bates, E., Dale, P.S., & Thal, D. (1995). Individual differences and their implications for theories of language development. In P. Fletcher and B. MacWhinney (Eds.), *The handbook of child language* (pp. 96–151).

Bateson, M. (1979). *The epigenesis of conversational interaction: A personal account of research development.* In M. Bullow (Ed.), *Before speech.* New York: Cambridge University Press.

Battison, R. (1992). Analyzing signs. Lexical borrowing in American Sign Language. Silver Spring, MD: Linstokz, Press.

Bebko, J.M. (1998). Learning, language, memory, and reading: The role of language automatization and its impact on complex cognitive activities. *Journal of Deaf Studies and Deaf Education, 3*(1), 4–14.

Beiter, A.L. & Brimacombe, J.A. (1998). Cochlear implants. In J.G. Alpiner and P. A. McCarthy (Eds.), *Rehabilitative audiology: Children and adults* (3rd ed.) (pp. 473–500). New York: Lippincott Williams and Wilkins.

Bell, A. (1883). Upon a method of teaching language to a very young congenital deaf child. *American Annals of the Deaf, 28,* 124–139.

Bender, R. (1981). *The conquest of deafness.* Danville, IL: Interstate Printers and Publishers.

Berger, K.W. (1980). History and development of hearing aids. In M.C. Pollack (Ed.), *Amplification for the hearing impaired* (2nd ed.) (pp. 1–19). New York: Grune and Stratton.

Bever, T.G. (1961). Prelinguistic behavior. Unpublished honors thesis. Harvard University Department of Linguistics: Cambridge, MA.

Blackwell, P., Engen, E., Fischgrund, J., Zarcadoolas, C. (1978). *Sentences and other systems: A language and learning curriculum for hearing-impaired children.* Washington, DC: Alexander Graham Bell Association for the Deaf and Hard of Hearing.

Bloom, L., Beckwith, R., Capatides, J., & Hafitz, J. (1988). Expression through affect and words in the transition from infancy to language. In P. Baltes, D. Featherman, and R. Lerner (Eds.), *Life-span development and behavior* (Vol. 8, pp. 99–127). Hillsdale, NJ: Lawrence Erlbaum Associates.

Bloom, L., & Lahey, M. (1978). *Language development and language disorders.* New York: John Wiley & Sons.

Bloome, D., & Knott, G. (1985). Teacher-student discourse. In D.N. Ripich and F.M. Spinelli (Eds.), *School discourse problems* (pp. 53–76). San Diego, CA: College-Hill Press.

Borkowski, J.G., & Burke, J.E. (1996). Theories, models, and measurements of functioning: An information processing perspective. In G.R. Lyon and N.A. Krasnegor (Eds.), *Attention, memory, and executive function* (pp. 235–262). Baltimore, MD: Paul H. Brookes.

Bornstein, M.H. (1989). Between caretakers and their young: Two modes of interaction and their consequences for cognitive growth. In M.H. Bornstein and J.S. Bruner (Eds.), Interaction in human development (pp. 197–214). Hillsdale, NJ: Lawrence Erlbaum Associates.

Bornstein, M.H., & Ruddy, M.G. (1984). Infant attention and maternal stimulation: Prediction of cognitive and linguistic development in singletons and twins. In H. Bouma and D.G. Bouwhuis (Eds.), *Attention and Performance X: Control of Language Processes.* London: Lawrence Erlbaum Associates.

Brentari, D. (1998). *A prosodic model of sign language phonology.* Cambridge, MA: The MIT Press.

Bowe, F. (1988). *Toward equality: Education of the deaf.* Washington, DC: Government Printing Office.

Bradley-Johnson, S., & Evans, L.D. (1991). *Psychoeducational assessment of hearing-impaired students: Infancy through high school.* Austin, TX: PRO-ED, Inc.

Brigance, A.H. (1991). *Brigance inventory of early development-Revised.* North Billerica, MA: Curriculum Associates.

British Broadcasting Corporation (BBC) (2000, April). Silent children, new language. Available: *http://www.bbc.cc.uk/horizon/silent.shtml.*

Brown, R. (1956). Language and categories: Appendix. In J. Bruner, J. Goodnow, and G. Austin (Eds.), *A study of thinking* (pp. 247–312). New York: John Wiley & Sons.

Brown, K., & Miller, J. (Eds.), (1999). *Concise encyclopedia of grammatical categories: Introduction.* New York: Elsevier.

Brownlee, S. (June, 1998). Baby talk. *U.S. News and World Report* [Online]. Available: http://www.usnews.com/usnews/issue/980615.

Bruner, J. (1971). *The relevance of education.* New York: W.W. Norton.

Bruner, J. (1973). *Beyond the information given.* New York: W.W. Norton.

Bruner, J. (1975). From communication to language—A psychological perspective. *Cognition, 3,* 255–288.

Bruner, J. (1981). The social context of language acquisition. *Language & Communication, 1,* 155–178.

Bruner, J. (1986). *Actual minds, possible worlds.* Cambridge, MA: Harvard University Press.

Bruner, J. (1990). *Acts of meaning.* Cambridge, MA: Harvard University Press.

Bruner, J., Goodnow, J., & Austin, G. (1956). *A study of thinking.* New York: John Wiley & Sons.

Buckler, M. (1968). Expanding language through patterning. *Volta Review, 70,* 89–96.

Bullard, C.S., & Schirmer, B.R. (1991). Understanding questions: Hearing-impaired children with learning problems. *The Volta Review, 93*(6), 235–245.

Caffi, C. (1998). Metapragmatics. In J. L. Mey and R.E. Asher (Eds.), *Concise encyclopedia of pragmatics* (pp. 581–586). New York: Elsevier.

Cacase, A.T., & McFarland, D.J. (1998). Central auditory processing disorders in school-aged children: A critical review. *Journal of Speech, Language, Hearing Research, 41*(2), 355–373.

Caissie, R., & Gibson, C. (1997). The effectiveness of repair strategies used by people with hearing losses and their conversational partners. *The Volta Review, 99*(4), 203–218.

Calderon, R. (2000). Parental involvement in deaf children's education programs as a predictor of child's language, early reading, and social-emotional development. *Journal of Deaf Studies and Deaf Education, 5,* 140–155.

Calderon, R., & Greenberg, M. (1997). The effectiveness of early intervention for deaf children and children with hearing loss. In M.J. Guralnick (Ed.), *The effectiveness of early intervention* (pp. 455–482). Baltimore, MD: Paul H. Brookes.

Calhoun, D. (1987). A comparison of two methods of evaluating play in toddlers. Unpublished master's thesis. Colorado State University: Ft. Collins, CO.

Calvert, D., & Silverman, S. (1983). *Speech & Deafness* (Rev. ed.). Washington DC: Alexander Graham Bell Association for the Deaf and Hard of Hearing.

Carney, A.E., & Moeller, M.P. (1998). Treatment efficacy: Hearing loss in children. *Journal of Speech, Language, Hearing Research, 41*, S61–S84.

Carrow-Woolfolk, E. (1985). *Test of Auditory Comprehension of Language-Revised* (1985). Austin, TX: PRO-ED, Inc.

Carston, R. (1998a). Conjunction and pragmatic effects. In J. L. Mey and R.E. Asher (Eds.), *Concise encyclopedia of pragmatics* (pp. 150–157). New York: Elsevier.

Carston, R. (1998b). Syntax and pragmatics. In J. L. Mey and R.E. Asher (Eds.), *Concise encyclopedia of pragmatics* (pp. 978–986). New York: Elsevier.

Chamot, A., & O'Malley, M. (1994). *The CALLA handbook.* Reading, MA: Addison-Wesley.

Cherkes-Julkowski, M., Sharp, S., & Stolzenberg, J. (1997). *Rethinking attention deficit disorders.* Cambridge, MA: Brookline Books.

Chermak, G.D., Hall, J.W. III, & Musiek, F.E. (1999). Differential diagnosis and management of central auditory processing disorder and attention deficit hyperactive disorder. *Journal of the American Academy of Audiology, 10*, 289–303.

Chomsky, N. (1965). *Aspects of the theory of syntax.* Cambridge, MA: MIT Press.

Chomsky, N. (1957). *Syntactic structures.* The Hague: Mouton.

Christensen, K. (1993). A multicultural approach to education of children who are deaf. In K. Christensen and G. Delgado (Eds.), *Multicultural Issues in Deafness.* White Plains, NY: Longman.

Christensen, K.M., & Delgado, G.L. (Eds.). (1993). *Multicultural issues in deafness.* White Plains, NY: Longman.

Clarke, B.R. (1983). Competence in communication for the hearing impaired: A conversation, activity, experience approach. *B.C. Journal of Special Education, 7*(1), 15–27.

Clement, C.J., & Koopmans-van Beinum, F.J. (1996, April). Influence of lack of feedback on infant vocalization in the first year. Abstract of the European Conference "The development of sensory, motor and cognitive abilities in early infancy: Antecedents of language and symbolic function" (p. 24). Girona, Spain: San Feliu de Ghuixols.

Cohen, O. (1993). Educational needs of African American and Hispanic deaf children and youth. In K. Christensen and G. Delgado (Eds.), *Multicultural Issues in Deafness* (pp. 45–68). White Plains, NY: Longman.

Cohen, O., Fischgrund, J. E., & Redding, R. (1990). Deaf children from ethnic, linguistic, and racial minority backgrounds: An overview. *American Annals of the Deaf, 135*, 67–82.

Collier, V. (1987). Age and rate of acquisition of second language for academic purposes. *TESOL Quarterly, 21*(4), 617–641.

Collins, G.M. (1977). Visual co-orientation and maternal speech. In H. Schaffer (Ed.), *Studies in mother-infant interaction.* New York: Academic Press.

Commission on Education of the Deaf. (1998). *Toward equality: Education of the deaf.* Washington, DC: Government Printing Office.

Compton, C. L. (1998). Assistive technology for the enhancement of receptive communication. In J.G. Alpiner and P. A. McCarthy (Eds.), *Rehabilitative audiology: Children and adults* (3rd ed.) (pp. 501–544). New York: Lippincott Williams & Wilkins.

Connor, C.M., Hieber, S., Arts, H.A., & Zowlan, T.A. (2000). Speech, vocabulary, and the education of children using cochlear implants: Oral and total communication. *Journal of Speech, Language, Hearing Research,* 43, 1185–1204.

Cooper, R., & Aslin, R. (1990). Preference for infant-directed speech in the first month after birth. *Child Development,* 51, 1584–1595.

Corina, D.P. (1998). Studies of neural processing in deaf signers: Toward a neurocognitive model of language processing in the deaf. *Journal of Deaf Studies and Deaf Education,* 3(1), 35–48.

Corina, D.P., Kritchevsky, M., & Bellugi, U. (1992). Linguistic permeability of unilateral neglect: Evidence from American Sign Language. *Proceeds of the 14th Annual Conference of the Cognitive Science Society* (pp. 384–389). Hillsdale, NJ: Lawrence Erlbaum Associates.

Crookston, I. (1999). *Verbs and verb phrases.* In K. Brown and J. Miller (Eds.), *Concise encyclopedia of grammatical categories* (pp. 400–406). New York: Elsevier.

Crutchfield, P. (1972). Prospects for teaching English Det + N structures to deaf students. *Sign Language Studies,* 1, 8–14.

Culatta, B., Long, J., & Gargaro-Larson, J. (1998). *Mathematics: An interactive discourse approach.* In D.D. Merritt and B. Culatta (Eds.), *Language intervention in the classroom* (pp. 331–362). San Diego, CA: Singular Publishing Group.

Cummins, J. (1980). Psychological assessment of immigrant children: Logic or intuition. *Journal of Multicultural Multilingual Development,* 1, 97–111.

Cummins, J. (1984). *Bilingualism and special education: Issues in assessment and pedagogy.* San Diego, CA: College-Hill Press.

Curtiss, S. (1977). *Genie: A psychological study of a modern-day wild child.* New York: Academic Press.

Dahl, O. (1998). Aspect. In J. L. Mey and R.E. Asher (Eds.), *Concise encyclopedia of pragmatics* (pp. 64–71). New York: Elsevier.

Dale, D.S. (1972). *Language development: Structure and function* (2nd ed.). New York: Holt, Rinehart, & Winston.

Daniels, M. (1997). *Benedictine roots in the development of deaf education: Listening with the heart.* Westport, CT: Bergin & Gravey.

D'Arc, J. (1958). The development of connected language skills with emphasis on a particular methodology. *Volta Review,* 60, 58–63.

Davis, J. (Ed.). (1990). *Our forgotten children: Hard of hearing pupils in the schools* (2nd ed.). Washington, DC: Self-help for the Hard of Hearing.

Davis, J. M., Elfenbein, J., Schum, R., & Bentler, R.A. (1986). Effects of mild and moderate hearing impairments on language, educational, and psychosocial behavior of children. *Journal of Speech and Hearing Disorders,* 51, 53–62.

Denckla, M.B. (1996). A theory and model of executive funtion: A Neuropsychological perspective. In G.R. Lyon and N.A. Krasnegor (Eds.), *Attention, memory, and executive function* (pp. 263–278). Baltimore, MD: Paul H. Brookes.

deVilliers, P.A. (1982). Later syntactic development: The contribution of semantics and pragmatics. Paper presented at the Convention of the New York State Speech-Language-Hearing Association.

deVilliers, J., & deVilliers, P. (1978). *Language acquisition*. Cambridge, MA: Harvard University Press.

deVilliers, P.A., & Pomerantz, S.B. (1992). Hearing-impaired students learning new words from written context. *Applied Psycholinguistics, 13*, 409–431.

Dixon, W.E., & Shore, C. (1997). Temperamental predictors of linguistic style during multiword acquistion. *Infant Behavior and Development, 20*(1), 99–103.

Dore, J. (1975). Holophrases, speech acts, and language universals. *Journal of Child Language, 2*, 21–40.

Easterbrooks, S.R. (1983). Literal and metaphoric understanding of four pairs of polar adjectives across four domains by hearing and hearing impaired children at two age levels. *Dissertation Abstracts International, 44*(8), 2437–Q. (University Microfilms No. DA 8326396).

Easterbrooks, S.R. (1999). Improving practices for student with hearing impairments. *Exceptional Children, 65*(4), 537–554.

Easterbrooks, S.R., & Baker-Hawkins, S. (Eds.) (1995). *Deaf and hard of hearing students: Educational services guidelines*. Washington, DC: National Association of State Directors of Special Education.

Easterbrooks, S. R., & Miller, D. L. (1986). Expanding the role of speech-language pathologists in instruction via Glasser's choice theory. *Journal of Children's Communication Development, 18*(2), 73–81.

Easterbrooks, S. R., & Mordica, J.A. (2000). Teachers' ratings of functional communication in students with cochlear implants. *American Annals of the Deaf, 145*(1), 54–59.

Easterbrooks, S.R., & O'Rourke, C.M. (in press). Gender differences in response to intervention in children who are deaf and hard of hearing. *American Annals of the Deaf.*

Easterbrooks, S.R., O'Rourke, C.M., & Todd, N.W. (2000). Child and family factors associated with deaf children's success in auditory-verbal therapy. *The American Journal of Otology, 21* (3), 1–4.

Ejiri, K. (1998). Synchronization between preverbal vocal behavior and motor action in early infancy: Its developmental change. *Japanese Journal of Psychology, 68*, 433–440.

Erting, C., Prezioso, C., & O'Grady-Hynes, M. (1994). The interactional context of deaf mother-infant interaction. In V. Volterra & C. Erting (Eds.), *From gesture to language in hearing and deaf children* (pp. 97–106). Washington, DC: Gallaudet University Press.

Estabrooks, W. (Ed.) (1994). *Auditory-verbal therapy for parents and professionals*. Washington, DC: Alexander Graham Bell Association for the Deaf and Hard of Hearing.

Evans, C., Zimmer, K., & Murray, D. (1994). *Discovery with words and signs: A resource guide for developing a bilingual and bicultural preschool programs for deaf and hard of hearing children*. Winnipeg, Manitoba, Canada: Sign Talk Development Project.

Falk, J. (1994). To be human: Language and the study of language. In V. Clark, P. Eschholtz, & A. Rosa (Eds.), *Language introductory readings* (pp. 49–76). New York: St. Martin's Press.

Fernandes, J. (1980). The gate to heaven: T.H. Gallaudet and the rhetoric of the deaf education movement. Unpublished dissertation. University of Michigan.

Field, T. (1990). *Infancy*. Cambridge, MA: Harvard University Press.

Fiese, B. (1990). Playful relationships: A contextual analysis of mother-toddler interaction and symbolic play. *Child Development, 61*, 1648–1656.

Fiez, J.A., Raife, E.A., Balota, D.A., Schwarz, J.P., Raichle, M.E., & Petersen, S.E. (1996). A positron emission tomography study of the short-term maintenance of verbal information. *Journal of Neuroscience, 16*, 808–822.

Finnegan, M. (1992). Bilingual-bicultural education. The method is message. *The Endeavor.* Silver Spring, MD: The American Society for Deaf Children.

Fitzgerald, E. (1929). *Straight language for the deaf.* Staunton, VA: McClure Co.

Fitzgerald, E. (1949). *Straight language for the deaf: A system of instruction for deaf children.* Washington DC: Alexander Graham Bell Association for the Deaf.

French, M. (1999). *Starting with assessment: A developmental approach to children's literacy.* Washington, DC: Gallaudet University Press.

Frith, U. (Ed.) (1991). Autism-Asperger syndromes. Cambridge, UK: Cambridge University Press.

Fryauf-Bertschy, H., Tyler, R.S., Kelsay, D.M.R., Gantz, B.J., Woodworth, G.G. (1997). Cochlear implant use by prelingually deafened children: The influence of age at implant and length of device use. *Journal of Speech, Language, and Hearing Research, 40,* 183–199.

Furth, H. (1969). Thinking without language. New York: Free Press.

Gallaudet University Outreach (1985). *Syntactic structures series.* Washington, DC: Gallaudet University Press.

Gallaudet, E.M. (1983). *History of the college for the deaf, 1857–1907.* Fischer, L., & de Lorenzo, D. (Eds.). Washington, DC: Gallaudet College Press.

Gallway, C., & Woll, B. (1994). Interaction and childhood deafness. In C. Gallaway & B.J. Richards (Eds.), *Input and interaction in language acquisition* (pp. 197–218). Cambridge, UK: Cambridge University Press.

Geers, A., & Moog, J. (1994). *Spoken language results: Vocabulary, syntax, and communication, 96*(5), 131–148.

Gesell, A. (1940). *The first five years of life.* New York: Harper & Row.

Gilbertson, M., & Kamhi, A.G. (1995). Novel word learning in children with hearing impairment. *Journal of Speech and Hearing Research, 38,* 630–642.

Glasser, W. (1998). *Choice theory in the classroom.* New York: Harper Perennial.

Gleason, J. (1993). Fathers and other strangers: Men's speech to children. In D. Dato (Ed.), *Developmental psycholinguistics: Theory and application.* Washington, DC: Georgetown University Press.

Golenkoff, R.M., Hirsch-Pasek, K., Bailey, L., & Wegner, N. (1992). Young children and adults use lexical principles to learn new nouns. *Developmental Psychology, 28,* 99–108.

Goldberg, J.P., & Bordman, M.B. (1975). The ESL approach to teaching English to hearing-impaired students. *American Annals of the Deaf, 120,* 22–27.

Goldsworthy, C. (1982). *Multilevel informal language inventory: Examiner's manual.* Columbus, OH: Charles E. Merrill.

Goodwyn, S., & Acredolo, L. (1993). Symbolic gesture versus word: Is there a modality advantage for onset of symbol use? *Child Development, 64,* 688–701.

Gregg, J., Roberts, K., & Colleran, M. (1983, October). Ear disease and hearing loss. Pierre, South Dakota: 1962–1982. *South Dakota,* 9–17.

Grice, H.P. (1975). Logic and conversation. In P. Cole and J.L. Morgan (Eds.), *Syntax and semantics 3: Speech acts* (pp. 41–58). New York: Academic Press.

Griffith, P.L., Johnson, H., & Dastoli, S. L. (1985). If teaching is conversation, can conversation be taught?: Discourse abilities in hearing impaired children. In D. Ripich and F. Spinelli (Eds.), *School discourse problems.* San Diego, CA: College-Hill.

Grimshaw, G., Adelstein, A., Bryden, M.P., & MacKinnon, G.E. (1998). First-language acquisition in adolescence: Evidence for a critical period for verbal language development. *Brain and Language, 63,* 237–255.

Groht, M. (1958). *Natural language for deaf children*. Washington, DC: Alexander Graham Bell Association for the Deaf and Hard of Hearing.

Grosjean, F. (1980). Spoken word recognition processes and the gating paradigm. *Perception and Psychophysics, 28,* 267–283.

Guralnick, D.B., & Friend, J.H. (Eds). (1966). Webster's New World Dictionary. New York: The World Publishing Company.

Gustason, G., Pfetzing, D., Zawolkow, E. (1980). *Signing exact English.* Silver Spring, MD: National Association of the Deaf.

Gutierrez, P. (1994). A preliminary study of deaf educational policy. *Bilingual Research Journal, 18*(3–4), 85–113.

Habib, M., Demonet, J.F., & Frackowiak, R. (1996). Cognitive neuroanatomy of language: Contribution of functional cerebral imaging. *Revue Neurologique,* 152(4), 249–260.

Handberg, T. (2000). *The making of a new subject—Norwegian Sign Language as a new language.* Paper presented at the World Congress of the Deaf, Brisbane, AU. 1999. Available: *http://www.ea.nl/Deaf2L/tonebritt_handberg.htm.*

Hargis, C. (1984). *English syntax* (2nd ed.). Springfield, OH: Charles C. Thomas.

Halliday, M. (1975). Learning how to mean. N. E. Lennenberg and E. Lennenberg (Eds.), *Foundations of language development: A multidisciplinary approach* (pp. 239–266). New York: Academic Press.

Hawkins, L. (1993). Option: full inclusion or isolation? *The Endeavor,* 2,7.

Hawkins, L., & Brawner, J. (1997). Educating children who are deaf or hard of hearing: Total communication. #559. Reston, VA: ERIC Clearinghouse on Disabilities and Gifted Education.

Hawkins, L., Harvey, S., Cohen, J. (1994). Parent's position on full inclusion for deaf children. *American Annals of the Deaf, 139,* 165–167.

Hawkins, L., & Harvey, S. (1995). Defining quality education for deaf and hard of hearing students. Washington, DC: Gallaudet University College for Continuing Education.

Haydon, D.M., Mann, N., & Fugate, G. (1995). Using conversation to enhance learning. *The Volta Review,* 97(5), 129–138.

Heidinger, V. (1984). *Analyzing syntax and semantics.* Washington, DC: Gallaudet College Press.

Hennon, J., & Ishiel, L. (2000). Everything old is new again. Paper presented at the 26th annual conference of the American College Educators of the Deaf and Hard of Hearing, New Orleans, LA, March 30–April 2.

Heward, W. (1996). *Exceptional children: An introduction to special education.* Englewood Cliffs, NJ: Prentice-Hall.

Hickock, G., Bellugi, U., & Klima, E.S. (1996). The neurobiology of sign language and its implications for the neural basis of language. *Nature, 381*(6584), 699–702.

Hiskey, M. (1966). *Hiskey-Nebraska Test of Learning Aptitude.* Lincoln, NE: Union College Press.

Hodgson, K. (1953). *The deaf and their problems.* New York: Philosophical Library.

Holden-Pitt, L. & Diaz, J. (1998). Thirty years of the annual survey of deaf and hard of hearing children and youth: A glance over the decades. *American Annals of the Deaf, 142*(2), 72–76.

Huttenlocker, P., & Dabholkar, A. (1997). Regional differences in synaptogenesis in human cerebral cortex. *Journal of Comparative Neurology, 387,* 167–178.

Hyerle, D. (1996). *Visual tools for constructing knowledge.* Alexandria, VA: Association for Supervision and Curriculum Development.

Individuals with disabilities Education Act amendments of 1997, P.L. 105–17, 105th Congress, 1st Session.

International Reading Association and National Council of Teachers of English (1994). *Standards for the assessment of reading and writing.* Newark, DE: Author.

James, S.L., & Seebach, M.A. (1982). The pragmatic function of children's questions. *Journal of Speech and Hearing Research, 25,* 2–11.

Jannedy, S., Poletto, R., & Weldon, T. (1994). *Language files: Materials for an introduction to language and linguistics.* Columbus: Ohio State University Press.

Jaworska, E. (1999). Prepositions and prepositional phrases. In K. Brown and J. Miller (Eds.), *Concise encyclopedia of grammatical categories* (pp. 304–311). New York: Elsevier.

Jeanes, R., Nienhuys, T., Rickards, F. (2000). The pragmatic skills of profoundly deaf children. *Journal of Deaf Studies and Deaf Education, 5,* 237–247.

Jenkins, J. R., Stein, M.L., & Wysocki, K. (1984). Learning vocabulary through reading. *American Educational Research Journal, 21*(4), 767–787.

Johnson, H. (1988). A sociolinguistic assessment scheme for the total communication student. In L. Kretschmer and R. Kretschmer (Eds.), Perspectives on language assessment with the hearing impaired. *Journal of the Academy of Rehabilitative Audiology, 21,* 101–127.

Johnson, H. (2000). Personal communication.

Johnson, H., & Dilka, K. (2000). Crossing the realities divide: Preservice teachers as "change agents" for the field of deaf education. U.S. Department of Education OPE Grant, CFDA No. 84.342.

Johnson, M.A., & Roberson, G.F. (1988). The language experience approach: Its use with young hearing-impaired students. *American Annals of the Deaf, 133* (3) 223–225.

Johnson, R., Liddell, S., & Erting, C. (1989). Unlocking the curriculum: Principles for achieving access in deaf education. Gallaudet Research Institute Working Paper 89–3. Washington, DC: Gallaudet University Press.

Jusczyk, P. (1997). *Discovery of spoken language.* Boston: MIT Press.

Kail, R., & Leonard, L.B. (1986). Word-finding abilities in language-impaired children. *ASHA Monograph Number 25.* Rockville, MD: American Speech-Language-Hearing Association.

Kantor, R. (1994). The acquisition of classifiers in American Sign Language. In M. McIntire (Ed.), *The acquisition of American Sign Language by deaf children* (pp. 39–56). Burtonsville, MD: Linstock.

Kemp, M. (1998). Why is learning American Sign Language a challenge? *American Annals of the Deaf, 143*(3), 255–59.

Kessler, C., Quinn, M., & Hayes, C. (1985). *Processing mathematics in a second language: Problems for IEP children.* Paper presented at the Delaware Symposium of Language Studies VII, University of Delaware, Newark.

Kelly, A. (1995). Fingerspelling interaction: A set of deaf parents and their deaf daughter. In C. Lucas (Ed.), *Sociolinguistics in deaf communities* (pp. 62–73). Washington, DC: Gallaudet University Press.

Kirk, K., Diefendorg, E., Riley, A., & Osberger, M. (1995). Consonant production by children with multichannel cochlear implants or hearing aids. *Advances in Oto-Rhino-Laryngology, 50,* 154–159.

Kisor, H. (1990). *What's that pig outdoors.* New York: Hill and Wang.

Klima, E., & Bellugi, U. (1966). Syntactic regularities in the speech of children. In J. Lyons & R. Wales (Eds.), *Psycholinguistic papers.* Edinburgh: Edinburgh University Press.

Koester, L., Brooks, L., and Traci, M.A. (2000). Tactile contact by deaf and hearing mothers during face-to-face interactions with their infants. *Journal of Deaf Studies and Deaf Education, 5,* 127–139.

Koester, L., Papoušek, H., & Papoušek, M. (1989). Patterns of rhythmic stimulation by mothers with three-month-olds: A cross-modal comparison. *International Journal of Behavioral Development, 12,* 143–154.

Koestner, L., Papoušek, H., & Smith-Gray, S. (2000). Intuitive parenting, communication, and interaction with deaf infants. In P. Spencer, C. Erting, and M. Marschark (Eds.), *The deaf child and the family and at school: Essays in honor of Kathryn P. Meadow-Orlans* (pp. 55–71). Mahwah, NJ: Lawrence Erlbaum Associates.

Kretschmer, R.R., & Kretschmer, L.W. (1997). Communication-based classrooms. *The Volta Review, 97*(5), 1–18.

Krifka, M. (1999). Mass expressions. In K. Brown and J. Miller (Eds.), *Concise encyclopedia of grammatical categories* (pp. 221–223). New York: Elsevier.

Landau, W.M., & Kleffner, F.R. (1957). Syndrome of acquired aphasia with convulsive disorder in children. *Neurology, 7,* 523–530.

Lane, H. (1976). *The wild boy of aveyron.* Cambridge, MA: Harvard University Press.

Lane, H. (1984). *The deaf experience: Classics in language and education.* Cambridge, MA: Harvard University Press.

Lane, H. (1989). *When the mind hears: A history of the deaf.* New York: Random House.

Lane, H. (1993, February/March). Cochlear implants: Boon for some—bane for others. *Hearing Health,* 19–23.

Lane, H. (1994). *The mask of benevolence.* New York: Alfred A. Knopf.

Lane, H., Hoffmeister, R., Behan, B. (1996). *Journey into the deaf-world.* San Diego, CA: Dawn Sign Press.

Laughton, J. (1983). The house/school that Jack/language built. *The Volta Review, 82*(6), 399–410.

Lederberg, A.R. (1993). The impact of deafness on mother-child and peer relationships. In M. Marsharck and M.D. Clark (Eds.), *Psychological perspectives on deafness* (pp. 93–119). Hillsdale, NJ: Lawrence Erlbaum Associates.

Lederberg, A.R., & Everhart, V. (1998). Communication between deaf children and hearing mothers: The role of language, gesture, and vocalization. *Journal of Speech, Language, and Hearing Research, 41,* 889–899.

Lederberg, A.R., & Mobley, C.E. (1990). The effect of hearing impairment on the quality of attachment and mother-toddler interaction. *Child Development, 61,* 1596–1604.

Lederberg, A.R., & Prezbindowski, A.K. (2000). Impact of child deafness on mother-toddler interaction: Strengths and weaknesses. In P. Spencer, C. Erting, and M. Marschark (Eds.), *The deaf child and the family and at school: Essays in honor of Kathryn P. Meadow-Orlans* (pp. 73–92). Mahwah, NJ: Lawrence Erlbaum Associates.

Lederberg, A.R., Prezbindowski, A.K., & Spencer, P. (2000). Word learning skills of deaf preschoolers: The development of novel word mapping and rapid word learning strategies. *Child Development, 71*(6), 1571–1585.

Lehmann, C. (1999). Aspectual types. In K. Brown and J. Miller (Eds.), *Concise encyclopedia of grammatical categories* (pp. 43–49). New York: Elsevier.

Lenneberg, E.H. (1967). *Biological foundations of language.* New York: John Wiley & Sons.

Levinson, S. (1998). Deixis. In J. L. Mey and R.E. Asher (Eds.), *Concise ncyclopedia of pragmatics* (pp. 200–205). New York: Elsevier.

Ling, D. (1976). Speech and the hearing impaired child: Theory and practice. Washington, DC: Alexander Graham Bell Association for the Deaf and Hard of Hearing.

Ling, D. (1989). *Foundations of spoken language for hearing-impaired children.* Washington, DC: Alexander Graham Bell Association for the Deaf and Hard of Hearing.

Livingston, S. (1997). *Rethinking the education of deaf students.* Portsmouth, NH: Heinemann.

Loban, W.D. (1963). *The language of elementary school children. NCTE Research Report No.1,* Urbana, IL: National Council of Teachers of English.

Loban, W.D. (1976). *Language development: Kindergarten through grade school.* Urbana, IL: National Council of Teachers of English.

Long, S.H., & Fey, M. E. (1991). *Computerized profiling* [computer program; Version 7.1]. Ithaca, NY: Computerized Profiling.

Lucas, E. (1980). *Semantic and pragmatic language disorders: Assessment and remediation.* Rockville, MD: Aspen Publishers.

Luetke-Stahlman, B. (1988). The benefit of oral English only as compared with signed input to hearing impaired students. *Volta Review, 90*(7), 349–361.

Luetke-Stahlman, B. (1988). Educational ramifications of various instructional inputs for hearing-impaired students. *Association of Canadian Educators of the Hearing-Impaired, 14*(30), 105–121.

Luetke-Stahlman, B. (1993). Research-based language intervention strategies adapted for deaf and hard of hearing children. *American Annals of the Deaf, 138*(5), 404–410.

Luetke-Stahlman, B. (1998). *Language issues in deaf education.* Hillsboro, OR: Butte Publications, Inc.

Luetke-Stahlman, B. (1998). Assessing the semantic language development of hearing impaired students. *ACEHI, 14*(1), 5–12.

Luetke-Stahlman, B. (1999). *Language across the curriculum.* Hillsboro, OR: Butte Publications, Inc.

Luria, A. (1966). *Higher cortical functions in man.* New York, Basic Books.

Lyman, H.B. (1998). *Test scores and what they mean* (6th ed.). Boston: Allyn & Bacon.

MacLeod-Gallinger, J. (1993). *Deaf ethnic minorities: Have they a double liability?* Paper presented at the Annual Meeting of the American Educational Research Association, Atlanta, GA, April 11–16.

MacLeod-Gallinger, J. (1993). *Deaf ethnic minorities: Have they a double liability?* Research/technical report. (ERIC Documents Reproduction Service #ED 408756).

Mahshie, S. (1995). *Educating deaf children bilingually.* Washington, DC: Gallaudet University Pre-College Programs.

Marschark, M. (1997). *Raising and educating a deaf child: A comprehensive guide to choices, controversies, and decisions faced by parents and educators.* New York: Oxford University Press.

Martin, R.P., Wisenbaker, J., Baker, J., & Huttunen, M.O. (1997). Gender differences in temperament at six months and five years. *Infant Behavior and Development, 20*(3), 339–347.

Marvelli, A. (1973). An historical examination and organizational analysis of the Smith College—Clarke School for the Deaf graduate teacher education program. Unpublished doctoral thesis. Amherst: University of Massachusetts.

Marmor, G., & Petitto, L. (1979). Simultaneous communication in the classroom: How well is English grammar represented? *Sign Language Studies, 23,* 99–136.

Masataka, N. (1992). Motherese in signed language. *Infant Behavior and Development, 15,* 453–460.

Masataka, N. (2000). The role of modality and input in the earliest stage of language acquisition: Studies of Japanese sign language. In C. Chamberlain, J. Morford, and R. Mayberry (Eds.), *Language acquisition by eye.* Mahwah, NJ: Lawrence Erlbaum Associates.

Mason, D., & Ewoldt (1996). Whole language and deaf bilingual-bicultural education—naturally! *American Annals of the Deaf* (141) 293–296.

Mauk, G.W., Barringer, D.G., & Mauk, P.P. (1995). Seizing the moment, setting the stage, and serving the future: Toward collaborative models of early identification and early intervention services for children born with hearing loss and their families. Part I: Early identification of hearing loss. *Infant–Toddler Intervention: A Transdisciplinary Journal, 5*(4), 367–393.

Mayne, A.M., Yoshinaga-Itano, C., Sedey, A.L., & Carey, A. (2000). Expressive vocabulary development of infants and toddlers who are deaf or hard of hearing. *The Volta Review, 100*(5), 1–28.

McAnally, P., Rose, S., & Quigley, S. (1994). *Language learning practices with deaf children* (2nd ed.). Austin, TX: PRO-ED, Inc.

McCarr, J. (1980). *Lessons in syntax.* Lake Oswego, OR: Dormac Publishing Company.

McIntire, M. (1994). *The acquisition of American Sign Language by Deaf children.* Burtonsville, MD: Linstook Press.

McNeill, D. (1970). *The acquisition of language.* New York: Harper & Row.

Meadow-Orlans, K. (1997). Effects of mother and infant hearing status on interactions at twelve and eighteen months. *Journal of Deaf Studies and Deaf Education, 2*(1), 27–36.

Meadow-Orlans, K. P., Sass-Lehrer, M., Scott-Olson, K., Mertens, D.M. (1998). Children who are hard of hearing: Are they forgotten? *Perspectives in Education and Deafness, 16*(3), 6–7, 24.

Meadow-Orlans, K., & Steinberg, A. (1993). Effects of infant hearing loss and maternal support on mother-infant interactions at 18 months. *Journal of Applied Developmental Psychology, 14,* 407–426.

Meier, R. (1991, January & February). Language acquisition by deaf children. *American Scientist,* 60–70.

Menyuk, P. (1969). *Sentences children use.* Cambridge, MA: MIT Press.

Menyuk, P. (1971). *The acquisition of development of language.* Englewood Cliffs, NJ: Prentice-Hall.

Mercer, N. (1998). Spoken language in the classroom. In J. L. Mey and R.E. Asher (Eds.), *Concise encyclopedia of pragmatics* (pp. 950–954). New York: Elsevier.

Merriman, W.E., Marazita, J., & Jarvis, L. (1995). Children's disposition to map new words into new referents. In M. Tomasello and W.E. Merriman (Eds.), *Beyond names for things: Young children's acquisition of verbs* (pp. 149–163). Hillsdale, NJ: Lawrence Erlbaum Associates.

Merritt, D.D., Barton, J., & Culatta, B. (1998). Instructional discourse: A framework for learning. In D.D. Merritt and B. Culatta (Eds.), *Language intervention in the classroom.* San Diego, CA: Singular Publishing Group.

Merritt, D.D., Culatta, B., & Trostle, S. (1998). Narratives: Implementing a discourse framework. In D.D. Merritt and B. Culatta (Eds.), *Language intervention in the classroom.* (277–330). San Diego, CA: Singular Publishing Group.

Mey, J.L. (1998a). Pragmatics. In J. L. Mey and R.E. Asher (Eds.), *Concise encyclopedia of pragmatics* (pp. 716–737). New York: Elsevier.

Mey, J.L (1998b). Pragmatic acts. In J. L. Mey and R.E. Asher (Eds.), *Concise encyclopedia of pragmatics* (pp. 701–703). New York: Elsevier.

Miller, J. (1981). *Assessing language production in children: Experimental procedures.* Baltimore, MD: University Park Press.

Miller, J., & Chapman, R.S. (1991). *Systematic anlaysis of language transcripts (SALT)* [Computer program: A. Nockerts, Programmer] Madison, WI: Language Analysis Laboratory, Waisman Center on Mental Retardation and Human Development.

Mindel, E., & Vernon, M. (1971). *They grow in silence.* Silver Spring, MD: National Association of the Deaf.

Mirsky, A. F. (1996). Disorders of attention: A neuropsychological perspective. In G.R. Lyon and N.A. Krasnegor (Eds.), *Attention, memory, and executive function.* Baltimore: Paul H. Brookes.

Moeller, M.P., Osberger, M.J., & Eccarius, M. (1986). Receptive language skills. In M. Osberger (Ed.), Language and learning skills in hearing-impaired children. [Monograph]. *ASHA Monographs, 23,* (pp. 41–53).

Mohay, H. (2000). Language in sight: Mothers' strategies for making language visually accessible to deaf children. In P.E. Spencer, C. J.Erting, and M. Marschark (Eds.), *The deaf child in the family and at school* (pp. 151–166). Mahwah, NJ: Lawrence Erlbaum Associates.

Moog, J.S., & Biedenstein, J.J.(1998). *Teacher assessment of spoken language.* St. Louis, MO: The Moog Oral School.

Moores, D. (2000). *Educating the deaf: Psychology, principles, and practices* (5th ed.). Boston: Houghton Mifflin.

Moores, D.F., & Oden, C.W. (1997). Educational needs of Black deaf children. *American Annals of the Deaf, 122*(3), 313–318.

Muma, J. (1978). *Language handbook: Concepts, assessment, intervention.* Englewood Cliffs, NJ: Prentice-Hall.

Muma, J.R. (1986). *Language acquisition. A functionalist perspective.* Austin, TX: PRO-ED, Inc.

Muma, J. R. (1998). *Effective speech-language pathology: A cognitive socialization approach.* Mahwah, NJ: Lawrence Erlbaum Associates.

Musselman, C., & Kircaali-Iftar, G. (1996). The development of spoken language in deaf children: Explaining the unexplained variance. *Journal of Deaf Studies and Deaf Education, 2*(1), 108–121.

Muysken, P. (1999). Nominalizations. In K. Brown and J. Miller (Eds.), *Concise encyclopedia of grammatical categories* (pp. 248–252). New York: Elsevier.

National Standards for Foreign Language Education Project (1996). *Standards for foreign language learning: Preparing for the 21st century.* Lawrence, KS: Allen Press Incorporated.

Neidle, C. (2000). SignStream, A tool for crosslinguistic analysis of signed languages. Seventh International Conference on Theoretical Issues in Sign Language Research. *(TISLR 2000).* Amsterdam, The Netherlands. July 23–27, 2000.

Neidle, C., Kegl, J., MacLaughlin, C., Bahan, B., & Lee, R.G. (2000). *The syntax of American Sign Language.* Cambridge, MA: The MIT Press.

Nelson, K. (1974). Concept, word, and sentence: Interrelations in acquisition and development. *Psychological Review, 81,* 267–285.

Nelson, K. (1981). Social cognition in a script framework. In J. Flavell and L. Ross (Eds.), *Social cognitive development.* New York: Cambridge University Press.

Nelson, K. (1985). *Making sense: The acquisition of shared meaning.* New York: Academic Press.

Nelson, K. (1993). Structure and strategy in learning to talk. *Monographs of the Society for Research in Child Development, 38,* No. 149.

Nelson, K. (1996). *Language in cognitive development.* New York: Cambridge University Press.

Nelson, K.E. (1998). Toward a differentiated account of facilitators of literacy development and ASL in deaf children. *Topics in Language Disorders, 18*(4), 73–88.

Nelson, N.W. (1998). *Childhood language disorders in context: Infancy through adolescence* (2nd ed.). Boston: Allyn & Bacon.

Neissar, A. (1983). *The other side of silence: Sign language and the deaf community.* New York: Alfred A. Knopf.

Newport, E.L. (1990). Maturational constraints on language learning. *Cognitive Science, 14,* 11–28.

Newport, E., & Meier, R. (1985). The acquisition of American Sign Language. In D. Slobin (Ed.), *The crosslinguistic study of language acquisition* pp. 881–938. Hillsdale, NJ: Lawrence Erlbaum Associates.

Newport, E., & Sapulla, T. (1990). A critical period effect in the acquisition of a primary language. Unpublished manuscript. University of Rochester, Rochester, NY.

Nover, S. (1995). Politics and language: American Sign Language and English in deaf education. In C. Lucas (Ed.), *Sociolinguistics in deaf communities* (pp. 109–163). Washington, DC: Gallaudet University Press.

Nover, S., & Andrews, J. (1998). Critical pedagogy in deaf education: Bilingual methodology and staff development. Star Schools Project. Washington, DC: U.S. Department of Education, Office of Educational Research and Improvement.

Nover, S., & Andrews, J. (1999). Critical pedagogy in deaf education: Bilingual methodology and staff development. Star Schools Project Grant no. R203A70030-97, Report No. 2. New Mexico School for the Deaf.

Nover, S., Christensen, K.M., & Cheng, L. (1998). Development of ASL and English competence for learners who are deaf. *Topics in Language Disorders, 18*(4), 661–72.

O'Donoghue, G.M., Nikolopoulos, T.P., Archbold, S.M., & Tait, M. (1999). Cochlear implants in young children: The relationship between speech perception and speech intelligibility. *Ear & Hearing, 20*(5), 419–425.

Oller, D. (1978). Infant vocalizations and the development of speech. *Allied Health and Behavior Sciences,* I, 523–549.

Osberger, M.J., Miyamoto, R.T., Zimmerman-Phillips, S., Kemink, J.L., Stroer, B.S., Firszt, J.B., & Novak, M.A. (1991). Independent evaluation of the speech perception abilities of children with the Nucleus 22-channel cochlear implant system. *Ear and Hearing, 12*(Suppl.), 66S–80S.

Osgood, C. (1957). Motivational dynamics of language behavior. *Nebraska Symposium on Motivation.* Lincoln: University of Nebraska Press.

Owens, R.E. (1996). *Language development: An introduction* (4th ed.). Boston: Allyn & Bacon.

Oyler, R. F., Oyler, A.L., & Matkin, N.D. (1998). Unilateral hearing loss: Demographics and educational impact. *Language, Speech, and Hearing Services in the Schools, 9*(2), 201–210.

Padden, C. (1989). The deaf community and the culture of deaf people. In S. Wilcox (Ed.), *American deaf culture* (p. 4–8). Burtonsville, MD: Linstok Press.

Padden, C., & Ramsey, C. (2000). American Sign Language and reading ability in deaf children. In C. Chamberlain, J. Morford, and R. Mayberry (Eds.), *Language acquisition by eye* (pp. 165–189). Mahwah, NJ: Lawrence Erlbaum Associates.

Palmer, F.R. (1999a). Mood and modality: Basic principles. In K. Brown and J. Miller (Eds.), *Concise encyclopedia of grammatical categories* (pp. 229–235). New York: Elsevier.

Palmer, F.R. (1999b). Mood and Modality: Further developments. In K. Brown and J. Miller (Eds.), *Concise encyclopedia of grammatical categories.* (pp. 235–239). New York: Elsevier.

Papoušek, H., & Papoušek, M. (1990). The art of motherhood. In N. Calder (Ed.), *Scientific Europe: Research and technology in 20 countries* (pp. 382–387). Maastricht, Holland: Scientific Publishers.

Parker, F., & Riley, K. (1994). *Linguistics for the non-linguist* (2nd ed.). Boston: Allyn & Bacon.

Paul, P. (1998). *Literacy and deafness.* Boston: Allyn & Bacon.

Paul, P., & Quigley, S. (1994). *Language and deafness* (2nd ed.). San Diego, CA: Singular Publishing.

Payne, J.R. (1999). Nouns and noun phrases. In K. Brown and J. Miller (Eds.), *Concise encyclopedia of grammatical categories* (pp. 258–266). New York: Elsevier.

Peet, H. (1869). The order of the first lesson in language for a class of deaf mutes. Proceedings of the Sixth Convention of the American Instructors of the Deaf (pp. 19–26). Washington, DC: U.S. Government Printing Office.

Pelley, S. (April, 2000). Birth of a language: Children without language so they invent one of their own. *60 Minutes II.* CBS Worldwide, Inc. Available: *http://www.cbsnews.cbs.com.*

Perkins, W.H., & Kent, R.D. (1987). *Functional anatomy of speech, language, and hearing: A primer.* Boston: College-Hill Publications.

Pettito, L., & Marentette, P. (1991). Babbling in the manual mode: Evidence from the ontogeny of language. *Science, 257,* 1493–1496.

Piaget, J. (1964). *The child's construction of reality.* New York: Basic Books.

Piaget, J. (1970). *Genetic epistemology.* New York: W.W. Norton.

Pillai, P. (1997). Understanding the needs of hard of hearing students in a mainstream setting. *Perspectives in Education and Deafness, 15*(5), 10–11.

Pinker, S. (1984). *Language learnabilty and language development.* Cambridge, MA: Harvard University Press.

Plann, S. (1993). Pedro Ponce de León: Myth and reality. In J. Van Cleve (Ed.), *Deaf history unveiled: Interpretations from the new scholarship* (pp. 1–12). Washington, DC: Gallaudet University Press.

Pollack, D. (1964). Acoupedics: A unisensory approach to auditory training. *Volta Review, 66*(7), 400–409.

Powers, A., Elliott, R., Fairbank, D., & Monaghon, C. (1988). The dilemma of identifying learning disabled hearing impaired students. *The Volta Review, 90,* 209–218.

Preisler, G.M. (1997). Sign language for hard of hearing children—A hindrance or a benefit for their development? *European Journal of Psychology in Education, 12*(4), 465–477.

Prelock, P.A. (1998). Language-based curriculum analysis: A collaborative assessment and intervention process. *Journal of Children's Communication Development, 19*(1), 35–42.

Prelock, P.A., Miller, B., & Reed, N.L. (1993). *Working with the classroom curriculum: A guide for analysis and use in speech therapy.* Tucson, AZ: Skill Builders.

Presneau, J. (1993). The scholars, the deaf, and the language of signs in France in the 18th century. In R. Fischer and H. Lane (Eds.), *Looking Back: A reader on the history of deaf communities and their sign language.* Hamburg: Signum Press.

Pressman, L.J., Pipp-Siegel, S., & Yoshinaga-Itano, C. (1998). The relation of hearing status and emotional availability to child language gain. Poster session at the International Conference for Infant Studies, Atlanta, GA.

Prinz, P.M., & Prinz, E. (1985). If only you could hear what I see: Discourse development in sign language. *Discourse Processes, 8*, 1–19.

Pugh, B.L. (1955). *Steps in language development for the deaf: Illustrated in the Fitzgerald Key.* Washington, DC: Volta Bureau.

Quigley, S., & Power, D. (1979). *TSA syntax program.* Austin, TX: PRO-ED, Inc.

Ramat, P. (1999). Negation. In K. Brown and J. Miller (Eds.), *Concise encyclopedia of grammatical categories* (pp. 241–248). New York: Elsevier.

Ramirez, A.G. (1995). *Creating contexts for second language acquisition: Theory and methods.* White Plains, NY: Longman.

Raphael, T.E., & McKinney, J. (1983). An examination of fifth- and eighth-grade children's question-answering behavior: An instructional study in metacognition. *Journal of Reading Behavior, 15*(3), 67–86.

Ratner, N.B., & Pye, C. (1984). Higher pitch in BT is not universal: Acoustic evidence from Quiche Mayan. *Journal of Child Language, 11*, 515–522.

Reed, R., & Bugen, C. (1985). *A process approach to developing language with hearing-impaired children.* Columbia, MO: General Printing Service.

Rehak, A., Kaplan, J.A., Weylman, S.T., Kelly, B., Brownell, H.H., & Gardner, H. (1992). Story processing in right-hemisphere brain-damaged patients. *Brain and Language, 42*(3) 320–336.

Reich, C., Hambleton, D., & Houldin, B. (1977). The integration of hearing impaired children in regular classrooms. *American Annals of the Deaf, 122*, 534–543.

Reilly, J., & Bellugi, U. (1996). Competition on the face: Affect and language in ASL motherese. *Child Language, 23*, 219–239.

Rittenhouse, R.K. & Kenyon, M.S. (1991). Conservation and metaphor acquisition in hearing-impaired children. *American Annals of the Deaf, 136*(4), 313–320.

Roberts, K. (1997). A preliminary account of the effect of otitis media on 15-month-olds' categorization and some implications for early language development. *Journal of Speech, Language, and Hearing Research, 40*(3), 508–518.

Roberts, I. (1999). Passive and related constructions. In K. Brown and J. Miller (Eds.), *Concise encyclopedia of grammatical categories* (pp. 284–290). New York: Elsevier.

Rogers, D.L., Perrin, M.S., & Waller, C.B. (1987). Enhancing the development of language and thought through conversations with young children. *Journal of Research in Childhood Education, 2*(1), 17–29.

Sabatino, D. (1983). The house that Jack built. *Journal of Learning Disabilities, 16*(1), 26–27.

Schacter, D. L. (1996). *Searching for memory: The brain, the mind, and the past.* New York: Basic Books.

Scheetz, N. (2001). *Orientation to deafness* (2nd ed.). Boston: Allyn & Bacon.

Schein, D., & Delk, M. (1974). *The deaf population in the United States.* Silver Spring, MD: National Association of the Deaf.

Schick, B., & Moeller, M.P. (1992). What is learnable in manually coded English? *Applied Psycholinguistics, 13,* 313–340.

Schildroth, A., & Hotto, S. (1996). Annual survey of hearing impaired children and youth: 1991–92 school year. *American Annals of the Deaf, 138*(2), 163–171.

Schirmer, B.R. (1984). Dynamic model of oral and/or signed language diagnosis. *Language, Speech & Hearing Services in Schools, 15,* 76–82.

Schirmer, B. R. (1985). An analysis of the language of young hearing-impaired children in terms of syntax, semantics and use. *American Annals of the Deaf, 15*–19.

Schirmer, B.R. (1989). Framework for using a language acquisition model in assessing semantic and syntactic development and planning instructional goals for hearing-impaired children. *The Volta Review,* 87–93.

Schirmer, B. (2000). *Language and literacy development in children who are deaf.* Boston: Allyn & Bacon.

Schirmer, B.R., Bailey, J., & Fitzgerald, S.M. (1999). Using a writing assessment rubric for writing development of children who are deaf. *Exceptional Children, 65*(3), 383–397.

Schirmer, B.R., & Woolsey, M.L. (1997). Effect of teacher questions on reading comprehension of deaf children. *Journal of Deaf Studies and Deaf Education, 2*(1), 47–56.

Schleper, D. (1997). *Reading to deaf children: Learning from deaf adults.* Washington, DC: Gallaudet University Pre-College National Mission Programs.

Schminky, M.M., & Baran, J.A. (1999). Central auditory processing disorders: An overview of assessment and management practices. *Deaf-Blind Perspectives, 7*(1), 1–6.

Schumaker, J.B., & Sheldon, J.B. (1999). *Proficiency in the sentence writing strategy: Instructor's manual.* Lawrence: University of Kansas.

Scouten, E. (1984). *Turning points in the education of deaf people.* Danville, IL: Interstate Printers and Publishers.

Sebba, M. (1999). Serial verbs. In K. Brown and J. Miller (Eds.), *Concise encyclopedia of grammatical categories* (pp. 344–347). New York: Elsevier.

Sergeant, J. (1996). A theory of attention: An information processing perspective. In G.R. Lyon and N.A. Krasnegor (Eds.), *Attention, memory, and executive function.* Baltimore, MD: Paul H. Brookes.

Shatz, M. (1987). Bootstrapping operations in child language. In K. Nelson and A. Van-Kleeck (Eds.), *Children's language* (Vol. 6). Hillsdale, NJ: Lawrence Erlbaum Associates.

Shaywitz, S.E., & Shaywitz, B.A. (1996). Unlocking learning disabilities: The neurologic basis. In S.C. Cramer and W. Ellis (Eds.), *Learning disabilities: Lifelong issues.* Baltimore, MD: Paul H. Brookes.

Shaywitz, B.A., Shaywitz, S.E., Fletcher, J.M., Pugh, K.R., Gore, J.C., Constable, R.T., Fulbright, R.K., Skudlarski, P., Liberman, A.M., Shankweiler, D.P., Katz, L., Bronen, R.A., Marchione, K.E., Holahan, J.M., Francis, D.J., Klorman, R., Aram,

D.M., Blachman, B.A., Stuebing, K.K., & Lacadie, C. (1997). The Yale Center for the Study of Learning and Attention: Longitudinal and neurobiological studies. *Learning Disabilities: A Multidisciplinary Journal, 8*(1), 21–29.

Shirai, Y., & Andersen, R. (1995). The acquisition of tense-aspect morphology: A prototype approach. *Language, 71*(4), 75–86.

Siegel, L. (2000). The educational and communication needs of deaf and hard of hearing children: A statement of principle on fundamental educational change. *American Annals of the Deaf, 145*, 64–77.

Singleton, J.L., & Tittle, M.D. (2000). Deaf parents and their hearing children. *Journal of Deaf Studies and Deaf Education, 5*(3), 221–236.

Singleton, J., Sapulla, S., Litchfield, S., Schley, S. (1998). From sign to word: Considering modality constraints in ASL/English bilingual education. *Topics in Language Disorders, 18,*(4), 16–29.

Smoski, W.J., Brunt, M.A., & Tannahill, J.C. (1992). Listening characteristics of children with central auditory processing disorders, *Language, Speech and Hearing Services in Schools, 23*(2), 145–152.

Snyder, L.S., & Yosinaga-Itano, C. (1998). Specific play behaviors and the development of communication in children with hearing loss. *The Volta Review, 100*(3), 165–185.

Spencer, P. (1993). Communication behaviors of infants with hearing loss and their hearing mothers. *Journal of Speech and Hearing Research, 36*, 311–321.

Spencer, P., & Gutfreund, M. (1990). Responsiveness in mother-infant interactions. In D. Moores and K. Meadow-Orlans (Eds.), *Educational and developmental aspects of deafness* (pp. 350–365). Washington, DC: Gallaudet University Press.

Spencer P., & Lederberg, A. (1997). Different modes, different models: Communication and language of young deaf children and their mothers. In L. Adamson and M. Romski (Eds.), *Communication and language: Discoveries from atypical development* (pp. 203–230). Baltimore: Paul H. Brookes.

Spencer, P., & Meadow-Orlans, K. (1996). Play, language, and maternal responsiveness: A longitudinal study of deaf and hearing infants. *Child Development, 67*, (3176–191).

Stephens, M. I. (1988). Pragmatics. In M.A. Nippold (Ed.), *Later language development.* New York: College-Hill.

Stickler, K.R. (1987). *Guide to analysis of language transcripts.* Eau Claire, WI: Thinking Publications.

Stokoe, W. (1995). On cats' eyes, flightless birds & home signs. *Sign Language Studies, 87*, 175–184.

Stone, P. (1988). *Blueprint for developing conversational competence: A planning instructional model with detailed scenarios.* Washington, DC: Alexander Graham Bell Association for the Deaf and Hard of Hearing.

Stredler-Brown, A. (1998). Early intervention for infants and toddlers who are deaf and hard of hearing: New perspectives. *Journal of Educational Audiology, 6*, 45–49.

Strong M. (Ed.). (1988). *Language learning and deafness.* New York: Cambridge University Press.

Subtelny, J.D. (1980). *Speech assessment and speech improvement for the hearing impaired.* Washington, DC: Alexander Graham Bell Association for the Deaf and Hard of Hearing.

Tabachnick, B.G., & Turbey, C.B. (1981). *WISC-R scatter and pattern in three types of learning disabled children.* Paper presented at the Western Psychological Association Conference. Los Angeles, CA, April 9–12, 1981.

Tattershall, S., & Creaghead, N. (1985). A comparison of communication at home and school. In D.N. Ripich and F.M. Spinelli (Eds.), *School discourse problems* (pp. 29–51). San Diego, CA: College-Hill Press.

Taylor, R.L. (1997). *Assessment of exceptional students* (4th ed.). Boston: Allyn & Bacon.

Thomas, S. (1958). A comparison of different approaches to vocabulary instruction. Unpublished doctoral dissertation. University of Wisconsin, Madison.

Thompson, M., Biro, P., Vethivelu, S., Pious, C., & Hatfield, N. (1987). *Language assessment of hearing-impaired school age children*. Seattle: University of Washington Press.

Togeby, O. (1998). Pragmatic principles. In J.L. Mey and R.E. Asher (Eds.), *Concise Encyclopedia of Pragmatics* (pp. 707–710). New York: Elsevier.

Tomblin, J.B., Spencer, L., Flock, S., Tyler, R., & Gantz, B. (1999). A comparison of language achievement in children with cochlear implants and children with hearing aids. *Journal of Speech, Language, and Hearing Research, 42*, 497–511.

Torgeson, J.K. (1996). A model of memory from an information processing perspective: The special case of phonological memory. In G.R. Lyons and N.A. Krasnegor (Eds.), *Attention, memory, and executive function* (pp. 157–184). Baltimore, MD: Paul H. Brookes.

Tough, J. (1977). *The development of meaning*. New York: John Wiley & Sons.

Tranthan, C.R., & Pedersen, J.K. (1976). Normal language development. Baltimore, MD: Williams & Wilkins.

Truffaut, B. (1993). Etienne de Fay and the history of the deaf. In R. Fischer and H. Lane (Eds.), *Looking back: A reader on the history of deaf communities and their sign languages*. Hamburg: Signum Press.

Tucker, J.A. (1985). Curriculum-based assessment: An introduction. *Exceptional Children, 52*, 199–204.

Tucker, B.P. (1998). Deaf culture, cochlear implants, and elective disability. *The Hastings Center Report, 28*(4), 6–14.

Tur-Kaspa, H., & Dromi, E. (1998). Spoken and written language assessment of orally trained children with hearing loss: Syntactic structures and deviations. *The Volta Review, 100*(3), 186–202.

Tyack, D. L., & Gottsleben, R. H. (1977). *Language sampling, analysis, and training: A handbook for teachers and clinicians*. Eau Claire, WI: Thinking Publications.

Tyack, D., & Ingram, D. (1977). Children's production and comprehension of questions. *Journal of Child Language , 4*, 211–224.

Tye-Murray, N. (Ed.). (1994). *Let's converse: A "how-to" guide to develop and expand conversational skills of children and teenagers who are hearing impaired*. Washington, DC: Alexander Graham Bell Association for the Deaf and Hard of Hearing.

Tyler, R. (1990). Speech perception with the Nucleus cochlear implant in children trained with the auditory/verbal approach. *American Journal of Otology, 11*, 99–107.

U.S. Office of Education. (1997). *To assure a free appropriate public education of children with disabilities: 19th annual report to Congress on the implementation of the Individuals with Disabilities Education Act*. Washington, DC: U.S. Government Printing Office.

U.S. Department of Education. (1998). *To assure the free appropriate public education of children with disabilities: 20th annual report to Congress on the implementation of the Individuals with Disabilities Education Act*. Washington, DC: U.S. Government Printing Office.

Valdes, G. (1995). The teaching of minority languages as "academic subjects." Pedagogical and theoretical challenges. *Modern Language Journal, 79*(3), 299–328.

Van Cleve, J., & Crouch, B. (1989). *Deaf history unveiled: Interpretations from the new scholarship.* Washington, DC: Gallaudet University Press.

Valade-Gabel, J.J. (1879). The institutions of the deaf and dumb in France. *American Annals of the Deaf* (Vol. 19, No. 1) (pp. 130–131).

Valli, C., & Lucas, C. (1995). *Linguistics of American Sign Language* (2nd ed.). Washington, DC: Gallaudet University Press.

van der Auwera, J. (1999). Adverbs and adverbials. In K. Brown and J. Miller (Eds.), *Concise encyclopedia of grammatical categories* (pp. 8–12). New York: Elsevier.

van Eijck, J. (1999). Determiners. In K. Brown and J. Miller (Eds.), *Concise encyclopedia of grammatical categories* (pp. 136–141). New York: Elsevier.

Vincent, N. (1999). Subordination and complementation. In K. Brown and J. Miller (Eds.), *Concise encyclopedia of grammatical categories* (pp. 352–358). New York: Elsevier.

Vygotsky, L. (1962). *Thought and language.* Cambridge, MA: MIT Press.

Vygotsky, L. (1978). *Mind in society.* Cambridge, MA: Harvard University Press.

Walker-Vann, C. (1998). Profiling Hispanic deaf children. *American Annals of the Deaf, 143*(1), 46–54.

Warren, S.F., & Kaiser, A.P. (1986). Incidental language teaching: A critical review. *Journal of Speech and Hearing Disorders,* 51, 291–299.

Watson, B. U., Sullivan, P.M., Moeller, M.P., & Jenson, J. K. (1982). Nonverbal intelligence and English language ability in deaf children. *Journal of Speech and Hearing Disorders, 47*(2), 199–204.

Wechsler, D. (1991). *Manual for the Wechsler intelligence scale for children—Third Edition.* San Antonio, TX: Psychological Corporation.

Weiss, A. (1986). Classroom discourse and the hearing-impaired child. *Topics in Language Disorders, 6*(3), 60–70.

Wells, G. (1985). *Language development in preschool years.* Cambridge, MA: Harvard University Press.

Wiig, L., & Semel, E.M. (1980). *Language assessment and intervention for the learning disabled.* Columbus, OH: Merrill.

Wix, T., & Supalla, S. (undated). *American Sign Language acquisition assessment.* Tucson, AZ: Arizona Schools for the Deaf and Blind.

Whitesell, K., & Klein, H.L. (1995). Facilitating language and learning via scripts. *The Volta Review, 97*(5), 117–128.

Wilbur, R. (1987). *American Sign Language, linguistic and applied dimensions,* (2nd ed.). Boston: College-Hill Press.

Wilcox, S. (1989). Breaking through the culture of silence. In S. Wilcox (Ed.), *American deaf culture.* Burtonsville, MD: Linstok Press.

Winfield, R. (1981). Bell, Gallaudet and the sign language debate. Unpublished doctoral dissertation. Harvard University School of Education.

Wolkomir, R. (1992). American Sign Language: It's not mouth stuff—it's brain stuff. *Smithsonian, 22*(4), 30–41.

Woll, B., & Kyle, J.G. (1998). Sign language. In J. Mey and R. Asher (Eds.), *Concise encyclopedia of pragmatics* (pp. 854–878). New York: Elsevier.

Wood, H.A., & Wood, D.J. (1984). An experimental evaluation fo the effects of five styles of teacher conversation on the language of hearing-impaired children. *Journal of Child Psychology and Psychiatry, 25*(1), 45–62.

Yoshinaga-Itano, C. (2000). Development of audition and speech: Implications for early intervention with infants who are deaf or hard of hearing. *The Volta Review, 100*(5), 213–236.

Yoshinaga-Itano, C., Snyder, L.S., & Day, D. (1998). The relationship of language and symbolic play in children with hearing loss. *The Volta Review, 100*(3), 135–164.

Zein, G., Say, K., Bellugi, U., Corina, D., & Reilly, J.S. (1993). The role of the right hemisphere for extra-syntactic aspects of ASL. Paper presented at the Academy of Aphasia, Tucson, Arizona, October, 1993.

Zieziula, F.R. (1982). *Assessment of hearing-impaired people. A guide for selecting psychological, educational, and vocational tests.* Washington, DC: Gallaudet College Press.

Zorfass, J.M. (1981). Metalinguistic awareness in young deaf children: A preliminary study. *Applied Psycholinguistics, 2,* 333–352.

Subject Index